"I am grateful for Dr. Jacob Teitelbaum's great work on FMS and CFS. His well-done, published research validates what many of us working in the trenches know: this works!"

—MARK HOCH, M.D.
Past President, American Holistic Medical Association

"[This] research and carefully designed program for patients suffering from CFS and fibromyalgia has given my patients relief from symptoms, improved sense of well-being, hope, and in many cases has facilitated a path to optimal health and full recovery."

—NANCY RUSSELL, M.D.
Medical Director, Combined Health Care Professionals, and
Founding Diplomat, American Board of Holistic Medicine

"As a psychiatrist and acupuncturist, I frequently see patients with chronic fatigue and soft-tissue pain. Dr. Teitelbaum's book *From Fatigued to Fantastic!* has been a fantastic resource for these individuals. They uniformly report to me that they found it helpful to them on many different levels. This book has clear benefit for anyone dealing with chronic fatigue or fibromyalgia."

—SCOTT SHANNON, M.D.
Past President, American Holistic Medical Association

"Dr. Teitelbaum's work and studies show us the way forward in treating this group of illnesses. They are a major advance on what we have here at present."

—ANDREW WRIGHT, M.D.
Editor, *Chronobiology* (UK)

"In the management of chronic fatigue syndrome, Dr. Teitelbaum's comprehensive approach is the most successful program available today. Practitioners and patients alike will find within the pages of *From Fatigued to Fantastic!* the rudiments of recovery, which offer hope to those afflicted with this disease."

—ROBERT A. ANDERSON, M.D.
Former President, American Board of Holistic Medicine

From
Fatigued *to*
Fantastic!

From
Fatigued to
Fantastic!

A Clinically Proven Program to Regain Vibrant Health

and Overcome Chronic Fatigue and Fibromyalgia

THIRD EDITION

Jacob Teitelbaum, M.D.

AVERY   *a member of Penguin Group (USA) Inc.*   *New York*

AVERY

Published by the Penguin Group

Penguin Group (USA) Inc., 375 Hudson Street, New York, New York 10014, USA • Penguin Group (Canada), 90 Eglinton Avenue East, Suite 700, Toronto, Ontario M4P 2Y3, Canada (a division of Pearson Penguin Canada Inc.) • Penguin Books Ltd, 80 Strand, London WC2R 0RL, England • Penguin Ireland, 25 St Stephen's Green, Dublin 2, Ireland (a division of Penguin Books Ltd) • Penguin Group (Australia), 250 Camberwell Road, Camberwell, Victoria 3124, Australia (a division of Pearson Australia Group Pty Ltd) • Penguin Books India Pvt Ltd, 11 Community Centre, Panchsheel Park, New Delhi–110 017, India • Penguin Group (NZ), 67 Apollo Drive, Rosedale, North Shore 0632, New Zealand (a division of Pearson New Zealand Ltd) • Penguin Books (South Africa) (Pty) Ltd, 24 Sturdee Avenue, Rosebank, Johannesburg 2196, South Africa

Penguin Books Ltd, Registered Offices: 80 Strand, London WC2R 0RL, England

"Effective Treatment of Severe Chronic Fatigue: A Report of a Series of 64 Patients" on pages 279–280 originally appeared in the *Journal of Musculoskeletal Pain* 3 (1995). Used courtesy Haworth Press. "Effective Treatment of Chronic Fatigue Syndrome and Fibromyalgia: A Randomized, Double-Blind Placebo-Controlled, Intent to Treat Study" originally appeared in the *Journal of Chronic Fatigue Syndrome* 8 (2) (2001). Appendix F is used with permission of Steven Krafchick, J.D.

Most Avery books are available at special quantity discounts for bulk purchase for sales promotions, premiums, fund-raising, and educational needs. Special books or book excerpts can be created for specific needs. For details, write Penguin Group (USA) Inc. Special Markets, 375 Hudson Street, New York, NY 10014.

Library of Congress Cataloging-in-Publication Data

Teitelbaum, Jacob.

From fatigued to fantastic! : a clinically proven program to regain vibrant health and overcome chronic fatigue and fibromyalgia / Jacob Teitelbaum.

p.   cm.

Includes bibliographical references and index.

ISBN 978-1-58333-289-4

1. Chronic fatigue syndrome—Popular works.   2. Fibromyalgia—Popular works.   I. Title.

RB150.F37T45   2007   2007028118

616'.0478—dc22

Printed in the United States of America

7   9   10   8

Neither the publisher nor the author is engaged in rendering professional advice or services to individual readers. Ideas, procedures, and suggestions in this book are not intended to substitute consulting with a physician. All matters regarding health require medical supervision. Neither the author nor the publisher shall be liable or responsible for any loss or damage allegedly arising from any information or suggestion in this book.

While the author has made every effort to provide accurate telephone numbers and Internet addresses at the time of publication, neither the publisher nor the author assumes any responsibility for errors, or for changes that occur after publication. Further, the publisher does not have any control over and does not assume any responsibility for author or third-party websites or their content.

To Laurie, my beautiful lady, my wife, and the love of my life;
my children, David, Amy, Shannon, Brittany, and Kelly,
who already seem to know so much of what I'm trying to learn;
my beautiful grandchildren, Payton and Bryce;
my mother, Sabina, and father, David,
whose unconditional love made this book possible;
The memories of Drs. Janet Travell, Hugh Riordan, and Billie Crook,
who were the pioneers in this field;
And to my patients, who have taught me more
than I can ever hope to teach them.

Acknowledgments

*S*o many special people helped make this book possible that I cannot possibly list them all. In truth, I have created nothing new; I have simply synthesized the wonderful work done by an army of hardworking and courageous physicians and healers.

I would like to extend my sincerest thanks to:

First and foremost, my staff. Their hard work, compassion, and dedication (and, I must admit, patience with me) are what made my work possible.

My research partner, Birdie (Barbara Bird). Her sense of humor and encouragement kept me going when I got tired. Her dedication to quality shines in every facet of her work. Cheryl Alberto, Denise Haire, Angie Borlik, Sue Marston, Amy Podd, and Mary Groom make everything run smoothly, no matter how much chaos I create.

The Anne Arundel Medical Center librarian, Joyce Miller. Over the last twenty-six years, I have often wondered when she would politely tell me to stop asking for so many studies. So far, she has not. In fact, she always smiles when I ask her for more.

Rev. Bren Jacobson and Dr. Alan Weiss, who keep me intellectually, emotionally, and spiritually honest while reminding me to reclaim my sense of humor.

My wonderful and dedicated publicists, Dean Draznin and Terri Slater, who are my teammates in making effective treatment and health available to everyone.

Bob Baurys and Sue Hrim, who took Bob's suffering and recovering from CFS as an opportunity to make effective treatment available for everyone by creating the Fibromyalgia & Fatigue Centers nationally (www.fibroandfatigue.com).

The publishers at Avery/Penguin books and my editor, Rebecca Behan.

My many teachers, the real heroes and heroines in their fields, whose names could fill this book. They include William Crook, Max Boverman, Brugh Joy, Janet Travell, William Jefferies, Hal Blatman, Jay Goldstein, Paul Levine, Leo Galland, Leonard Jason, George Mitchell, Lloyd Lewis, Michael Rosenbaum, Murray Susser, Charles Lapp, Paul Cheney, James Brodsky, Melvyn Werbach, Sherry Rogers, Sheri Lieberman, Robert Ivker, Tony Lebro, and Alan Gaby.

The many chronic fatigue syndrome and fibromyalgia support groups. These are easily the best patient support groups I have ever seen.

And finally, God and the universe, for the guidance and infinite blessings I have been given and for using me as an instrument for healing.

Contents

Introduction

I remember 1975. I was in my third year of medical school, doing my pediatrics rotation. I had always excelled, having finished college in three years. Now I was the second-youngest in a class of more than two hundred students, and I was continuing to perform well. My approach to life was to move quickly—"full speed ahead." But then, a nasty viral illness hit me and made it hard for me to even get out of bed for my morning pediatrics lecture. I cannot forget walking into an auditorium full of medical students, the professor saying, "Teitelbaum, why are you . . ." As he said "late?" I just about collapsed on the steps.

Although I was barely able to function, I spent the next four weeks working in the electron microscopy and research labs. The work I performed there was considered low-key—good tasks for a medical student trying to recuperate. But my brain fog made even these duties impossible, and by the end of the month, I was finding it impossible to even get out of bed before noon. I wanted to push forward and try harder. Though it was not what I wanted to hear, one wise professor advised me that this was not a time to push forward but rather a time to take a leave of absence and "regroup." I am still thankful for this teacher's guidance.

My illness seemed to close a door to one chapter of my life and open other doors to whole new possibilities of self-exploration. As I had to drop out of medical school and had no more scholarship or work-study, and was too ill to work, I was also homeless. Taking off in my '65 Dodge Dart, I had the novel experience of having no agenda, no plans. I was to meet many teachers on my journey. Most important, I was taking time to get to know myself.

With my family's and friends' help and support and my own inner work, as well as what I learned from people I met while I was homeless, I recovered my energy and strength and went on to finish medical school and residency. Though I did well, I continued to intermittently suffer the many diverse symptoms seen in fibromyalgia. My experiences with chronic fatigue syndrome and fibromyalgia left me with an appreciation of the impact of these illnesses. The symptoms that persisted—such as fatigue, achiness, poor sleep, and bowel problems—acted as the arena in which I learned how to help other people overcome these illnesses. It also taught me that it helps to have a sense of humor to survive this illness.

If you have chronic fatigue syndrome (CFS), fibromyalgia syndrome (FMS), myalgic encephalomyelitis (ME), or another disabling chronic fatigue state, you have been through a difficult journey. I remember being told that I was depressed. I *was* depressed. I was unable to function. Most people with chronic fatigue syndrome have to struggle just to get compassion and understanding.

Building on what I have learned since 1975, my research partner, Barbara Bird, and I initially completed an open study (in 1993) of sixty-four patients with disabling chronic fatigue.[1] In 1999, we completed a randomized, double-blind follow-up study, and appreciate the assistance given by National Institutes of Health researchers in developing the study protocol. This study showed that 91 percent of you can improve with proper treatment, and half of those with fibromyalgia were pain free at ninety-nine days.[2] Our recently published study showed an average 45 percent increase in energy in CFS/FMS by simply taking ribose (see Chapter 2).[3] My staff and I have treated more than three thousand CFS/FMS patients, and tens of thousands more have been treated by doctors at the Fibromyalgia & Fatigue Centers (www.fibroandfatigue.com) and by many other physicians worldwide. More than 50 percent of our patients are much better—that is, their symptoms are no longer a major problem—with our treatment, while most of the remainder have shown significant, albeit incomplete, improvement. Only 10 to 15 percent have had no significant improvement.

We have found that, on average, patients begin to feel better in two to three months.[1, 2]

If you suffer from CFS, FMS, or ME, this book will provide you with the tools and information you need to move beyond fatigue and into wellness. If you are a physician, it will teach you how to help—often dramatically—your patients who experience chronic exhaustion, including those frustrating cases in which no treatment has thus far been successful.

If you have researched chronic fatigue and immune dysfunction syndrome (CFIDS—also called chronic fatigue syndrome, or CFS, and I use CFS and CFIDS interchangeably), you will find some information here that is familiar, but you will also discover much that is new. For instance, to restore energy production and recover, it is usually necessary to treat many different problems simultaneously. Most sufferers of chronic exhaustion have a mix of at least five or six underlying problems (out of more than a hundred possible problems), which vary from person to person. This occurs because each problem can cause several others. You may have found some relief in the past by treating one, or a few, of these problems; I think you will be pleasantly surprised at what happens when you treat all your underlying problems simultaneously.

Certainly, we still have much more to learn in this area. However, we have now crossed a threshold and can effectively treat the illness. As the *Journal of the American Academy of Pain Management* noted in an editorial, "This study by Dr. Teitelbaum et al confirms what years of clinical success have shown—that the treatment approach described in Chapter 4 of *The Trigger Point Manual* (by Dr. Janet Travell) is effective, that subclinical abnormalities are important, and that the comprehensive and aggressive metabolic approach to treatment in Teitelbaum's study is highly successful and makes fibromyalgia a very treatable disorder. The study by Dr. Teitelbaum et al and years of clinical experience makes this approach an excellent and powerfully effective part of the standard of practice for treatment of people who suffer from FMS and MPS [myofascial pain syndrome]—both of which are common and devastating syndromes. It is very exciting that this research helps to usher in a new, more effective era in medical care by treating the patient and not only the laboratory tests!"[4]

It's time for you to get well! Ready?

PART 1

*Your Body's
Energy Crisis*

A curious thing happened during the rigorous process I went through to become a physician. By the time I completed my formal training, I presumed that if an important treatment existed for an illness I had been taught about it in medical school. I understood, of course, that physicians need to continue their education to stay abreast of new information and treatments. But I felt sure that if someone claimed he or she could effectively treat a "nontreatable" disease, that person was a quack.

I was wrong.

As I have developed as a physician and have spent countless hours exploring the scientific literature, taking notes of effective treatments for a wide range of illnesses, and observing the often flawed process that prescription drugs go through as they become commonly used in the United States, I've discovered that natural remedies can work just as well as prescriptions and with fewer or less serious side effects and at a significantly lower cost to the consumer. I've also learned that some natural remedies and prescription drugs can work better together than either one can alone.

My preference is to practice what is called "comprehensive medicine," which uses the best of natural and pharmaceutical therapies. It's like having a complete tool kit at your disposal. The approach you will learn about in *From Fatigued to Fantastic!* is well-grounded in the scientific literature and patient practice. The program within these pages treats the underlying, perpetuating factors of your illness that keep you from feeling better.

Although readers with chronic fatigue syndrome and those with fibromyalgia will find that this book feels like it was written just about them, those of you with general fatigue without CFS will also find that this book will help you to restore your vitality and regain control over your life.

What Are Chronic Fatigue Syndrome and Fibromyalgia?

1

*C*hronic fatigue and immune dysfunction syndrome (abbreviated CFIDS or CFS) is a group of symptoms associated with severe, almost unrelenting fatigue. Some of the more common symptoms are:

- poor sleep
- difficulties with short-term memory, concentration, word finding, word substitution, and orientation (a group of symptoms collectively known as brain fog)
- increased thirst
- bowel disorders
- recurrent infections and sinusitis
- exhaustion after minimal exertion

A related problem, fibromyalgia syndrome (FMS), is present if you also have widespread pain and achiness. If this sounds like you, I would assume that you have CFS/FMS unless it can be proven otherwise. For most people, fibromyalgia and CFIDS/CFS are the same illness, so I use the terms CFIDS and CFS interchangeably to refer to all of these. Myalgic encephalomyelitis and myalgic encephalomyelopathy (ME) are other names sometimes used to refer to these syndromes.

How Is Chronic Fatigue Syndrome Defined?

The U.S. Centers for Disease Control and Prevention (CDC) has put together an updated list of criteria for the diagnosis of chronic fatigue syndrome (see the box on page 7). Although the CDC's criteria have helped researchers define groups for studies, its original criteria for chronic fatigue syndrome excluded all but about five thousand to twenty thousand people in the United States.[1-3] However, more than 25 million Americans have severe fatigue, lasting at least one month, at any given time.[4] Of these, around 6 million people currently suffer from fibromyalgia.[5] Research has shown that people with disabling fatigue who do not fit the CDC criteria often have the same immunologic changes and responses to treatment as those who do fit.[6] My experience, too, suggests that the underlying causes of patients' chronic fatigue and their responses to treatment are not affected by whether they strictly meet the CDC guidelines.[7]

Because of problems defining chronic fatigue syndrome and fibromyalgia, I prefer to use the following definition: Unexplained fatigue that significantly interferes with your functioning and is associated with any two of the following symptoms:

1. Brain fog
2. Poor sleep
3. Diffuse achiness
4. Increased thirst
5. Bowel dysfunction and/or
6. Recurrent and/or persistent infections or flu-like feelings

If this describes how you are feeling, then you probably have CFS. If any of the above symptoms are accompanied by widespread pain, you may have FMS, as well.

What Chronic Fatigue Syndrome and Fibromyalgia Feel Like

Chronic fatigue syndrome and fibromyalgia occur in varying degrees of severity. Many people have mild to moderate fatigue with achiness and

CDC Criteria for Chronic Fatigue Syndrome

A case of chronic fatigue syndrome is defined by the presence of the following:

1. Clinically evaluated, unexplained, persistent, or relapsing chronic fatigue that is of new or definite onset (has not been lifelong); is not the result of ongoing exertion; is not substantially alleviated by rest; and results in substantial reduction in previous levels of occupational, educational, social, or personal activities.

2. Concurrent occurrence of four or more of the following symptoms, all of which must have persisted or recurred during six or more consecutive months of illness and must not have predated the fatigue:

   A. Self-reported impairment in short-term memory or concentration severe enough to cause substantial reduction in previous levels of occupational, educational, social, or personal activities
   B. Sore throat
   C. Tender cervical [neck] or axillary [underarm] lymph nodes
   D. Muscle pain
   E. Multijoint pain without joint swelling or redness
   F. Headaches of a new type, pattern, or severity
   G. Unrefreshing sleep
   H. Postexertional malaise lasting more than twenty-four hours

Adapted from Annals of Internal Medicine *121 (14 December 1994). Used with permission.*

poor sleep. Often, these people attribute the symptoms simply to aging or stress—for example, they may say they feel like they're fifty years old when they're only thirty. Others have fatigue so disabling that they cannot even get out of bed, let alone participate in regular daily activities.

The most common complaints among chronic fatigue and fibromyalgia patients are:

- *Overwhelming fatigue.* Most of these patients are fatigued most or all of the time. Occasionally, they experience short periods during which they feel better. However, after several hours or days of feeling energetic, they typically crash back down into severe fatigue.

Most CFS patients wake up feeling tired and often have the most energy between 10 p.m. and 4 a.m., in part because their day/night cycles are reversed. In addition, exercise often makes the fatigue worse. When CFS patients try to exercise, they feel worse that day and as if they were "hit by a truck" the next. The postexertional fatigue occurs because they can't make enough energy to condition their bodies when they exercise, simply depleting their energy instead. This causes further deconditioning and discouragement. A better approach is to walk as much as you can, but only to the point where you feel "good tired" after the exercise and better the next day. After approximately ten weeks of gentle, slow walking, most people find that they can start to increase their walking by up to one minute a day as their energy levels increase with the treatments we'll discuss. Once they can walk for about an hour a day, they then can start slowly increasing the intensity of exercise through an activity such as biking, rowing, or tennis.

- *Frequent infections.* Many CFS patients have recurrent sinus or respiratory infections, sore throats, swollen glands, bladder infections, and/or vaginal, bowel, or skin yeast infections. These are usually best treated without antibiotics (see "Treating Infections without Antibiotics," page 126). Some also have a recurrent rash that is resistant to treatment. Abdominal gas, cramps, and bloating are also very common, as is alternating diarrhea and constipation. These digestive complaints are attributed to spastic colon, and are often triggered by bowel yeast or parasitic infections. People often find that their rash, as well as the sinusitis and spastic colon, goes away for the first time in years when they have their bowel fungal overgrowth treated (see Chapter 5). Poor food absorption and food sensitivities may also play significant roles in bowel symptoms and go away with treatment (see Chapter 9).

- *Brain fog.* Chronic fatigue patients often suffer from poor short-term memory, difficulty with word finding and word substitution, and, occasionally, brief episodes of disorientation, lasting thirty seconds to two minutes, that occur despite being in a familiar place. Brain fog is one of the most frustrating symptoms for some people and is often the scariest. Many people are afraid that they are developing Alzheimer's disease, but this is not the case. A simple way to differentiate between brain fog and dementia is that with brain fog you may constantly forget where you left the keys. However, with Alzheimer's you may forget how to *use* your keys. They are not the same, and brain fog also routinely resolves with treatment.

- *Achiness.* Achiness in both muscles and joints is also common in chronic fatigue patients. For most, this achiness comes from disordered sleep, low thyroid function, yeast infections, and nutritional deficiencies. It is important to remember that pain is your body's way of telling you that something desperately needs attention—kind of like the oil light on your dashboard. When you give your body what it needs, you'll find that the pain often disappears—just as the oil light goes out when you add needed oil to a car. This does not mean that you have to put up with pain, however, while you treat the underlying causes of chronic fatigue and fibromyalgia. We will also discuss how to use both natural and prescription therapies to keep you comfortable.

- *Increased thirst.* Because of hormonal problems, people with chronic fatigue and fibromyalgia often have decreased fluid retention, which increases urine output and thirst. A classic description of a CFS/FMS patient is that they "drink like a fish and pee like a racehorse." Drinking a lot of water, therefore, becomes important. In fact, many CFS patients find that they may need to drink up to four times as much liquid as the average person. When people ask me how many glasses of water to drink a day, I tell them a much better approach is simply to check your mouth and lips. If they are dry you need to drink more water.

  It is important to note that dry eyes and dry mouth that do not improve when you drink more water (called sicca syndrome) are also common. These symptoms can often be resolved by taking fish-oil supplements, B vitamins, and magnesium.

- *Allergies.* Fatigue patients often have a history of being sensitive to many foods and medications. Fortunately, severe environmental sensitivity is much less common. I find that food sensitivities and other sensitivities usually improve when the adrenal insufficiency and yeast or parasitic overgrowth are treated. Desensitization techniques can also be helpful (more about this in Chapter 9).

- *Anxiety and depression.* Approximately 12 percent of people with CFS have marked anxiety, with palpitations, sweating, and other signs of panic. These symptoms, too, often improve with treatment. We will discuss how to treat these naturally in Chapters 8 and 10.

- *Weight gain.* Despite no change in diet, studies done in our research center show that people with CFS and fibromyalgia gain an average of thirty-two pounds with their illness. I suspect this occurs because of changes in metabolism caused by low thyroid function, yeast over-growth, a deficiency of acetyl-L-carnitine, insulin resistance, and poor sleep. Many patients are thrilled not only to feel better and have their pain go away, but also to find their weight dropping (see Chapter 11).

• *Decreased libido.* When I ask CFIDS patients how their libido is, most answer, "What libido?" In addition to pain and a general "yucky" feeling, hormonal deficiencies also contribute to this symptom. However, libido often also improves with treatment, though it often takes about six months.

You may have recognized yourself as you read through this list. If you did, please be assured that you are not alone. You are part of a large group of more than 50 million people worldwide. Many support groups exist, including the National Fibromyalgia Association (www.fmaware.org) and the International Coalition for the Advancement of Fibromyalgia/Chronic Fatigue Syndrome Treatments (ICAF; www.icafcoalition.org). For support groups around the world, see Appendix E: Resources.

What Is Fibromyalgia?

We often talk about chronic fatigue syndrome and fibromyalgia together, because the two syndromes often coexist and share many of the same symptoms. Fibromyalgia is basically a sleep disorder characterized by many tender knots in the muscles. These tender knots, called tender points and trigger points, are a major cause of the achiness that fibromyalgia and CFIDS patients feel. For most patients, it is easier to consider fibromyalgia and CFIDS as the same illness. However, in addition to fatigue, pain is a major and defining symptom in fibromyalgia. Fibromyalgia is a cousin to other muscle diseases, called myofascial pain syndromes.

The diagnostic criteria developed in 1990 by the American College of Rheumatology[8] are much more clinically useful than the chronic fatigue diagnostic criteria the CDC developed, which were meant largely for research. The criteria for fibromyalgia are as follows:

• Feeling pain both above and below the waist in both the left and right sides of the body

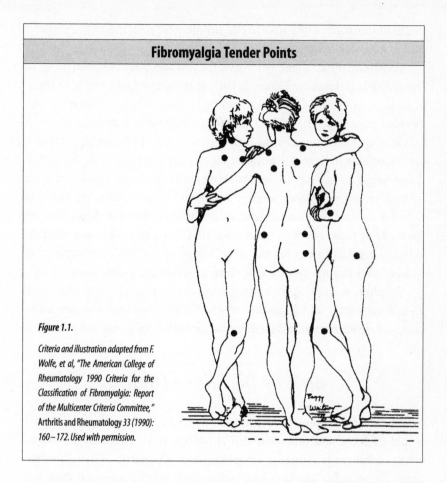

Fibromyalgia Tender Points

Figure 1.1.

Criteria and illustration adapted from F. Wolfe, et al, "The American College of Rheumatology 1990 Criteria for the Classification of Fibromyalgia: Report of the Multicenter Criteria Committee," Arthritis and Rheumatology 33 (1990): 160–172. Used with permission.

- Feeling pain somewhere down the middle of the body (e.g., headache, back, chest, or abdominal pain)
- Being tender in eleven out of eighteen arbitrarily chosen locations on the body, called *tender points*

Unfortunately, most doctors don't know how to find and check the tender points, which are not necessarily the same as trigger points. And many of the major researchers in the field are recognizing that there is an intermediate form of fibromyalgia where people have fewer than eleven of the eighteen tender points. The tender-point exam will probably be eliminated when we have a good blood or urine test for FMS available.

The good news is that the pain can usually be eliminated, or at least markedly improved, by using the SHIN protocol, as discussed in this book. In our studies, the majority of people were pain free at the end of a ninety-nine-day treatment period.[7, 9]

As with chronic fatigue syndrome, the first and foremost component of fibromyalgia is disordered sleep. If you are not getting seven to nine hours of solid, uninterrupted sleep, you will be in pain. When we sleep, we usually have periods during which we stop moving and go into deep, very restful slumber. Unfortunately, the little muscle knots of fibromyalgia make it uncomfortable to lie in one position for an extended time, and people with fibromyalgia do not stay in the deep stages of sleep (stages 3 and 4) that are integral to renewing one's energy. Although a fibromyalgia patient may sleep for twelve hours every night, he or she may not have slept *effectively* for many of those hours. A good indication that you are not experiencing enough deep-stage sleep is a morning "hangover" feeling. A critical part of making your pain go away will be correcting your sleep deficiency.

In addition, treating underlying infections (especially yeast infections), an underactive thyroid (regardless of whether the blood tests are normal or not), and deficiencies of magnesium and ribose will be key to your recovery.

So Why Do I Have Pain?

When muscles do not have enough energy you might think that they would go loose and limp, but that is not the case. Think about writer's cramp, when your muscles stop getting enough energy. When this happens, the muscles become tight—often stiff as a board—and they will hurt. The multiple little painful knots (called trigger points) are in the belly of the muscles where they have bunched up. As you feel pain from these knots, your muscles will start shifting your weight to take the strain off the uncomfortable areas. Unfortunately, this puts more strain on other areas, and the pain starts moving around your body. In addition, when you're not able to get deep sleep your muscles do not heal from the day's activities, and this also contributes to pain. To add insult to injury, once you develop this chronic pain, the brain actually starts to amplify the pain signal, and can become the source of much of the pain you feel. This is called "central sensitization." You'll be amazed at how dramatically your pain can be decreased and usually eliminated as you get eight to nine hours of deep sleep a night, restore energy production in your muscles, and stop sending excessive pain signals to your brain.

PERPETUATING FACTORS

It never ceases to amaze me how quickly a case of fibromyalgia can resolve once the underlying problems are treated. In fact, the duration of the disease does not seem to affect how responsive it is to treatment. Two of the top authorities on muscle pain, Drs. Janet Travell and David Simons, have devoted much of their study to trigger points, their causes, and their resolutions. They have noted in their talks and writings that hormonal, nutritional, infectious, and even major structural problems, such as a short leg or short hemipelvis (an uneven pelvis), as well as other factors cause the trigger points to persist.[10]

I have found that my fibromyalgia patients tend to recover when *all* of the major underlying perpetuating factors are treated.[7, 9] It is important to understand that fibromyalgia is *both* a common endpoint for many of the problems we have discussed thus far *and* a cause for these problems. Infections, nutritional deficiencies, and hormonal deficiencies can all, individually and in concert, trigger and perpetuate fibromyalgia. Fibromyalgia can also cause the hormonal and immune dysfunctions and, perhaps by leading to malabsorption, the nutritional deficiencies. Fibromyalgia becomes self-perpetuating as soon as sleep is disrupted. Even if the underlying trigger, such as a trauma that occurred years before, has resolved, the sleep deprivation of the illness can cause suppression of the hypothalamus (discussed in Chapter 3).

What Causes CFS/FMS?

I do not view these syndromes as the enemy. Rather, I see them as attempts on the body's part to protect itself from further harm and damage in the face of any of a number of overwhelming stresses. A simple way to look at fibromyalgia and CFS would be to view them as circuit breakers in a house. These breakers disconnect the electricity from the home's wiring when electrical systems become overstressed. To solve the problem, you just reset the breakers. Your body's "circuit breaker" does much the same thing, resetting after a stress with rest and proper nutrition. In CFS/FMS, however, it is as if a major circuit breaker, in this situation the master gland in the brain called the hypothalamus, has gone off-line and is not able to reset itself. When this occurs, rest is no longer enough to restore proper function. The ensuing fatigue forces the person to use less energy without the accompanying benefits that rest brings to a healthy individual.

Just as there are hundreds of ways that you can blow an electrical fuse in a house, there are also many diverse triggers that can cause these syndromes in the body. Nonetheless, most patients' symptoms seem to come from a common endpoint—decreased energy production or increased energy needs with secondary dysfunction or suppression of the hypothalamus.[11–14]

HYPOTHALAMIC DYSFUNCTION

You've no doubt heard the old story of the blind men who stumbled upon an elephant. One felt its trunk and believed it was a snake. Another felt its leg and thought it was a tree trunk. Yet another, missing the elephant entirely, was certain nothing was there and told his friends they must be crazy. This seems to be the current state of affairs in our understanding of CFS/FMS.

Even so, we are lucky to be at a point where we have as many pieces of the puzzle as we do. Let's examine what we do know, beginning with two assumptions that I believe to be true:

1. CFS/FMS are the same illness in most cases.
2. CFS/FMS represent a common endpoint of a large number of possible underlying triggers—that is, many different things can trigger these syndromes. Once triggered, the process is similar and self-perpetuating, regardless of what the triggers were and whether or not the triggers are now gone. For example, either an auto accident or a viral syndrome can trigger CFS/FMS in different people.

Furthermore, we know that several processes are common in people with CFS/FMS:

- Disordered sleep
- Hormonal dysfunction
- Infection and immune dysfunction
- Autonomic nervous system dysfunction, with neurally mediated hypotension (NMH), a problem with blood pressure regulation that results in weakness and dizziness when rising
- Low body temperature

Things simplify a bit when one realizes that all of the above processes are controlled or affected by the hypothalamus—our bodies' master gland, controlling the activity of most other glands in the body. Let's look at each of these problems individually.

DISORDERED SLEEP

When we look at sleep-deprivation research, several things stand out. Among other things, sleep deprivation can cause:

- *Immune dysfunction, with multiple opportunistic infections.*
- *Decreased metabolic activity, specifically in the hypothalamus, limbic system, and thalamus.* This, as well as low estrogen levels, could account for the decreases in blood flow to the brain, causing brain fog.
- *Autonomic and temperature-regulation dysfunction.* When given the choice, sleep-deprived test animals will often choose a higher room temperature. Higher nighttime room temperatures may further worsen sleep quality.

Chapter 3 discusses sleep problems in detail.

HORMONAL DYSFUNCTION

The effects of hypothalamic dysfunction on the body's hormone levels can include:

- *Low thyroid hormone.* This can cause decreased metabolism, with weight gain and low body temperature, which can cause poor enzyme and metabolic function.
- *Low vasopressin (antidiuretic hormone).* This causes decreased ability to hold onto fluid, resulting in frequent urination and increased thirst.
- *Low growth hormone.* This also causes low levels of dehydroepiandrosterone (DHEA), a hormone produced by the adrenal glands. DHEA is used by the body to make other hormones, including estrogen and testosterone, and is tied to energy levels and a general feeling of well-being.
- *Decreased cortisol.* Low levels of this stress hormone cause immune dysfunction, hypotension, and the tendency to "crash" in stressful situations.
- *Low ovarian and testicular function.* Low estrogen can contribute to the decreased blood flow to specific areas in the brain that is seen in CFS/

FMS. Low testosterone in both males and females can cause immune dysfunction. Although total testosterone levels are often normal, the levels of active (free, or unbound, serum) testosterone are suboptimal in the majority of people with CFS/FMS. In both women and men, bringing free testosterone levels back to mid- to high-normal often dramatically improves symptoms after two months.

Chapter 4 discusses hormonal deficiencies in detail.

INFECTION AND IMMUNE DYSFUNCTION

Chronic fatigue patients typically have multiple opportunistic infections, that is, infections caused by organisms that usually do not cause illness in most people, as well as other recurrent infections. These persistent infections are probably a result of immune dysfunction. Hypothalamic dysfunction, poor digestion, a "leaky gut," and poor sleep likely play major roles in suppressing the immune system. The resulting infections can cause CFS/FMS to persist. Some common types of infections that affect people with CFS/FMS are:

- *Yeast (candida) overgrowth.* This overgrowth, along with secondary bacterial infections, then can cause chronic sinusitis.
- *Bowel infections.* These types of infections are major players in CFS/FMS. Parasitic, fungal, and bacterial overgrowths are common in the bowel, and often account for irritable bowel syndrome. They can cause CFS/FMS and contribute to the nutritional deficiencies by causing malabsorption and a leaky gut. The liver and the immune system then must detoxify and break down many large molecules that would otherwise have been properly digested in the stomach and intestines. These problems in turn can lead to food, chemical/environmental, and medication sensitivities; immune dysfunction; decreased adrenal function; and liver overload.
- *Infections caused by rickettsia, mycoplasma, chlamydia, and other unusual organisms.* Several organisms that are difficult to test for may both trigger and perpetuate CFS/FMS. Antibiotics such as minocycline (Minocin), azithromycin (Zithromax), or ciprofloxacin (Cipro) given for anywhere from six months to years at a time may eradicate these, but also may cause yeast overgrowth, necessitating the use of an antifungal medication.

- *Viral infections.* Some viruses can cause hypothalamic suppression. Although in most people this resolves when the virus goes away, if you have CFS/FMS, it may not. Because many patients get well without antiviral treatments, I suspect that the triggering viral infection is often long gone by several months after the illness begins, or is eliminated when the immune suppression is treated and resolves. In other cases, antiviral therapy may be needed. Post-polio syndrome, herpesvirus 6 (HHV-6), cytomegalovirus (CMV), and the Epstein-Barr virus are four of many suspected culprits.
- *Chronic prostatitis.* This is common in men with CFS.

Chapter 5 addresses how to eradicate infections and boost the immune system in more detail.

Autonomic Nervous System Dysfunction

The autonomic (sympathetic/parasympathetic) nervous system, the part of the nervous system that controls such basic bodily processes as circulation and sweating (among others), is controlled by the hypothalamus. Improper functioning of the autonomic nervous system can cause a variety of problems, among them:

- *Neurally mediated hypotension (NMH).* This can cause dizziness and weakness, especially when rising.
- *Night and day sweats.* The night sweats can disrupt sleep.

Low Body Temperature

A low body temperature causes the body's energy and enzyme systems to work inefficiently, as enzyme function is temperature-sensitive. If the body temperature is returned to 98.6°F (using different types of thyroid hormones), people often feel better.[15] Stress, including that caused by infection or dieting, may trigger persistently low levels of triiodothyronine (T_3), the active form of thyroid hormone, and cause low body temperature. Unfortunately, since T_3 is mostly made inside the cells, low T_3 levels often do not show up on standard blood tests for thyroid function. Altered temperature regulation may also further contribute to impaired sleep.

(For a visual representation of the interrelationships among all these factors, see Figure 1.2, The CFIDS/FMS Cycle.)

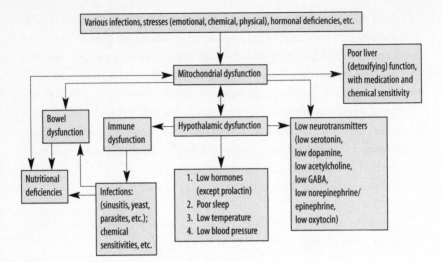

FIGURE 1.2. *The CFIDS/FMS Cycle*

THE GOOD NEWS

As you see, hypothalamic dysfunction can cause a cascade of problems that may account for many, if not most, of the abnormal findings seen in CFS/ FMS. These processes can then perpetuate hypothalamic suppression. They also explain the multitude of symptoms seen in these illnesses.

The good news is that everything I have discussed above is treatable. The trick is to sort out which problems are most active in each individual and to treat them all. We certainly have much more to learn. I really do not think we have defined "the whole elephant" yet. As we continue to integrate what we learn, we may begin to see the whole picture. Nonetheless, hypothalamic dysfunction, secondary to your body's energy crisis, explains why people with CFS/FMS can't sleep, have low body temperatures, gain weight, and are prone to multiple and recurrent infections. The hypothalamic dysfunction by itself can therefore cause most of the symptoms we see in chronic fatigue and fibromyalgia.

I suspect that the root cause of the hypothalamic suppression can be found in the mitochondria, or the "energy furnaces" in the cells. The good news is that restoring adequate energy production using the treatments discussed in Chapter 2 can jump-start your healing process by getting at the root of the problem. We will then discuss how to use sleep and hormonal, anti-infectious, and nutritional support to further restore function in the hypothalamic circuit breaker, allowing it to resume functioning. There is no single magic bullet to get well, however. People who suffer from CFS/FMS usually have a combination of several different problems. The exact combination varies considerably from individual to individual. There are dozens of major underlying factors, with individual people typically displaying more than five or six factors each. It is important to look for and treat all of the factors simultaneously. Chronic fatigue and fibromyalgia are unusual in that each separate problem can trigger other problems. Because of this, it is rare to need to treat only one single underlying problem.

So How Can I Tell What Triggered My Illness?

Although there are infinite ways to "blow your fuse," many common subsets and patterns are seen. One of the most helpful clues is whether your illness began suddenly or gradually. Think back to what stresses were going on in your life when the illness began, and what symptoms you had at the onset of the illness. For example, if you had high fevers you probably had an infectious trigger. If you received antibiotics, especially several courses, and have spastic colon or sinusitis, you probably had a candida or yeast-overgrowth trigger. If you were traveling overseas and had diarrhea, you may have had a bowel-infection trigger such as parasitic infection.

Below are some of the most common triggers to consider if your illness began suddenly:

1. Viral, parasitic, or antibiotic-sensitive infections
2. Injury
3. Pregnancy (usually beginning soon after the baby is born)
4. Toxic exposures (especially if others around you also got sick)

If your illness came on gradually, consider:

1. Yeast (candida) overgrowth—especially if you have sinusitis/nasal congestion and/or spastic colon
2. Hormonal deficiencies (even if your blood tests are normal)—especially low thyroid or perimenopause
3. Chronic stress, including both at work and within relationships. These syndromes commonly affect hardworking "adrenaline junkies."

4. Autoimmune disorders (e.g., lupus, rheumatoid arthritis, Sjögren's syndrome)
5. Anything that disrupts sleep, including sleep apnea, restless leg syndrome, or a spouse who snores

Let's look more closely at a few of the most common triggers.

INFECTIONS

SUDDEN ONSET—THE DROP-DEAD FLU

The most notorious pattern seen in severe chronic fatigue states is one in which a person who is feeling fine suddenly comes down with a brutal flu-like illness that never goes away. In most of these CFS patients, an underlying viral or other infection is suspected.[16-24] These infections can directly suppress the hypothalamus.[25] For most people, the suppression of the hypothalamus ends when the flu is over. Dr. William Jefferies, a retired endocrinologist and assistant professor of medicine at Case Western Reserve University, has theorized that people who remain chronically ill after an infection have long-term hypothalamic suppression. He explains that the flu causes suppression of adrenocorticotropic hormone (ACTH), which is the hormone that causes the adrenal gland to make adrenal hormone. If the adrenal gland is suppressed and cannot make sufficient adrenal hormone, a variety of fatigue symptoms can result. Dr. Jefferies has found that treating such instances of adrenal suppression with additional adrenal hormone can safely bring about marked improvement, as long as those doses are normal for the body and do not exceed natural adrenal levels.[25]

What makes treatment complicated, however, is that even if a gland is underactive, blood testing can often mistakenly suggest that the gland is technically normal, albeit in the low range (more on this in Chapter 4). Patients are then often told that their thyroid and/or adrenal glands are healthy when indeed they are not. You'll find more information on finding a doctor who can correctly interpret blood tests and identify subclinical hormonal deficiencies in Chapter 12.

The drop-dead flu also causes many people to develop poor immunity, facilitating repeated bladder, respiratory, or sinus infections. I have found that patients who then take repeated courses of antibiotics for any reason often end up with an overgrowth of yeast in the bowel. Bowel parasites and other infections are also common in CFIDS patients.[7, 9] Some of these infections can sneak up on you slowly. Suppressed hypothalamic function from chronic infections can then trigger disordered sleep, continuing the fatigue cycle.

Gradual Onset—Yeast / Candida Overgrowth

If you have chronic sinusitis/nasal congestion or spastic colon (gas, bloating, diarrhea, or constipation), you probably have yeast or candida overgrowth. This overgrowth may have triggered your CFS/FMS. In other cases, the immune suppression caused by the illness may result in the yeast overgrowth itself. Most of the overgrowth occurs in the bowels. In my experience, it is worth treating everybody who has chronic fatigue syndrome and/or fibromyalgia for possible yeast/candida overgrowth.

Poor Sleep

As discussed earlier, chronic fatigue and fibromyalgia sufferers may not have slept effectively for several years. I suspect that poor sleep further suppresses the hypothalamus. Poor sleep can then cause immune suppression, with secondary bowel infections.[26–28]

Many people enter the fatigue cycle directly through disrupted sleep. Chronic fatigue syndrome and fibromyalgia can be triggered by anything that suppresses the hypothalamus, disrupts sleep, or causes tight muscles. These include a trauma, such as an accident; a parasitic or other infection; chronic emotional or physical stress; hormonal imbalances; and/or recent childbirth. They can also be triggered by a number of other problems, such as an anatomic problem (for example, having legs of different lengths) or temporomandibular joint (TMJ) syndrome, which is characterized by tenderness and clicking in the jaw.

The Autoimmune Triad and Hormonal Deficiencies

Another common pattern seen in severe chronic fatigue states is the autoimmune triad. In autoimmune disorders, the body mistakes parts of itself for outside invaders. The autoimmune triad seen in CFIDS patients involves the thyroid and adrenal glands, as well as the cells in the body that assist in the absorption of vitamin B_{12}. When the body attacks these "invaders," the resulting low levels of thyroid and adrenal hormones and vitamin B_{12} trigger fibromyalgia and poor sleep. This can then suppress the hypothalamus gland, setting the fatigue cycle in motion. Multiple other hormonal problems, especially low estrogen in the ten to fifteen years before one is "officially" in menopause, can also trigger CFIDS/FMS.

So How Do I Determine
Which Treatments I Need?

Fill out the questionnaires I've placed at the end of many chapters. Based on the answers, you will be directed to check off certain treatments on the SHIN Treatment Worksheet in Appendix B. This will tailor a treatment protocol based on your symptoms. If you have lab results, the educational program on my Web site (www.vitality101.com) can analyze both your symptoms and lab results to help you and your physician determine which treatments are likely to be needed in your case.

Because the best results seem to come from treating all of the symptoms of CFS/FMS simultaneously, it can sometimes be difficult to tell exactly which treatment is producing the main benefit. However, once you are feeling better, you and your doctor can taper off the treatments to see which ones are still needed. If you would like to go more slowly with your treatment, especially if you have a history of being very sensitive to natural or prescription therapies, be sure to let your health-care practitioner know.

Why Have CFS and Fibromyalgia
Been Ignored by Doctors?

Many pieces of the CFIDS/FMS puzzle are still missing. The outlook is bright, however, with new research continually providing important clues on how to improve treatment. For the vast majority of people with CFS/FMS-related symptoms, effective treatment is now available. Unfortunately, the medical community often refuses to acknowledge an illness until there is a definitive test for it. In the early days of polio, for example, before a blood test was developed, some physicians intimated that the children on iron lungs were simply having a psychosomatic illness. The same thing occurred with lupus, even though many women died of the disease. Indeed, relief came for lupus sufferers only when a blood test was developed. The same thing is now occurring with CFS and fibromyalgia. Fortunately, the CDC and the National Institutes of Health (NIH), the two main governmental agencies responsible for CFS and fibromyalgia research, are now getting more serious about making it clear to physicians that these are very real and devastating syndromes—and not simply psychosomatic. The CDC is spending millions of dollars in advertising to help correct misimpressions about CFS and to educate both physicians and the public about how real and devastating these syndromes are. This recognition is coming just in time, as the prevalence of these syndromes is skyrocketing.

You're Not Alone

Let's look at the numbers. Fibromyalgia was conservatively estimated to affect 6 million Americans in a major study published in 1995.[29] However, in our study sixty-nine of seventy-two patients with fibromyalgia (approximately 95 percent) also had CFIDS. In another study by Dr. Dedra Buchwald, 64 percent of her FMS patients also had CFIDS. By extrapolating these percentages, you might expect at least 4 to 5 million cases of CFIDS. In addition, about 10 to 20 percent of CFIDS patients do not have fibromyalgia, so again using these figures, there should be almost 6 million cases of CFIDS. Yet some researchers still believe that only a few hundred thousand people are affected by these syndromes.

To show that CFS/FMS is much more common than the current estimates of five hundred thousand to 1 million Americans, let's break it down further. A study by Dr. Leonard Jason, the world's foremost epidemiologist for CFS, found[4] that:

- 11.9 percent of the population currently had "severe fatigue, extreme tiredness, or exhaustion" lasting more than one month.
- 4.2 percent had these symptoms for more than six months.
- 2.2 percent also had no other medical or psychological diagnosis that could cause fatigue (approximately 2 percent of Americans have FMS).
- 0.4 percent is all that was left over after doctors and a psychiatrist looked for any problems that could be used as an excuse to account for fatigue (now or in the past).

These numbers suggest a CFIDS-related illness likely affects at least 2 to 4 percent of the population, and perhaps as much as 12 percent. However, when Dr. Jason applied the rigid criteria that the CDC uses, which rules out cases where other possible causes of fatigue may be present, he found that less than one million Americans would be diagnosed with CFIDS.

Chronic fatigue and fibromyalgia appear to be becoming much more common. Four studies published in 2006 suggest that, using the same diagnostic criteria, fibromyalgia has gone from affecting approximately 2 percent of the European and African population ten years ago[30–34] to approximately 8 percent just a decade later. When individual country data from these studies are analyzed, the surge in diagnoses tops 400 percent. It seems that effective treatment has arrived just in time.

Important Points

- Chronic fatigue syndrome (CFS or CFIDS) is characterized by the paradox of the inability to sleep despite being exhausted, brain fog, and, if fibromyalgia (FMS) is also present, widespread pain. You may have a variety of other symptoms as well. Common symptoms include increased thirst, weight gain, low libido, spastic colon, nasal congestion/sinusitis, and frequent infections.
- Chronic fatigue syndrome and/or fibromyalgia occur when you expend more energy than you can make. This overloads your circuits, causing you to "blow a fuse" called the hypothalamus. This gland controls sleep, hormonal function, autonomic function (blood pressure, pulse, sweating), and temperature regulation. In essence, although the symptoms can be devastating, chronic fatigue syndrome and fibromyalgia keep you from causing yourself any permanent harm when you've overdrawn your body's energy account.
- "Blowing a fuse" can occur because of overwork, infections, poor sleep, hormonal problems, toxic work or home situations, pregnancy, injury, or many other causes.
- Research shows that effective therapy is available for 91 percent of patients with CFIDS/FMS by simply treating symptoms with the SHIN (Sleep, Hormones, Infections, and Nutrition) protocol.

Create Your Individual Treatment Protocol— Beginning with Ribose for Energy Production

2

*A*lthough many physicians use this book as a guide, *From Fatigued to Fantastic!* is for you, the person suffering from chronic fatigue syndrome and/or fibromyalgia. After giving an overview of the possible causes and patterns of chronic fatigue states in Chapter 1 and discussing how they represent an energy crisis in your body, we will then teach you how to get well, starting at the end of this chapter.

As discussed in Chapter 1, it's good that you have a circuit breaker to keep you from "burning out your wiring" and hurting yourself, but it doesn't do you much good if you don't know how to turn your circuit breaker back on. This requires optimizing energy production and eliminating the things that are draining your energy. We call this the SHIN protocol, which stands for the four main treatment areas:

1. Sleep
2. Hormonal deficiencies
3. Infections
4. Nutritional deficiencies

Our placebo-controlled study shows that when you treat these four building blocks of health, 91 percent of you can improve your energy levels and decrease your pain—often dramatically.[1, 2] Part 2 will go into the specifics of each treatment area, and in Part 3, you'll learn how to overcome other problems, such as chronic pain, weight gain, low libido, pregnancy concerns, and mind-body issues. Several appendices offer additional or supporting information, including an overview of this illness for your physician and a treatment checklist that you can use as you read the book to help you tailor a treatment protocol to your specific case.

Your doctor may not be familiar with the research on effective treatment of chronic fatigue and fibromyalgia. If this is the case, you may want to show your doctor Appendix G: For Physicians (which I wrote specifically for medical professionals) and the abstracts of my clinical studies that are available in Appendix A and on my Web site. The full text of two of the studies done in our research center using the treatments discussed in this book can also be found at www.vitality101.com. These will be helpful to your physician. Feel free to download the studies from the Web site and give him or her a copy.

If you are looking for a new doctor, turn to Chapter 12 for more information on what to look for and how to choose a practitioner. In addition, I have become the medical director of the national Fibromyalgia & Fatigue Centers, which use the protocol described in this book. More information can be found in Chapter 12 and Appendix E: Resources.

Regardless of which physician you choose, it is essential that you work with a doctor to monitor your treatment, guide your use of natural remedies, and help implement the strategies you're going to read about here.

If you finish the book and find yourself wishing for more information, check my Web site (www.vitality101.com):

1. For more detailed information on many of the topics covered in this book, go to the *From Fatigued to Fantastic!* notes and use the password FFTF;
2. Visit the question-and-answer section, where you can see the answers to thousands of questions and ask your own questions;
3. Sign up for the free e-mail newsletter so you can stay on the cutting edge of new research information;
4. Sign onto the computer program that can do a more detailed analysis of not only your symptoms, but also your lab tests, to help you tailor a treatment protocol specific to your case. If you like, you can even use the "long program" to make a complete medical record of your case for your doctor (so he or she can use your appointment time far more effectively);
5. Visit the Web site shop for useful products.

How to Follow the SHIN Protocol

As you read this book, you'll find questions at the end of most chapters; answer the questions and check off the appropriate numbers on the SHIN Treatment Worksheet (see Appendix B). When you are done reading the book, you will have a treatment protocol tailored to your specific case. A fair number of treatments will be a recommended. Each treatment will be marked by level of importance as a top, middle, or low priority. This way, you can choose how aggressively you want to proceed. You'll want to bring this treatment worksheet to a doctor specializing in CFS/FMS and consult with him or her on how best to proceed.

Once you are ready to begin your treatment, you can follow this basic timeline, adjusting as needed.

WEEKS 1 THROUGH 3

- Nutritional therapies, specifically vitamin and ribose supplementation
- Treatments for pain if needed
- Sleep aids

WEEKS 4 THROUGH 8

- Hormonal therapies, continuing to use nutritional therapies and sleep aids

WEEKS 9 THROUGH 20

- Anti-infection treatments, adding one new treatment every one to three days, if necessary. Continue nutritional therapies, sleep aids, and hormonal therapies as needed.

You should continue this regimen for six months or until you begin to feel better. Then, slowly lower the doses of your treatments, without compromising how you feel. You may find that you need to continue some treatments, such as vitamin and ribose supplementation, indefinitely. In each chapter, I will discuss natural therapies first, as these are safer and often highly effective. However, it is helpful to have prescriptions available as well, and these will also be discussed.

Before we begin the SHIN protocol, however, let's jump-start our energy and set ourselves up for success.

Jump-Starting Your Body's Energy Furnaces

As we will discuss throughout this book, CFS and fibromyalgia reflect an energy crisis in your body. Although it can have numerous causes, the energy crisis will then trigger a host of downstream effects, including hypothalamic dysfunction ("blowing a fuse"), which causes multiple other problems, including muscle pain, insomnia, hormonal deficiencies, infections, poor liver detoxification, and decreased heart function. Although going after these many triggers and problems is important, it is also critical to go to the heart of the problem and treat your body's "energy furnaces." We will begin our discussion of treatments with those that directly increase energy production.

Each cell in your body contains structures called mitochondria, the tiny furnaces in each cell that produce energy by burning calories. Many problems, including Epstein-Barr viral infections, can suppress your energy furnaces.[3] In this chapter, I will discuss treatments that can help your mitochondrial furnaces work properly, and explain how you can use this information to feel better.

THE ROLE OF ENERGY PRODUCTION

We simply can't overcome fatigue if the cells and tissues in our bodies don't have enough energy. Medical research shows there are many conditions that drain energy from the body, leaving us fatigued and with frequent complications such as muscle pain, heart problems, and even depression.

Of course athletes who participate in high-intensity, endurance-type exercise often face the fatigue and muscle pain associated with energy depletion. Typically, a few days' rest will allow an athlete's muscles to recharge with energy. For the rest of us, however, the physiological factors that drain the heart and muscles of energy are not as easily overcome. It is amazing how a special simple sugar, called D-ribose, can help the body restore energy, giving the heart and muscles the power they need to fully recharge, so they can recover from fatigue and chronic muscle pain.

As we age, our bodies go through many changes that affect our ability to efficiently metabolize energy. For some, these changes occur more rapidly and are more pronounced, while for others the impact is seemingly absent. People with fibromyalgia and CFS have almost 20 percent less energy in their muscles than normal, and this lack of energy causes poor exercise tolerance and lack of endurance, making it hard to perform even the most basic of life's daily activities.[4, 5]

The metabolic changes that occur in our bodies over time or with the onset of disease are varied. Many patients experience thickening of the walls of capillaries that feed blood to muscles. These thickened capillary walls make it harder for oxygen to move from the blood to the muscle tissue, reducing the oxygen tension of the muscle and slowing the rate of energy synthesis.[6, 7]

In some, the mitochondrial energy furnaces are defective and cannot keep up with the energy demand of cells and tissues as they work through daily activities.[8–10] For others, cells and tissues are deficient in certain nutrients that are needed to process food into energy, leaving the tissues energy-starved.[11–13] In the most difficult conditions, the muscle itself is affected, leaking vital cellular constituents that include energy compounds and the fuels needed to restore energy levels in affected tissues.[14]

No matter the cause, the impact of energy depletion is to propel a downward spiral of fatigue, muscle pain, and stiffness that will not stop until the energy in the affected tissue can be restored. As energy is used faster than it can be restored, muscles become more painful, stiff, and fatigued. This causes even more energy to be used as the muscle struggles to recover, causing more fatigue, soreness, and stiffness,[15–17] and the cycle continues. If the conditions leading to energy depletion are not arrested in time, the fatigue can become overwhelming and debilitating—as occurs in CFS/FMS.

The Consequences of Mitochondrial Dysfunction

A large number of clinical findings common in CFS/FMS can be explained by mitochondrial furnace malfunction.

- *Hypothalamic suppression.* Particularly severe changes in the hypothalamus have been seen in mitochondrial dysfunction syndromes.[18]
- *Brain fog.* Mitochondrial dysfunction can cause decreases in levels of neurotransmitters in the brain, specifically low dopamine and acetylcholine, and possibly low serotonin.

- *Sensitivities and allergies.* Decreased ability of the liver to eliminate toxins and medications could contribute to sensitivities to both medications and environmental factors, as well as food sensitivities.
- *Postexertion fatigue.* Low energy production and accumulation of excessive amounts of lactic acid in muscles could inhibit recovery after exercise.
- *Poor digestion.* Mitochondrial dysfunction could also cause the bowel-related problems that plague so many people with chronic fatigue syndrome and fibromyalgia.
- *Weak immune system.* With problems in the mitochondria, you would expect to see poor white blood cell function and therefore a decreased ability to fight infection.
- *Heart dysfunction.* Based on research by Dr. Paul Cheney, mitochondrial dysfunction may weaken the heart muscle, requiring increased antioxidant and energy levels through supplementation.
- *Kidney function.* Poor kidney function resulting from mitochondrial dysfunction may cause a defect in the filtration and detoxification process.

Thus, mitochondrial dysfunction might well be the root cause of—or at least a contributing factor to—the hypothalamic, immune, neurotransmitter, nutritional, detoxification, sleep, and other disorders seen in CFS/FMS. (For a visual representation of the interrelationships among all these factors, see Figure 1.2, The CFIDS/FMS Cycle, page 18.)

Improving Mitochondrial Function

If mitochondrial dysfunction is an underlying or contributing cause to CFS/FMS, the next question is whether anything can be done to make your cellular energy furnaces work better. Several natural treatments are available to do just that. Let us now look at some of the treatments that can improve mitochondrial energy production. We'll begin with D-ribose, the key to energy production.

D-RIBOSE—THE NATURAL BODY ENERGIZER

Regarding energy production, it helps to look at the "energy molecules" such as ATP, NADH, and FADH. These represent the energy currency in your body, and are like the paper that money is printed on. You can have all the fuel you want, but if it cannot be converted to these molecules, it is useless.

For years, I talked about the importance of B vitamins, which are a key component of these molecules. These helped to a degree, but it was clear that another key component was missing. In looking at the biochemistry of these energy molecules, we saw that they were also made of two other key components—adenine and ribose. Adenine is plentiful in the body, and supplementing with adenine did not help CFS. We then turned our attention to ribose, which is made in your body in a slow, laborious process and cannot usually be found in food. We knew that CFS/FMS causes the body to dump other key energy molecules like acetyl-L-carnitine. We then found that the body did the same with ribose, making it hard to get your furnaces working again even after the other problems were treated.

This was like one of those "Eureka!" moments, when things come together. Not having ribose would be like trying to build a fire without kindling—nothing would happen. We wondered if giving ribose to people with CFS would jump-start their energy furnaces. The answer was a resounding yes!

Our recently published study (see the study abstract in Appendix A) showed an average 45 percent increase in energy after only three weeks (improvement began at twelve days) and an average overall improvement in quality of life of 30 percent. Two-thirds of the CFS/FMS patients felt they had improved.[19] Usually a 10 percent improvement for a single nutrient is considered excellent. A 45 percent increase left us amazed, and I am now recommending ribose for all of my CFS/FMS patients, for athletes, and for anyone with pain, fatigue, or heart problems. Ribose recently became available over the counter, and is one of the few natural products actually starting with physicians and then moving into health food stores.

It is critical to use the proper dose, which is 5 grams (5,000 milligrams) three times a day for the first three weeks. It can then be dropped to twice a day. I recommend the CORvalen form of ribose, as it is the least expensive and highest quality, and is packaged with a 5-gram dosing scoop in it. One 280-gram container will be enough to tell you if it will work. CORvalen M (which has ribose plus magnesium and malic acid) is also available, but if you are also taking the Energy Revitalization System vitamin powder (see Chapter 6), you are already getting the magnesium and malic acid, and the regular CORvalen is a better deal financially. Bioenergy, which makes

CORvalen, also conducts almost all of the research on ribose, knows the most about it, and has outstanding customer service in case you have any questions. Because of its importance, it's worth looking at energy production and ribose in greater detail. Having had the chance to explore the research and speak with a number of the researchers, here is what I've learned from them.

D-RIBOSE ACCELERATES ENERGY RECOVERY

D-ribose (which is what I am referring to when I say ribose) is a simple, five-carbon sugar (known as a pentose by biochemists) that is found naturally in our bodies. But ribose is not like any other sugar. Sugars we are all familiar with, such as table sugar (sucrose), corn sugar (glucose), milk sugar (lactose), honey (predominantly fructose), and others are used by the body as fuel. These sugars are consumed and, with the help of the oxygen we breathe, are "burned" by the body as fuel. Because they are used excessively, they can also be toxic, as we discuss in Chapter 6. Ribose, on the other hand, is special. When we consume ribose, the body recognizes that it is different from other sugars, and preserves it for the vital work of actually making the energy molecules that power the heart, muscles, brain, and every other tissue in the body.

A key molecule, called adenosine triphosphate (ATP, for short), is known as the energy currency of the cell because the amount of ATP we have in our tissues determines whether we will be fatigued or will have the energy we need to live vital, active lives. Ribose provides the key building block of ATP, and the presence of ribose in the cell stimulates the metabolic pathway our bodies use to actually make this vital compound. If the cell does not have enough ribose, it cannot make ATP. So, when cells and tissues become energy-starved, the availability of ribose is critical to energy recovery.

Normal, healthy heart and muscle tissues have the capacity to make all the ribose they need. When normal tissues are stressed by overexertion, several days' rest will usually allow full recovery. The muscles may be sore during recovery, as we frequently see for the three or four days after a hard day of yard work or after a weekend pickup football game, but eventually energy levels will be restored and the soreness will disappear. But when the muscles are chronically stressed by disease or conditions that affect tissue energy metabolism, the cells and tissues simply cannot make enough ribose quickly enough to recover. The heart and muscles just don't have the metabolic machinery they need to make ribose very efficiently. The result is chronic and persistent pain, stiffness, soreness, and overwhelming fatigue that may never go away.

THE LINK AMONG RIBOSE, ENERGY, AND FATIGUE

Clinical and scientific research has repeatedly shown that giving ribose to an energy-deficient heart and muscles stimulates energy recovery. One important study involved healthy athletes participating in high-intensity endurance exercise over the course of one week. After exercise, the energy level in the athletes' muscles was reduced by almost 30 percent. Giving 10 grams of ribose per day for three days following exercise restored muscle energy levels to normal, while treatment with a placebo provided virtually no effect.[20] This study clearly showed that ribose stimulated the energy recovery pathways in the body, helping the muscles rebuild their energy supply quickly and completely. Even after three days' rest, muscle that was not treated with ribose remained energy-starved and fatigued.

Two very interesting studies in animals showed how dramatic the effect of ribose could be on energy recovery in fatigued muscle. These studies were conducted by Dr. Ron Terjung, one of the top muscle physiologists in the United States. In their research, Dr. Terjung and his coinvestigators found that ribose administration in fatigued muscle increased the rate of energy recovery by 340 percent to 430 percent, depending on which type of muscle was tested.[21] He also found that even very small amounts of ribose had the effect of helping the muscle cell preserve energy, a process known as energy salvage, and the higher the ribose dose, the more dramatic the effect on energy preservation.[22] Although this groundbreaking research was done in animals, it was instrumental in defining the biochemistry and physiology associated with the use of ribose in overcoming heart and muscle fatigue. But most of us with CFS and FMS are neither top athletes nor animals, so the question remains: "How will ribose affect me?"

Research in ribose and CFS/FMS began with a case study that was published in the prestigious journal *Pharmacotherapy* in 2004.[23] This case study told the story of a veterinary surgeon diagnosed with fibromyalgia. For months, this dedicated doctor found herself becoming more and more fatigued, with pain becoming so profound that she was finally unable to stand during surgery. As a result, she was forced to all but give up the practice she loved.

Upon hearing that a clinical study on ribose in congestive heart failure was under way in the university where she worked, she asked if she could try the ribose to see if it might help her overcome the mind-numbing fatigue she experienced from her disease. After three weeks of ribose therapy, she was back in the operating room, practicing normally with no muscle pain or stiffness, and without the fatigue that had kept her bedridden for many months.

Being a doctor, she was skeptical, not believing that a simple sugar could have such a dramatic effect on her condition. Within two weeks of stopping the ribose therapy, however, she was out of the operating room and back in bed. So, to again test the theory, she began ribose therapy a second time. The result was similar to her first experience, and she was back doing surgery in days. After yet a third round of stopping (with the return of symptoms) and starting (with the reduction of symptoms) the ribose therapy, she was convinced, and has been on ribose therapy since that time.

I found this report intriguing, and decided to design the larger study in patients with fibromyalgia or chronic fatigue syndrome, which I began to discuss earlier. Along with two research collaborators, I recently published a scientific paper describing the results of this research. The study we designed was intended to determine whether or not ribose would be effective in relieving the overwhelming fatigue, pain, soreness, and stiffness suffered by patients having this debilitating condition. Our study included forty-one patients with a diagnosis of fibromyalgia or chronic fatigue syndrome who were given ribose at a dose of 5 grams three times per day for an average of three weeks. We found the ribose treatment led to significant improvement in energy levels, sleep patterns, mental clarity, pain intensity, and well-being. Of the patients participating in the study, 66 percent experienced significant improvement while on ribose, with an average increase in energy of 45 percent and overall well-being of 30 percent—remarkable results from a single nutrient.[19] The only significant side effects were that two people felt too energized and hyper/anxious on the ribose. This is dealt with by simply lowering the dose and/or taking it with food.

To further validate these findings, we are currently conducting a much larger placebo-controlled study. Interestingly, one of our study patients had an abnormal heart rhythm called atrial fibrillation. Ribose is outstanding in the treatment of heart disease as well, because it restores energy production in the heart muscle. Because of this, it was not surprising that this man's atrial fibrillation also went away with the ribose treatment and he was able to stop his heart medications as well. Because of its importance

Ribose—A Powerful Tool for Healing

Several of the patients participating in the study have contacted me regarding the relief they found with ribose therapy. Most importantly, they speak to the profound joy they felt when they were able to begin living normal, active lives after sometimes years of fatigue, pain, and suffering. Here is a sample of what one patient, Julie (Minnesota), an elementary teacher, wrote:"I had so much pain and fatigue I thought I was going to have to quit teaching. When I take [ribose], I feel like a huge weight is being lifted from my chest, and I'm ready to take on those kids again!" The relief patients feel with ribose therapy is heartwarming, and goes directly to the dramatic impact ribose has on increasing energy, overcoming fatigue, enhancing exercise tolerance, and raising the patient's quality of life.

and the research showing marked heart muscle dysfunction because of low energy in CFS, let's look at ribose and the heart in more detail.

RIBOSE AND THE FATIGUE ASSOCIATED WITH HEART DISEASE

Decades of research have shown that ribose has a profound effect on heart function in patients with congestive heart failure, coronary artery disease, and cardiomyopathy (a weakened heart muscle). Like the muscles in patients with fibromyalgia, sick hearts are energy-starved.[24] This energy deprivation keeps the heart from relaxing between heartbeats, making it impossible for the heart to completely fill with blood[25] (it surprisingly takes more energy for the heart muscle to relax than to contract). Because the heart does not fill completely, less blood is pumped to the body with each heartbeat. The heart then gets stiff, and it strains to contract. Ultimately, the heart becomes enlarged, a condition known as hypertrophy, and it is unable to pump normally.

You can compare this to the effect of weight training on the muscles in the biceps of the upper arm. Over time, weight training against more and more weight makes the muscle larger and harder. Similarly, when the heart becomes stiff, it is forced to contract less efficiently, making the heart muscle grow. While in the case of the biceps this muscle enlargement may be a desirable outcome, in the heart it can be deadly. In contrast to the biceps muscle, the heart must remain supple so that it can fill properly and empty fully with each contraction. If the heart cannot pump normal volumes of blood, muscles of the arms, legs, and brain tissue become oxygen-starved.

The result is fatigue; pain on standing or walking; loss of interest in, or the ability to perform, any physical activity; brain fog; and depression. In the end, the heart cannot pump enough blood to even supply itself with life-giving oxygen, and a heart attack can be the result.

Using ribose to restore the energy level in the heart allows it to fully relax, fill, and empty completely to circulate blood to the outer reaches of the body.[26] Circulating more blood means muscles in the arms, legs, and brain tissues get the oxygen they need to function normally. This result was made evident in several important studies in patients with congestive heart failure and angina.

In one study conducted at the University of Bonn, in Germany, patients with congestive heart failure were treated with either 10 grams of ribose or a sugar placebo every day for three weeks.[27] They were then tested for heart function, exercise tolerance, and quality of life using a questionnaire designed for this purpose. In this study, ribose therapy had a significant effect on all measures of diastolic heart function, showing that increased energy in the heart allowed the heart to relax, fill, and pump more normally. Patients in the study were also much more tolerant to exercise when they were on ribose and, through their responses to the questionnaire, showed that they had a higher quality of life as a result.

Two additional studies went on to help explain how ribose therapy in congestive heart failure may affect fatigue and exercise tolerance.[28, 29] These studies showed that ribose treatment increased ventilatory and oxygen utilization efficiency, a medical way of saying that the patients were able to use the oxygen they inhaled more efficiently. Improving the patient's ability to use oxygen means more oxygen is available to the tissues. Having more oxygen available allows the muscles to burn fuel more efficiently, helping them keep pace with their energy demand. The result is less fatigue, a greater ability to tolerate exercise, and a higher quality of life. An added benefit to improving ventilatory efficiency is that it is a dominant predictor of mortality in congestive heart failure. Increasing ventilatory efficiency with ribose therapy is, therefore, a direct correlate to prolonging life in this patient population.

There are few nutritional therapies that can legitimately boast of having this profound an effect on the tissues they target. None, other than ribose, can claim such an effect in cell or tissue energy metabolism. Ribose is a unique and powerful addition to our complement of metabolic therapies in that it is completely safe, proven by well-designed clinical and scientific evidence, natural, and fundamental to a vital metabolic process in the body.[30–34] I have added a few more study references for those who would like more information about ribose.[35–56]

Ribose regulates how much energy we have in our bodies, and for those suffering from fatigue, muscle soreness, stiffness, and a host of related medical complications, the relief found in energy restoration can be life changing. This is why I recommend that all CFS/FMS patients begin with 5 grams of D-ribose (1 scoop of CORvalen) three times a day for two to three weeks, then twice a day. It is critical to take three scoops a day for the first few weeks to see the optimal effects. Although many of the treatments in this book take six to twelve weeks to start working, most people feel the difference by the end of a single 280-gram container of ribose. The few who don't may retry it twelve to sixteen weeks into the other treatments we discuss. You'll be glad you did.

Although ribose is the most promising energy nutrient, others are also worth looking at. Most of these only need to be taken for four to nine months, though some people choose to take them longer: I take my ribose every day even though I feel great. It makes me feel even better! You will know whether to keep taking them by how you feel on them.

These other energy boosters are discussed at length in the notes section of my Web site (www.vitality101.com) and include:

- *Aspartates and malic acid.* Aspartates and malic acid are compounds that are needed to "rescue" part of the Krebs energy cycle, a series of chemical reactions that take place in the body's cells and allow glucose to be used for the production of energy. Malic acid is a compound that occurs naturally in foods, in fruits in general, and in especially high levels in apples. (Remember the old saying: An apple a day keeps the doctor away.) When levels of malic acid and the other compounds discussed in this chapter are low, the body often has to shift to an inefficient anaerobic means of generating energy. This causes muscle pain, achiness, and fatigue. Malic acid and magnesium can easily be found in several vitamin powders, as discussed in Chapter 6.
- *L-carnitine and acetyl-L-carnitine.* Low levels of the carnitine compound acylcarnitine in the blood or muscles of people with CFS/FMS have been found by two different research centers.[57, 58] Carnitine plays many roles in the body. It has the critical function of preventing the mitochondria from being shut down when the system backs up. Also,

without sufficient carnitine, the body cannot burn fat (and, in fact, makes excess fat), resulting in large weight gains. L-carnitine is a naturally occurring form of carnitine that is only found in animal flesh (think "carni-vore"), and any brand is fine as long as it is pure acetyl-L-carnitine. Although you may not see a marked effect, it helps lay the foundation for your getting better and may help you lose any weight you have gained. Take 500 milligrams twice a day for four months.

- *NADH.* Because of the cost, hassle, and modest effectiveness, I rarely use NADH and prefer to simply use ribose. I will sometimes consider it for those with pure CFS without pain who have failed other treatments.
- *Coenzyme Q_{10}.* Coenzyme Q_{10} is critical for the electron transport system (ETS) to do its job of harvesting more than 75 percent of the ATP energy from food. Because of this, it is important in energy production. Although a lot is found in the diet, it can become depleted during periods of excessive energy demands. Levels of coenzyme Q_{10} are also significantly lower in women who use oral contraceptives[59] or Premarin and Provera, which may in turn increase the risk of cardiovascular disease.[60] In addition, most cholesterol-lowering drugs deplete coenzyme Q_{10}.[61] This is especially tragic because this deficiency can cause or aggravate the congestive heart failure (CHF) seen in some patients with heart disease—and doctors are largely unaware of this, simply blaming it on the heart disease. Giving ribose, coenzyme Q_{10}, magnesium, and acetyl-L-carnitine should be done routinely in almost everyone with heart disease. In fact, a review of more than a dozen studies showed that coenzyme Q_{10} increases heart function significantly in heart-failure patients.[62, 63] I have seen patients on the heart transplant list (or even too sick to make it that far) go back to normal function with these nutrients.

In addition to helping energy and heart disease, studies have demonstrated that coenzyme Q_{10} can:

- Enhance immune function.[64–69]
- Assist weight loss when dieting.[70]
- Decrease the frequency of migraine headaches.[71]
- Raise low sperm counts.
- Help slow Parkinson's disease.

- Improve exercise tolerance in sedentary people.[72]
- Decrease allergies.[73]

Treating Mitochondrial Dysfunction Summarized

To sum up, following is my recipe for treating mitochondrial dysfunction and jump-starting your body's energy production. The supplements are listed in order of priority, if cost is an issue (some of them can be expensive).

1. Take D-ribose (CORvalen) 5,000 milligrams three times a day for three weeks, then two times a day. It's a powder that looks and tastes like sugar and does not act as food for yeast. It can be added to food or drinks, even hot tea.
2. Take the Energy Revitalization System vitamin powder (by Enzymatic Therapy) or a similar multivitamin with B-complex vitamins.
3. Take 500 to 1,000 milligrams of acetyl-L-carnitine a day for four to nine months, and then as needed.
4. Take 200 milligrams of coenzyme Q_{10} daily for four months (Vitaline, Enzymatic Therapy, or Ultraceuticals brand).

I would recommend the first two for everyone, and I'd take them long term (this is what I still take daily). Add the acetyl-L-carnitine for three to four months. If you can afford the cost, add the coenzyme Q_{10} for a three- to four-month trial. If you do not feel better in six to nine months, consider adding magnesium-potassium aspartate and NADH.

Important Points

- Like blowing a fuse, CFS and fibromyalgia actually protect your body from harm. Unfortunately, if you don't know how to "turn your circuit breaker back on," this doesn't do you much good.
- Solid research has shown that more than 91 percent of people on the SHIN protocol report significant improvements.

1. *Sleep.* Because your sleep center is not working, you need aggressive treatment to be sure that you can get at least eight hours of deep sleep each night.
2. *Hormonal support.* This includes treatment with bioidentical hormones for thyroid, adrenal, and ovarian/testicular support—even if your blood tests (which are very unreliable) are normal.
3. *Infections.* Because your immune system is working poorly, there are many infections present that need to be treated.
4. *Nutritional support.* Make nutritional support easy without taking handfuls of supplements throughout the day by taking the Energy Revitalization System vitamin powder (see Chapter 6) and D-ribose powder.

- At the end of each chapter, fill out the relevant questionnaire. It will tell you which treatments to check off in Appendix B: SHIN Treatment Worksheet. When you finish reading the book, you will have tailored a treatment protocol to your specific case.
- Many of the treatments will be natural remedies that you can use on your own. However, to get the full benefit, you should apply the SHIN protocol with the help of a physician. (See Chapter 12)
- The mitochondria are the energy furnaces in your cells that burn food for energy. Many studies and findings suggest that these furnaces are functioning inefficiently in CFS/FMS.
- Due to mitochondrial dysfunction, a person with CFS/FMS becomes unable to make the "tools" the furnace needs to work well—a problematic cycle that occurs throughout the body, affecting the brain (fatigue, brain fog), liver (chemical and other sensitivities), bowel (malabsorption of nutrients), and muscles (pain and postexertional fatigue).
- D-ribose (CORvalen) supplementation can jump-start the body, getting it ready for the SHIN protocol. Take 5,000 milligrams CORvalen or CORvalen M three times a day for three weeks, then lower the dose to twice a day. Take it at least four months, though many people choose to take it long term.
- Take 500 to 1,000 milligrams acetyl-L-carnitine a day for four to nine months, and 200 milligrams coenzyme Q_{10} daily for four months.

Questionnaire (Items to be checked off are in Appendix B.)

1. Do you have CFS/FMS, pain, or fatigue? If yes, check off #10.

2. Are you on cholesterol-lowering medications (related to Mevacor)? If yes, check off #9, and consider switching to natural cholesterol-lowering herbs instead (see Chapter 8).

3. Do you have any heart problems? If yes, check off #8, 9, and 10.

4. Have you gained weight you don't want? If yes, check off #8.

PART 2

Restore Energy Production with the SHIN Protocol

As we discussed earlier, chronic fatigue syndrome and fibromyalgia represent a bodywide energy crisis. As the hypothalamus uses more energy for its size than any other area in your body, it malfunctions first. This results in insomnia, hormonal deficiencies, low body temperature, and low blood pressure. Inadequate energy also may contribute to immune dysfunction and your muscles getting stuck in the shortened position—resulting in chronic pain. As energy runs all of your body systems, other problems such as immune dysfunction and difficulties with detoxification are also common. Restoring optimal energy production and eliminating those things that drain your energy are critical to your recovery. Your checklist for doing this and getting well is the acronym SHIN.

Sleep
Hormonal deficiencies
Infections
Nutritional support

Sleep is where we recharge our batteries and restore immune function. It is also critical for tissue repair, and therefore the elimination of pain. Hormonal control is also essential. For example, the thyroid acts like your body's gas pedal. If it is sluggish, you will simply not produce adequate energy. In addition, most of you will find that there are numerous infections that you picked up over the years because of your immune dysfunction, and all of these can drag you down. The most important of these in treating CFS/FMS is the chronic candida/fungal/yeast overgrowth (same infections, many names). Treating candida not only will help resolve your chronic fatigue and fibromyalgia, but also will likely resolve other chronic conditions like sinusitis and spastic colon. Nutrition, of course, is the key to health and energy production. We will teach you how to get outstanding and optimized nutritional support—without taking handfuls of tablets for the rest of your life.

At this point, you're already aware of the importance of ribose supplementation and have started filling out the SHIN Treatment Worksheet (see Appendix B). The next section of the book will lead you through the steps to getting well.

3 S—Sleep: The Foundation of Getting Well

*T*he most effective way to eliminate fatigue and pain in CFS/FMS is to get eight to nine hours of solid, deep sleep each night on a regular basis. Disordered sleep is, in my opinion, one of the key underlying processes that drive CFS/FMS. Usually, when I lecture, I ask, "How many of you who have CFS/FMS can get at least seven to nine hours of solid sleep a night without medications?" Generally, out of three hundred to four hundred people in the audience, only one or two people, if any, raise their hands. When I speak with these people later, I usually find that they have sleep apnea, narcolepsy, or another treatable cause for their fatigue besides CFS/FMS. Research shows that poor sleep quality is reported by 99 percent of fibromyalgia patients, and the degree of poor sleep quality was able to predict the degree of pain, fatigue, and poor social functioning in patients with FMS.[1]

Hypothalamic dysfunction affects sleep, as well as blood pressure, hormonal systems, and temperature regulation. In animals with hypothalamic dysfunction, sleep is either disordered or, in very severe cases, simply no longer occurs. In animal studies done by Carol Everson, Ph.D., at the University of Tennessee, sleep deprivation resulted in immune suppression, resulting in multiple infections (including yeast overgrowth in the gut).[2, 3] Many other abnormalities also occurred based on the sleep disorder. These same processes seem to occur in people with CFS/FMS.[3] Other sleep disorders are also common in CFS/FMS, including sleep apnea, upper airway resistance syndrome (UARS), and restless leg syndrome (RLS). These will be reviewed after the discussion of natural and prescription sleep aids.

Disordered sleep was first demonstrated by Dr. Harvey Moldofsky, a Canadian researcher, who noted that the quality of deep sleep in fibromyalgia was poor.[4] This was described as alpha wave intrusion into delta wave sleep. To put this into English, sleep has its own architecture and is not a single state. REM sleep, a light-sleep period during which we have our dreams, is the best-known part of the sleep architecture. There are other stages of sleep, designated simply by number. Stages 1 and 2 sleep are fairly light stages, while stages 3 and 4 (or delta wave) sleep are the deeper stages of sleep. My experience, and that of many other clinicians, suggests that stages 3 and 4 sleep are inadequate in CFS/FMS. This is supported by Robert Bennett's research at the University of Oregon Health Services Center. Bennett is one of the world's foremost researchers in fibromyalgia. He found that growth-hormone deficiency occurred in fibromyalgia, and that treating this deficiency resulted in improvement of symptoms after four to five months. However, he felt uncomfortable recommending routine growth-hormone treatment for fibromyalgia because of its high cost (approximately fifteen thousand dollars per year). What is interesting, though, is that growth hormone is released during stages 3 and 4 sleep. Therefore, the loss of these deep stages of sleep may be a significant contributor to the growth-hormone deficiency that has been observed. My own suspicion is that not only does hypothalamic dysfunction cause disordered sleep, but that the poor sleep then further suppresses the hypothalamus. It is because of this that breaking the cycle of poor sleep and maintaining quality sleep for at least six to nine months is critical to breaking the cycle of CFS and fibromyalgia.

Growth hormone is responsible for many of the repair processes that go on in our muscles and in the rest of our body. It may be that it is the loss of this repair function, which normally occurs during deep sleep, that contributes to the pain of fibromyalgia. Several studies have shown that if you wake people up whenever they go into deep sleep, or even shake them lightly, so that they go from deep sleep into light sleep, they will develop classic fibromyalgia-like pain within one to two weeks and often within one night.[4, 5]

In addition to causing growth-hormone deficiency (which we will discuss in more detail in Chapter 4), pain, and immune dysfunction, poor sleep also contributes to the average thirty-two-pound weight gain most patients with CFS and fibromyalgia report. In a study of 68,183 women, followed over sixteen years, those sleeping five or fewer hours per night had a 32 percent increased risk of gaining thirty-three pounds relative to those who slept seven hours per night.[6]

It is absolutely critical that people with CFS/FMS get eight to nine hours of solid sleep each night, without waking or without feeling "hungover" the next day. Sound sleep is the goal and, hard as this may be to believe, it is attainable using the suggestions I will give you in this chapter.

The Basics: Good Sleep Hygiene

Although poor sleep hygiene is not a major problem for most people with this disease, it is the major cause of poor sleep for most Americans, and it is important to address this first. The following are some things to consider:

- Consume little or no alcohol before bedtime.
- Do not consume any caffeine after 4 p.m.
- Do not use your bed for problem solving or doing work. If you are in the habit of using your bed for doing work, it is best to change your work area to another area of the house. If it helps you to fall asleep, you can watch relaxing television (perhaps on a timer that turns the television off if you fall asleep while watching) or read a relaxing book in bed until you can no longer stay awake.
- Take a hot bath before bed.
- Keep your room cool.
- If your mind races because your brain thinks it is daytime when it is really nighttime, continually focus your thoughts on things that feel good and do not require much "thinking energy." If you find that you cannot help but continue to problem-solve, get out of bed and write down all your problems on a piece of paper until you can think of no more—then set them aside and go back to bed. Do this as often as you need to. It may be helpful to schedule thirty minutes of "worry time" early in the afternoon or evening when you can update a checklist of your concerns.

  As CFS/FMS patients, we seem to think that we're responsible for making everything happen, like making our bodies heal. That stress and anxiety can make a good night's sleep difficult to come by. I certainly struggle with this and have devised a simple strategy that works for me. You may find something similar to be useful as well. When I feel overcome by details, I list my problems and projects on the left side of a page, and what I eventually plan to do about them (if anything) in the middle of the page. I consider these two columns to be what I leave in the hands of God, the universe, or whatever you wish to call it. Every so often, I move a problem from the "universe's" columns over to a third ("my") column on the right side. The items in the third column are the one or two things that I want to work on right now. I am constantly amazed at how the things that I leave in the "universe's" hands progress (on their own) as quickly as the things that I've put in "my" column.

I also have a separate list for day-to-day errands. I put a star by those items that must get done soon. I do other items if and when I feel like it. It is helpful to remember that neither you nor anyone else will ever get everything done. Just do those things that feel good to do on any given day, even if it's nothing. It will usually feel good to do the things that really have to get done. When I was doing general hospital internal medicine, I never heard a dying patient bemoan not having worked enough, or not having completed all the errands on his or her checklist.

- If your partner snores, get a good pair of earplugs and use them. The wax plugs that mold to the shape of the ear are often the best ones. It may also be useful to have either a sound generator that makes nature sounds or, better yet, a tape that induces stage 4 sleep (more about this later). Spouses of people with sleep apnea and/or snoring often also have severely disturbed sleep. You may need to sleep in a separate bedroom (after tucking in or being tucked in by your partner) until you find a way to sleep soundly through the snoring.

- If you frequently wake up to urinate during the night, do not drink a lot of fluids near bedtime. Most patients with CFS/FMS have frequent waking during the night. Like most people, their bladders are full at night. Because of a full bladder, they think they are waking up because they have to urinate. This is not the case. They are waking up because of their CFIDS/FMS.

   If you were to wake up your spouse when you woke up and asked, "Honey, is your bladder full?" he or she would moan, "Uh-huh," and roll over and go back to sleep. Unfortunately, most people have learned to get up and go to the bathroom when they wake up at night.

The bladder is kind of like a baby—if you teach the baby to wake up to play in the middle of the night (that is, if you go to the bathroom frequently), pretty soon it will wake you up to play at night. There is a simple way to remedy this problem. If and when you wake up during the night and you notice your bladder is full, just talk to it (in your mind, so your spouse doesn't think you're nuts) and tell it, "Nighttime is for sleeping. We will go to the bathroom in the morning when it is time to wake up." Then roll over and go back to sleep. If you still have to urinate five minutes later, then you can go to the bathroom. Most of you will find that your bladder will happily go back to sleep, and when you wake up in the morning, you won't even have to urinate as badly as you did when you woke up in the middle of the night.

Because of the bladder muscle spasticity that is common in fibromyalgia, you may be afraid that you will wet yourself if you don't get up to urinate. The large majority of people with CFS/FMS will not experience incontinence. If this concerns you, the first couple of nights you may want to use an incontinence protection product such as a Depend undergarment just so you don't worry about wetting yourself. After a few nights, you will be comfortable sleeping without protection. Although this sounds like a low-tech approach to treating a sleep problem, you will be amazed at how beneficial it is. Try it and see.

- Put the bedroom clock out of arm's reach and facing away from you so you can't see it. Frequently looking at the clock aggravates sleep problems and is frustrating.

- Decrease the amount of time you spend in bed. Although you might think that you would increase your deep sleep time by spending extra time in bed, this is not what happens. When people routinely stay in bed longer than they need to, they may get their usual deep sleep in the beginning of the night and then have long awakenings and very shallow sleep during the middle of the night. Then they may sleep soundly again when it is time to wake up. When such people consistently decrease the amount of time spent in bed to the length actually needed for sleep, they gradually squeeze out the long middle-of-the-night awakenings. Two of the medications discussed later in this chapter (Ambien and Sonata) are especially helpful for this.

- Have a light snack before bedtime. Hunger causes insomnia in all animals, and humans are no exception. Adding foods high in the amino acid tryptophan, such as milk and turkey, also contributes to sleep.

- Get out of bed at the same time each morning, even after a poor night's sleep. Regular rising supports a healthy circadian (day/night) rhythm and can be helpful. You can nap up to one and a half hours a day, but try not to nap much after 2 p.m. if possible. Set an alarm clock for one to one and a half hours of nap time and splash cold water on your face when you wake up.

If you follow the suggestions above, you can be sure that poor sleep hygiene is not your problem. This is important because your doctor may want to blame your insomnia on poor sleep hygiene. It is important to let him or her know that your problem is not poor sleep hygiene; it is hypothalamic sleep-center suppression. In addition, there are often diagnosable sleep disorders that may be affecting your sleep, such as sleep-disordered breathing, restless leg syndrome, and narcolepsy. These may resolve themselves once you take care of the hypothalamic sleep-center suppression, so I've included basic information on the most common disorders and how to treat them at the end of this chapter.

Sleep Medications and Remedies

The hypothalamic sleep disorder in CFS/FMS is usually too severe to be dealt with by any single prescription or natural remedy. What works best is to mix these until you find a combination that gives you eight to nine hours of solid sleep a night without a hangover. Natural remedies can be very helpful, and in general, I much prefer natural remedies to prescription medications. Although you'll likely need a mix of natural and prescription therapies, the natural remedies can decrease the amount of medication you need, and therefore the cost and side effects.

In addition, once you come off sleep medications (usually after nine to eighteen months, although they can be used indefinitely, if needed) you may find that all you require are the natural remedies. Whatever treatments you use, though, it is important that they not only increase the duration of sleep but also maintain or improve the deep stages (stages 3 and 4) of sleep. Unfortunately, many sleeping pills in common use—for example, Dalmane, Halcion, and Valium—actually worsen the quality of sleep by increasing the amount of light-stage sleep and decreasing the amount of deep-stage sleep even further. You want to be certain that the treatments and medications you use leave you feeling better the next day, not worse.

There are several approaches to using sleep treatments in CFIDS/FMS. Some doctors prefer to use a single medication or treatment and push it up to its maximum level. If that works, great; if not, they stop that medication and switch to another. Other doctors prefer to use low doses of many different treatments together until the patient is getting good, solid sleep regularly. I strongly prefer the latter approach, for two main reasons. First, my experience is that people with CFS and fibromyalgia can be medication-sensitive if high doses are used. Most of a medication's benefits occur at low doses and most of the side effects at high doses. Second, each medication is cleared out of the body on its own schedule, regardless of whether it is taken with other medications. If you take a low dose of a sleep medication, so that it is out of your body when it is time to wake up eight hours later, the blood level may not be high enough to keep you asleep all night. If you increase the dose to the level at which it does keep you asleep all night, it may not be cleared out of your body until 2 p.m. the next day, leaving you feeling very hungover. If, however, you combine low doses of four or five different sleep aids, each of them will be cleared out of your body by morning. Meanwhile, the effective blood levels that you have during the middle of the night from each treatment are additive and will keep you asleep. Because of this, most people find that it takes anywhere from three to seven different treatments combined to get eight to nine hours of solid sleep each night without waking prematurely or being hungover.

Getting Started

My "long-form" treatment checklist at www.vitality101.com lists more than twenty-five natural and prescription sleep aids. Depending on your preference, you may want to start with the natural sleep aids, see how those work, and then add the prescription ones as needed. Because of the severity of the sleep problem in CFS/FMS, my preference is to start with at least one of the sleep medications (Ambien and/or Desyrel) combined with some of the natural remedies—but this is a decision to be made by you and your physician. However you choose to do it, on the first night simply begin with one of the remedies at the lowest recommended dose.

For all of the treatments recommended (except 5-HTP), you will know the effects (both positive and negative) that the treatment is going to have by the next morning. In rare cases, some of these treatments have the opposite of their intended effect, activating you instead of putting you to sleep. If this happens, don't use that treatment. In addition, approximately 3 percent of people find that all sleep treatments stop working after three days to a month. If you are one of these patients, simply rotate groups of treatments that work—going back to the first ones when you've finished the last ones on your list.

Once you have tried a low dose of a single treatment, increase the dosage each night until you either get eight to nine hours of solid sleep without a hangover, until you get side effects (for example, next-day sedation), or until you are at the maximum dose noted on the checklist. It is worth noting the lowest dose that gives you the most benefit. In other words, you may find that 50 milligrams of Desyrel is just as effective as 150 milligrams, in which case there is no need to take the higher dose. Once you have tried one treatment, you can go ahead and add in a second one in the way I just discussed, and then a third one, and so on. You may also initially drop the earlier treatments, using each of the new ones by it-self so you can see what each one does by itself. Or you may choose to add one treatment to the next. Basically, you are trying the treatments on to see what "fits," in the same way you would try on shoes to see which ones feel the best. Once you have found the combination of treatments that feels the best, you can simply stay on that combination. You can even safely take most of the medications on the checklist together if needed to get eight to nine hours of solid sleep a night. Your doctor should be able to provide guidance as you find the best treatments.

It is not uncommon to see your sleep worsen again during periods of increased stress—whether physical or emotional—and the flaring of your illness. During these times, increase the treatments as needed to maintain seven to eight hours of solid sleep without waking prematurely or being hungover. I find that patients do not have a problem with continually hav-ing to escalate the dose, so don't worry about increasing the treatments during periods of stress or flaring of your illness. The best way to need less medication in the long run is to use as much as it takes to get eight hours of solid sleep each night for six months. When you are sleeping well and feeling better for six months, you can then decrease the treatments as long as you continue to get eight hours of solid sleep each night. Most people find that they can taper off all sleep medications after about eighteen months. Other people need to take some of the sleep treatments for years. This is okay.

Side Effects of Sleep Aids

For all of the medications listed in this section, any side effects that you may notice will occur the same day that you take the medication. I have not seen any "fly now, pay later" side effects from prolonged use. The exception is that less than 1 percent of people who take Ambien for more than a year develop an unusual depression, which dramatically resolves one to three days after stopping the sleep medication. In these rare situations I simply leave the person off Ambien. I have not seen Ambien worsen symptoms in patients with preexisting depression. I've also seen sleepwalking and eating in approximately one patient per thousand. These side effects only occurred when the individuals were taking at least 15 milligrams a night. Although we have been aware of this for many years, it has just recently received media attention. I suspect that this is largely because two new sleep medications, Lunesta and Rozerem, came out and we're seeing the battle for market share between these companies. I have not found these two new medications to be very effective in treating disordered sleep in my CFS and FMS patients.

I tend to be highly opinionated and very picky about what I find works well and what does not work as well. Because there is so much marketing out there for both natural and prescription remedies, it is hard for most nonexperts to tell what works. I decided more than fifteen years ago that my position would be that of a patient advocate and that I work for you. Because of this, to maintain both credibility and objectivity, I accept no money from either pharmaceutical or natural products companies and direct that all royalties for products that I design be donated to charity.

Natural Sleep Remedies

Most of the natural sleep remedies discussed here are not sedating, yet they help you fall asleep and stay in deep sleep. The good news is that many natural remedies that are effective for sleep also directly help pain because they are muscle relaxants and may also improve libido.[7–11] The first six herbs listed below are available in a combination formula as well.

My favorite natural sleep aids:

SUNTHEANINE

Theanine, an amino acid (protein) that comes from green tea, has been shown not only to improve deep sleep, but also to help people maintain a calm alertness during the day. L-theanine likely plays a role in the formation of gamma-aminobutyric acid (GABA). This inhibitory neurotransmitter is critical for sleep, and is what is stimulated by many medications that help improve sleep. L-theanine also directly stimulates the production of alpha brain waves during the day.[12-13] These brain waves are associated with an awake yet relaxed (almost meditative) state.[14] L-theanine is also often used in weight-loss products, as studies show that green tea helps with weight loss, and the animal model studies suggest that the theanine in the green tea contributes significantly to this.[15] Green tea also is helpful as an immune stimulant and has many other benefits; however, the amount of L-theanine present in green tea is not enough to advocate drinking it as a sleep aid.

The only form of theanine that I use and recommend is called Suntheanine (pure L-theanine), as most other brands include inactive forms of the theanine that block its effectiveness. In fact, Suntheanine is the only form that most companies that maintain high quality standards will use in their products. In Chapter 8, "More Natural Remedies," I discuss Suntheanine at length in the section on how to treat anxiety without worsening brain fog. As the FDA just approved its use as a food additive in the United States (it's been used in drinks in Japan for decades for its calming effects), it may just be a matter of time until the barista at the local Starbucks asks, "One pump of Suntheanine or two?"

Take 50 to 200 milligrams at bedtime, although you can also use it several times a day for anxiety.

WILD LETTUCE

Traditionally, wild lettuce has been found to be effective for anxiety and insomnia, as well as for headache, muscle, and joint pain. Wild lettuce may also decrease restless leg syndrome.

Take 30 to 120 milligrams at bedtime.

JAMAICAN DOGWOOD

This extract acts as a muscle relaxant and also helps people to fall asleep while calming them.[7] According to tradition, Jamaican dogwood was once used by Jamaican fishermen. Large amounts were thrown in the water. The fish would then fall asleep and be easy to net.

Take 12 to 48 milligrams of the extract at bedtime.

HOPS

The hops plant is a member of the hemp family, and the female flowers are used in beer making. It also has some hormonal activity, suppressing breast, colon, and ovarian cancer in test-tube studies, and has been reported to reduce hot flashes in menopausal women. Hops also has antibiotic and antifungal activity and a long history of being used as a mild sedative for anxiety and insomnia. A study showed an improvement in insomnia, with effectiveness similar to that of the Valium family medications. It is considered safe.[8] As any beer-drinking college student can tell you, hops helps your muscles relax and promotes sleep, as well.

Take 30 to 120 milligrams of a hops extract at bedtime.

PASSIONFLOWER (*PASSIFLORA*)

This herb is commonly used throughout South America as a calming agent, even present as an ingredient in sodas. A number of studies support its having a calming effect. Herbalists have also used it to treat muscle spasms, colic, dysentery, diarrhea, anxiety, and menstrual pain, and it may also increase men's libidos, all problems often associated with CFS/FMS.[9] Passionflower has other pain-management benefits. In one animal study, it was shown that it decreases morphine tolerance, so that less medication is needed, as well as decreasing morphine withdrawal symptoms.[10] Passionflower may help decrease the pain of fibromyalgia.

Take 90 to 360 milligrams of the extract at bedtime.

VALERIAN

Commonly used as a sleep remedy for insomnia, valerian has many benefits, as shown in a number of studies, including an improvement in deep sleep, speed of falling asleep, and quality of sleep without next-day sedation. The benefits were most pronounced when people used valerian for extended periods of time, as opposed to simply taking it for one night. Valerian's effectiveness has been compared to that of a Valium family medication (oxazepam), without the "hungover" feeling present with most Valium medications.

A review of multiple studies found that "valerian is a safe herbal choice for the treatment of mild insomnia and has good tolerance. . . . Most studies suggest that it is more effective when used continuously rather than as an acute sleep aid."[11] Clinical experience shows that for around 10 percent of people, valerian is energizing and may keep them up. If this happens to you, you can use valerian during the day instead of at night, as valerian does have a calming effect and can be used during the day for anxiety as well.

Take 200 to 800 milligrams of the extract at bedtime.

These herbs may be used in any combination at the suggested doses above. Because I have found these herbs to be dramatically helpful in patients with disordered sleep, anxiety, and/or chronic pain, I worked with Enzymatic Therapy to develop the Revitalizing Sleep Formula, a supplement that contains optimum doses of all six herbs. If you prefer, take one to four capsules at bedtime to help you sleep or take the same dosage one to three hours before bedtime if the main problem is one of falling asleep. As with the individual doses of the herbs above, these capsules can also be used during the day for anxiety and pain. Some CFS/FMS patients have also reported an increase in their libido while taking this combination.

Your doctor can also prescribe a combination supplement of these herbs (also called the Revitalizing Sleep Formula) made by Integrative Therapeutics. See Appendix E: Resources for more information.

You may find, however, that the above sleep aids are not adequate by themselves. Other natural remedies include:

- *D-ribose* (see Chapter 2). Helps sleep while increasing energy.[16]
- *Magnesium and calcium.* Taking at least 75 to 150 milligrams of magnesium at night is a good idea because it can help you sleep. Lower the dose if it causes diarrhea. Taking 600 milligrams of calcium at bedtime also may improve the quality of your sleep, and you may wish to take the two supplements together.
- *Lemon balm.* A double-blind research study showed that taking 80 to 160 milligrams of lemon balm (also known as melissa) in combination with 180 to 360 milligrams of valerian a night improved deep-stage sleep,[17] without being sedating.

- *5-Hydroxy-L-Tryptophan (5-HTP).* Your body uses 5-HTP to make serotonin, a neurotransmitter that helps improve the quality of sleep. A double-blind, placebo-controlled study looked at the effectiveness of 5-HTP or placebo in fifty people with fibromyalgia. After four weeks, there was improvement in pain, stiffness, anxiety, fatigue, and sleep.[18] In addition, it often helps people lose weight. Take 100 to 400 milligrams at night.

  The one caution I would note with 5-HTP is that if you are taking a number of treatments that increase serotonin (these include antidepressants like Prozac, Saint John's wort, Ultram, Desyrel, and the like), taking doses higher than 200 milligrams of 5-HTP can result in serotonergic syndrome, a life-threatening reaction caused by a too-high level of serotonin. Because of this, discuss the use of 5-HTP with your holistic doctor. This is a rare problem, however, and I have never seen a serious reaction myself. Mild serotonergic syndrome can more often be associated with a constant fast heart rate. But when it gets more severe and potentially dangerous, it can be associated with a fever and feels like "the panic attack from hell." Common in CFS/FMS, most panic attacks are not caused by excessive serotonin. However, if a reaction does happen, you should be checked out in a hospital emergency room to be safe. If you are taking any of the serotonin-raising treatments, it is reasonable to limit the 5-HTP to 200 milligrams at night. For anyone whose heart rate is constantly above 90, even if you are not taking 5-HTP, it is worth considering whether you are on too many treatments that raise serotonin and discussing lowering these with your doctor. If the rapid heart rate is coming from these treatments, it should come down within a few days of lowering treatments.

- *Melatonin.* This is a hormone made by the pineal gland. Although it is natural and available over the counter, this does not mean that it is without risk. My concern with any hormone is that although it might be quite safe when used within the body's normal range, I worry about toxicity when people take more than the body would normally make. For most people, all it takes to restore melatonin to normal levels is ⅓ milligram. The usual dose you find in stores, however, is 3 milligrams, which is ten times the level I recommend. Except for a small subset of people, who likely have trouble absorbing it properly, 0.5 milligram is every bit as effective for sleep as higher doses. Moreover, high levels of melatonin may raise the level of another hormone, prolactin, which is often already high in people with CFS/FMS, aggravating the risk of depression or infertility. Although I don't know of any danger yet from using melatonin in higher doses—and it may even have immune-stimulating and antioxidant effects that could well be beneficial—I would only use a dose higher than 0.5 milligram under the supervision of your holistic doctor.

- *Delta-wave sleep-inducing compact discs or cassettes (www.vitality101.com).* To fall asleep and stay in deep sleep, you can play the tapes or CDs and they will help your brain waves attune to and stay in the delta-wave frequency of deep sleep. If you wake up during the night, you can push your sound system's replay button. Better yet, get a CD or tape player that can replay continuously throughout the night.
- *Cuddle Ewe mattress pad.* Lying on this cushioning sheepskin pad can help relieve pain when it interferes with sleep (800-328-9493).

Prescription Medications

Although I prescribe medications in different orders for different people, depending on their symptoms, the most common order I use is the one below. If something is mentioned as especially good for a certain condition, you may want to try that medication first. A physician specializing in CFS can help you find the best combination. Do not drive or operate hazardous equipment if you are sedated from the medications. Also, as with almost any medication and most herbs, do not get pregnant during treatment.

As we've discussed, CFS/FMS patients usually do better with combining low doses of several medications than with a high dose of just one. If you had to use only one medication at a high enough dose to keep you out all night, you'd likely be hungover until two the next afternoon. If you use several different medications, however, each of them is cleared out of your body individually, so by morning you are not hungover. Fortunately, the positive effects of the multiple treatments are combined during the night. Most people find they may need a mix of anywhere from three to seven different natural and prescription sleep aids to get the eight hours of solid sleep that they need each night. Although in my experience it is quite uncommon, even for CFS/FMS patients, it is possible to get unusual reactions from combining these medications. If a medication causes recurring nightmares, change the dose or medication.

With hypothalamic sleep-center dysfunction, it is inappropriate to stop taking your sleep medications prematurely. Just as with high blood pressure, it is reasonable to stay on your sleep medications for years, if needed. Fortunately, after people are feeling better for six months they usually find that they can lower the dose of sleep medication as the sleep center (in the hypothalamus) recovers. Keep in mind that if you use adequate medication to get eight to nine hours of solid sleep a night for six to nine months, you will likely need less sleep medication in the long run.

Let's look at the prescription sleep medications that work best in CFS/FMS:

* *Zolpidem (Ambien).* This is my first choice of sleep medication for treatment in CFS/FMS because it is usually effective and well tolerated. Because Ambien is short acting (that is, it is out of your body after six hours), it is less likely to cause side effects than many other medications, but it also may not keep you asleep all the way through the night. Five to 15 milligrams will likely give you at least four to six hours of good, solid sleep as a foundation.

   If you wake up in the middle of the night with the Ambien, switch to the newer Ambien CR (sustained release) 6.25 to 12.5 milligrams at bedtime. Around half of our patients prefer the sustained-release form over the original form of Ambien. However, the older form is now available as a generic, and is much less expensive. If you use the older, short-acting form, you can take an extra one half to one tablet (leave it by your bedside) and chew it if you wake during the night. Any sedation has usually worn off by the time you are ready to wake up in the morning. If you find that taking an additional dose in the middle of the night leaves you hungover, try Sonata (see zaleplon, page 64) when you wake instead.

   Do not take more than 15 milligrams of Ambien at one time. I usually don't see improved sleep with the higher doses, and I have seen a case of sleepwalking that occurred when a patient took 20 milligrams as a single dose. Rarely, some people even eat while sleepwalking. Despite media attention, these are both unusual occurrences. Studies have not shown a wearing-off effect with Ambien or Sonata in most people, nor have they found addiction with long-term Ambien use.[19] What does occur, though, is rebound insomnia when you stop using this medication—that is, the need to use something else to assist your sleep for about a week. Because of this need for sleep assistance, if you have taken Ambien for more than two months, when you stop it, use one of the other medications or natural sleep remedies discussed in this chapter for a week or so to assist sleep during the adjustment period. In my experience, Ambien can also be helpful for restless leg syndrome.

- *Trazodone (Desyrel)*. Desyrel is marketed as an antidepressant, but its main use in CFS/FMS is to treat disordered sleep. It has the added benefit of being helpful for anxiety, and can be used during the day for this as well. Desyrel comes in 50-milligram tablets, and the usual recommendation is to take one half to six at bedtime (most patients need no more than two). If you take more than two, you can get Desyrel in 150- to 300-milligram tablets as well, decreasing the number of pills you'll need to take. Your total daily dose should not exceed 450 milligrams.

    If you are on other antidepressants, limit the dosage to 150 milligrams a day to avoid the risk of excessive serotonin levels discussed on page 59. The main side effects of Desyrel are next-day sedation (if this happens, either lower the dose or take it earlier in the evening) and, in males, priapism, a condition characterized by a painful erection that does not go away. The latter side effect is rare, and I have never had a patient experience this, despite prescribing Desyrel hundreds of times. Most men find that while it causes an improvement in the strength of their erections, it does so at a comfortable level, as opposed to an erection that will not go away after a normal amount of time. If you develop an erection that does not go away after an hour (despite a cold bath), stop taking the medication and go to a hospital emergency room. If the erections are not lasting extraordinarily long but seem to be even the least bit uncomfortably long, you should stop the Desyrel and switch to other medications.

- *Clonazepam (Klonopin)*. Although in the Valium family, and therefore potentially addictive, Klonopin can be very helpful for people with restless leg syndrome or for those whose sleep is disrupted by pain. When used at doses of less than 1 to 2 milligrams at night, we've seen no problem with addiction. Most people do not need to go above this dose. Start with half of a 0.5-milligram tablet and work your way up slowly as needed. The main side effect is next-day sedation, which is fairly common. If this occurs, take a lower dose several hours before bedtime, or switch to its shorter-acting cousin Xanax (see

Alprazolam, page 66). Most people find that they can slowly increase the dose over time, if needed, as the next-day sedation wears off. Because it is potentially addictive, do not suddenly stop taking Klonopin if you have been on it for more than six weeks. Instead, taper off by decreasing the dosage by 0.25–0.5 milligrams a day every few weeks as symptoms allow.

- *Gabapentin (Neurontin), tiagabine (Gabitril), or pregabalin (Lyrica).* These three medications work by increasing the calming, sleep-inducing neurotransmitter gamma-aminobutyric acid (GABA). Although the three are related, one will often work and be well tolerated even if the others are not. They are likely all effective for pain and restless leg syndrome, and can markedly improve deep sleep. The main side effects are sedation, dizziness, and gastric upset. Lyrica may also cause weight gain. These are also discussed in Chapter 7. Take 300 milligrams of Neurontin, 2 milligrams of Gabitril, or 50 milligrams of Lyrica.

- *Doxylamine (Unisom for Sleep).* This is an antihistamine that is available over the counter. It is worth trying, especially if you tend to have a stuffy nose that interferes with your sleep. However, if you have trouble with severe dry eyes and mouth, this may not be a good medication for you because it can aggravate these symptoms. Some people find that the effect wears off with continued use and that it works best when used intermittently (for example, two days on, then two days off). The standard dose is 25 milligrams at nighttime.

- *Carisoprodol (Soma).* This is predominantly a muscle relaxant, and I recommend using this medication earlier in treatment if you experience severe pain because of your CFS/FMS. Soma is potentially addictive, although I have never seen this in patients who are only using one to two tablets at bedtime (as opposed to people taking it four times a day for pain). The usual dose is half to one 350-milligram tablet at bedtime. The main side effect is sedation.

- *Doxepin (Sinequan).* In high doses this medication is used as an antidepressant, and it is also a powerful antihistamine. As a sleep aid, I recommend taking 5 to 30 milligrams, or taking 10 mg/cc of doxepin liquid at bedtime. Some people, however, get the greatest benefit with the least next-day sedation using a dose of less than 5 milligrams a night. Since it is always best to take the lowest dose possible, you should start with this amount. If you are sensitive to medications, you should start with a lower dose of the doxepin liquid, about one to three drops nightly, but the dose can be increased up to 100 milligrams, if needed. This medication is related to Elavil; however, I recommend doxepin because it causes much less dry mouth, weight gain, next-day sedation, and other side effects often seen with Elavil.

- *Cyclobenzaprine (Flexeril).* This medication is a muscle relaxant, and can be helpful for people who experience severe muscle pain with fibromyalgia. The usual dose is half to one 10-milligram tablet at bedtime, but some people need to take two. Flexeril is also related to Elavil, and does pose some risk for people with abnormal heart rhythms. Rarely, it leads to weight gain, and can also cause dry mouth and eyes.

- *Tizanidine (Zanaflex).* Although unrelated to cyclobenzaprine, zanaflex is another sleep aid that relieves pain (for more information, see Chapter 7). Stop the medication if it causes nightmares, and do not take it while on the antibiotic Cipro, as it raises blood levels of zanaflex too high. Take half to two tablets at bedtime for sleep, not to exceed 8 milligrams.

- *Zaleplon (Sonata).* Sonata is a comparatively new sleep medication. It helps people fall asleep, and the sedating effect generally wears off within four hours, making next-day hangover uncommon. It is best used in the middle of the night if you wake up and need something to help you fall back to sleep, or if you have trouble falling asleep but not staying asleep. Sonata is not like any other medication—that is, it is the first drug in its class, and therefore of a unique type. It affects receptors for the neurotransmitter gamma-aminobutyric acid (GABA). This makes it seem very promising for people with CFS/FMS.

In research studies on patients who were awakened four hours after taking the medication, they showed no evidence of impairment of waking function. The most common side effects are headache, dizziness, or sedation, but these were found to occur as frequently in patients taking this drug at low dose as in people taking a placebo. There is no evidence of withdrawal symptoms, even if the medication is stopped abruptly. The recommended dose is one to two 10-milligram capsules. Most FMS patients require 20 milligrams (two capsules). It is recommended that Sonata not be taken with, or immediately after, a high-fat or heavy meal, as this decreases its effectiveness. If you are taking the antacid medication Tagamet, you may need to take a lower dose of Sonata because it is cleared out of the body more slowly while on Tagamet. This can, however, be a good thing, if you find yourself waking easily while taking Sonata.

If Other Sleep Medications
Do Not Give Eight Hours of Sleep

- *GHB, gamma hydroxybutyrate (Xyrem).* Xyrem is the most effective way known to increase deep sleep and raise growth hormone—thereby decreasing pain for fibromyalgia sufferers. However, because of DEA claims that it was being used as a "date rape" drug, it is now tightly regulated and expensive, and must come from a special pharmacy with special paperwork. For this reason, I do not recommend it as highly as some other natural and prescription treatments. However, if all else fails, Xyrem can be helpful. Take 9 cc (4.5 grams) at bedtime and repeat approximately four hours later, if needed. The first night you use Xyrem, take it by itself without other sleep medications. In our practice, if the Xyrem is not adequately effective by itself, we then add one low-dose tablet of any other sleep medication with each Xyrem dose until the patient is getting good sleep for at least four hours with each dose or for eight hours a night. Be sure to rinse well with water and swallow after taking liquid. If the medication is left in your mouth, it can dissolve enamel and damage teeth. The FDA has approved it for narcolepsy, but a number of studies are being done to evaluate its effectiveness in treating fibromyalgia, and hopefully it will soon be approved for this use as well. This approval will make it more likely that insurance companies will pay for it.
- *Eszopiclone (Lunesta)—2 to 3 milligrams at bedtime.* Initial studies suggested that this would be very promising. Unfortunately, it was not very effective clinically, with approximately 80 percent of patients preferring Ambien. Nonetheless, it can be helpful in a small subset of patients. Its main side effect, besides next-day sedation, is a bad taste left in your mouth during the day. If taken with Sporanox, Nizoral, Diflucan (antifungals), or the antibiotic Zithromax, a lower dose may be needed.
- *Mirtazapine (Remeron).* This medication is unrelated to any of the other medications discussed above. One doctor has noted that it seems to be especially helpful in patients who seem to "hibernate" during the day. Generally, Remeron causes more next-day sedation and weight gain than most other sleep medications. The usual dosage is one to three 15-milligram tablets, taken at bedtime.

- *Amitriptyline (Elavil).* Technically an antidepressant, Elavil was one of the first medications studied for fibromyalgia and was found to be effective. It is also the only medication that many doctors have heard of for treating fibromyalgia. Although Elavil can be very helpful, it has been moved to the bottom of my list because of its significant side effects. These include weight gain, dry mouth, sedation, aggravation of restless leg syndrome, neurally mediated hypotension, and abnormal heart rhythms. However, for people who suffer from nerve pain, vulvodynia (pain in the vulvar area), and interstitial cystitis (severe urinary frequency and burning without infection), amitriptyline is effective even in very low doses. You can take one-half to five 10-milligram tablets at bedtime. If you take more than two tablets, it should be tapered off and not stopped suddenly. I rarely recommend more than 80 milligrams at bedtime because of the aforementioned side effects.

- *Alprazolam (Xanax).* Although alprazolam is related to Valium, it produces much more desirable effects: a good three to five hours of sleep with fewer morning hangovers and improved sleep quality. It is good for anxiety as well, and tends to be well tolerated. It can be addictive, however, so you'll want to monitor this prescription closely with your doctor. The usual dosage is half to four 0.5-milligram tablets at bedtime or during the night.

- *Quetiapine (Seroquel) and Olanzapine (Zyprexa).* These two antischizophrenic medications can be helpful for sleep as last resorts. The main problems are a flattening of emotion and sometimes dramatic weight gain. If absolutely necessary, take 12.5 to 50 milligrams at bedtime.

In addition to the prescription medications above, the serotonin-raising antidepressants known as SSRIs can help improve sleep, and often have many other benefits for CFS/FMS, even if there is no depression present. If depression, low blood pressure, and/or pain are problematic, these can also be helpful. They include fluoxetine (Prozac), paroxetine (Paxil), and sertraline (Zoloft). Experience suggests that by lowering elevated levels of the pain transmitter called substance P, they can decrease pain. SSRIs (specifically Prozac and Zoloft) also improve neurally mediated hypotension (NMH), which is often seen in these diseases.[20] They take about six weeks to start working. Most patients find that these antidepressants energize them and do best taking the medication in the morning. Occasionally, the increased energy interferes with sleep. Other patients find the medication sedating, and these patients should take it at night.

By using a combination of the treatments discussed above, almost all people with CFS/FMS can get eight to nine hours of solid sleep a night without waking prematurely or having a hangover. It can take a lot of trial and error to find out exactly what is best for you, but it is worth being persistent. Once you are feeling well for six to nine months, or you find you need less medication to get eight to nine hours of solid sleep without waking prematurely or having hangover, you can go ahead and decrease the medication. If I have a patient who has been feeling better and then finds his or her fatigue or pain coming back, one of the first things I ask is, "How is your sleep?" The usual answer is, "Not good." Many people, because of fear of addiction and having to use constantly escalating doses of sleeping pills, are afraid to take enough medication to get adequate sleep. They are so grateful to get five hours of sleep a night that they settle for that. That's a bad idea. I recommend taking whatever is necessary to get eight to nine hours of solid sleep without waking prematurely or having a hangover, even if this means taking several of these medications at one time. Your CFS/FMS specialist should be able to address any concerns you may have about taking natural and/or prescription sleep medications.

After you're better, you may also occasionally find that your sleep worsens for a while during physical and/or emotional stresses. If this occurs, increase or resume your sleep medications for as long as you need and then taper them back down or stop them when the problem is resolved. Sometimes poor sleep persists, and when this happens there is usually an underlying cause. If the cause of your sleep disruption is not obvious, you may have recurrent yeast overgrowth, which we talk about more in Chapter 5. Please be sure to do what you can to achieve the goal of adequate good-quality sleep. You'll be very happy you did.

Other Critical Sleep-Related Disorders

In addition to poor sleep caused by hypothalamic dysfunction, there are four other sleep-related disorders that contribute significantly to the insomnia and other sleep-related symptoms seen in CFS/FMS. The first two fall into the category of sleep-disordered breathing (SDB) and the other two are restless leg syndrome (RLS) and narcolepsy. Treating these can markedly improve your symptoms.

SLEEP-DISORDERED BREATHING (SDB)

Problems can occur anywhere from air entering our nose to the pipes that carry air into our lungs. During sleep we are designed to breathe through our nose. However, there are several reasons why some people find it difficult to breathe through their nose during sleep. These include the size of the nostrils, obstruction of the air passageways, and nasal congestion caused by yeast overgrowth secondary to excess sugar and antibiotic use (see Chapter 5). In addition, if the tissues are prone to collapsing anywhere along the path air is carried, this can also prevent you from getting the air you need while you're sleeping. If oxygen is unable to be delivered around the body and in particular to the brain during sleep, sleep quality is affected and can cause not just excessive sleepiness during the day, but also many of the symptoms seen in chronic fatigue syndrome and fibromyalgia.

If the breathing problem occurs in the upper airway (e.g., the nose) it is called "nasal resistance," which can contribute to sleep-disordered breathing by causing upper airway resistance syndrome (UARS), snoring, and obstructive sleep apnea (OSA). These syndromes are part of the spectrum of sleep-disordered breathing. When the breathing problem is mild, it manifests as UARS, and most standard sleep studies will not detect it unless specifically looking for it. When the blockage of air is more severe, as more often occurs lower down in the airway, it manifests as sleep apnea. Paradoxically, the symptoms of UARS may be more severe than those of sleep apnea, and are more likely to mimic CFS and fibromyalgia. Just as it is common to find that people with CFS/FMS have sleep-disordered breathing, the reverse is also true. In a study of those with sleep-disordered breathing, half of the women and 6 percent of the men were also found to have fibromyalgia.[21]

Although both UARS and sleep apnea are caused by blocked airflow while sleeping, there are many critical differences in the problems they cause: [22]

- Chronic insomnia with frequent awakenings and the inability to fall back asleep tends to be more common in patients with UARS than those with sleep apnea. [23]

- Patients with sleep apnea tend to fall asleep easily during the day (such as when driving), while patients with UARS are more likely to complain of fatigue than sleepiness.
- Patients with sleep apnea tend to be overweight, while those with UARS can be any weight.
- About 50 percent of patients with UARS are women, while only 8 percent of those with sleep apnea are female.
- Upper airway resistance syndrome is often accompanied by a spastic colon and low blood pressure with light-headedness on standing,[24, 25] while sleep apnea is usually associated with high blood pressure.[26]
- People with UARS usually have cold hands and feet and other symptoms of hypothyroidism and a brain-wave pattern called alpha intrusion into delta sleep, which often also occurs in CFS and fibromyalgia.

Upper Airway Resistance Syndrome (UARS)

UARS is often misdiagnosed as chronic fatigue syndrome, fibromyalgia, or even attention deficit disorder/hyperactivity[27] and may be a key contributor to CFS and fibromyalgia. The sleep disorder was first recognized in children in 1982,[28] but the term UARS was not used until adult cases were reported in 1993.[29] With use of newer techniques, it has become easier to identify subtle changes in breathing patterns during sleep, and recently UARS has been linked to not just CFS and fibromyalgia but also to ADD and chronic insomnia.

Unfortunately, there is no good way to diagnose UARS without going to a sleep lab that specializes in looking for it. Unlike sleep apnea, which actually prevents air from getting into your body and causes the oxygen levels in your blood to drop, UARS does not cause this or necessarily even a decrease in airflow. It is simply the increased work of breathing that tends to repeatedly disrupt sleep during the night. If you are going to have a sleep study, check with the lab before doing so to be sure that they will be checking for UARS. Although in the past the gold standard for doing this testing required putting a small tube down into the esophagus, newer technologies that look for pressure changes in your nose or even alterations in breathing or pulse wave signals are already making this testing more user-friendly.

If you are unable to go to a sleep clinic, there is a ssimple nose test to see if you are suffering from nasal resistance. Looking in a mirror, press the side of one nostril to close it. With your mouth closed, breathe in through your other nostril. If the nostril tends to collapse, try holding it open with the flat side of a toothpick. Test both nostrils. If breathing is easier with one nostril held open, using nasal dilators or strips when sleeping (see below) may help.

TREATMENT FOR UARS

Although a mild decrease in airflow while sleeping may not seem like a big problem, it has been shown to disrupt sleep enough to cause and/or perpetuate CFS/FMS. Therefore, keeping your airways open can be critical.[30]

Over the years, a simple nasal dilator called Nozovent (available online) has proved to be one of the most popular and easy-to-use devices to enhance nasal breathing. This device is not just for snorers, but can also be used by anybody who suffers from nasal resistance. Another easy option is Breathe Right nasal strips, which are available at most pharmacies and many supermarkets. Also, a product called the Sinusitis Nose Spray, which combines itraconazole (Sporanox), xylitol, mupirocin (Bactroban), and dexamethasone, is available by prescription from the ITC compounding pharmacy (see Appendix E: Resources) and is often very effective at treating the nasal congestion and sinusitis that can trigger UARS.

I would recommend trying each of these for one month and even all three together, if necessary, and seeing how you feel. If they help, suggesting the presence of UARS, you may wish to consider CPAP or an oral appliance, which are even more effective.

Continuous Positive Airway Pressure (CPAP) is often one of the first recommendations a doctor will make for this condition. The CPAP delivers air into your airway through a specially designed nasal mask that prevents your nasal passages from collapsing. Oral appliances to move the jaw forward can also help, and in some severe cases, surgery on the soft palate or even to widen narrowed jawbones may be necessary.

SLEEP APNEA

Sleep apnea is a condition in which you repeatedly stop breathing during the night. There are two main types of sleep apnea. One is obstructive, in which the pipe that carries air into the lungs gets blocked intermittently; the other is central, which means that the brain trigger that controls breathing stops working intermittently. Obstructive sleep apnea (OSA) is the condition that we are most concerned with in CFIDS/FMS.

In OSA, the pharynx (throat) repeatedly collapses during sleep. The person with OSA fights to breathe against a blocked airway, resulting in decreased oxygen levels in the blood. Eventually, the sense of suffocation wakes the person, the throat muscles contract, the airway opens, and air rushes in under high pressure. When the airway is opened, the rushing air allows the patient to once again drift back into sleep, but creates a loud gasping sound. People with OSA are generally not aware that this is happening, although their partners often have severely disrupted sleep from the snoring and gasping. This cycle repeats itself many times throughout the night, and this constant waking from deep sleep, as well as the loss of oxygen in the blood, can cause next-day sleepiness, brain fog, poor concentration, and mood changes. Another side effect of OSA is high blood pressure (in contrast to low blood pressure in UARS). I generally recommend that any CFS/FMS patient who has high blood pressure, snores, and is overweight consider testing for sleep apnea.

There is a lot of controversy about how common OSA is. As is the case for other illnesses, there is not even an agreement about how to define it. Generally, if the throat closes off for at least ten seconds with no airflow, it is considered to be an apneic episode. This lack of breathing for ten seconds is enough to cause the oxygen level to drop in the blood and to cause one to go from deep sleep into light sleep. Many sleep specialists define sleep apnea as having five or more episodes of decreased breathing per hour in association with daytime sleepiness. Although some specialists estimate that OSA is present in only 3 percent of the adult population, a recent study of all patients in five general medicine doctors' offices suggested that approximately 17 percent of adults had clinically significant sleep apnea, which is defined as having at least fifteen episodes an hour of nonbreathing during sleep. This study suggests that sleep apnea may be much more common than previously thought, and the numbers of diagnosed individuals will rise when a doctor specifically looks for the disorder.[31] In one study, sleep apnea was present in almost 50 percent of patients with CFS.[32] Although sleep apnea is diagnosed by a positive overnight sleep study, fewer than eight of ten thousand patients are referred for sleep studies, though it would be expected that as many as seventeen hundred of each ten thousand patients will have sleep apnea. This is because doctors simply have not been trained to look for OSA. In fact, as noted in an editorial in the *Annals of Internal Medicine*, "Physicians have been shown to receive, on average, a total of only 2.1 hours of formal education in sleep medicine during their medical school training. Sleep history is typically skipped in the general history."[33] When physicians did receive training about sleep apnea, the number of patients they sent for sleep-apnea testing increased dramatically.

CAUSES OF SLEEP APNEA

The main cause of OSA is being overweight. Just as fat deposits develop elsewhere in the body, they also occur in the tissue surrounding the throat. When lying down, the angle of the head can actually cause compression of the pipe that carries air into the lungs. As noted above, because of the often large weight gain caused by the metabolic disturbances in CFIDS/FMS, OSA can occur and complicate treatment of these illnesses. The primary symptoms associated with sleep apnea are snoring and daytime sleepiness. Having a neck circumference of seventeen inches or more also predisposes one to OSA. And because we inherit certain physical characteristics of the throat, there also appears to be a genetic predisposition to sleep apnea.

There are other problems that occur besides the daytime sleepiness in sleep apnea. As noted above, high blood pressure is common. Studies have also shown that patients with severe sleep apnea are at a two- to sevenfold increased risk of having an automobile accident, as they tend to fall asleep while driving. There is also a possible risk of heart and lung damage as a result of untreated OSA. Although some doctors do not consider OSA to be significant until there are fifteen or more apneic episodes per hour of sleep, evidence suggests that even five or more episodes per hour are associated with increased risk of auto accidents and high blood pressure.

DIAGNOSING SLEEP APNEA

Symptoms that suggest sleep apnea are snoring, being overweight, hypertension, daytime sleepiness, periods where breathing stops at night, and frequent auto accidents. If you have several of these symptoms, you should have an overnight sleep study done. During this test, several aspects of sleep are measured. An electroencephalogram (EEG) measures the brain-wave patterns that tell the depth of sleep and gives a printout of how much time is spent in the various stages of sleep. It can also tell how long it takes to fall asleep, how many times you wake during the night, and how many actual hours of sleep you get. Respiratory monitors can measure airflow and tell if the blood oxygen level is dropping, which demonstrates the apnea. The test should also be able to check for leg movements to look for restless leg syndrome (more about this later in this chapter) and to monitor for UARS as well.

This test can be expensive, running approximately $2,000 dollars. Because of the cost, insurance companies are sometimes hesitant to pay for it. It is a good idea to have the sleep laboratory get preauthorization from your insurance company before the test is done. To minimize the high costs, it is common and a good idea to have what is called a split-night study. When this is done, technicians spend the first half of the night looking for evidence of clinically important sleep apnea. If they find it, they put a mask on you that gently maintains the pressure in your throat, which in turn keeps your airway from collapsing. This is like gently blowing into a balloon to keep the opening open. They will do a CPAP titration to determine the optimum mask pressure needed to keep your airway open.

For sleep testing, the lab will often recommend that you be off all sleep medications for several nights before doing the test. If you have not yet started sleep medications, this is reasonable. However, I recommend that patients who have been on sleep medications stay on them during the test. I suggest this for three reasons. First, because most CFS/FMS patients need the sleep medications, as a doctor I need to know whether they are developing sleep apnea from the medication. The second is that, during testing, it is often difficult to fall asleep hooked up with wires in a strange environment and hearing the noise of the technician. It is not uncommon to have inadequate sleep studies where the person is simply not able to sleep for a significant amount of time during the night. The result is an expensive and useless study, which, at best, the doctor recognizes was not effective. At worst (because the person did not sleep much and therefore had no periods when he or she stopped breathing), the lab incorrectly concludes that sleep apnea is not present. The third reason I recommend staying on whatever sleep aid you might be taking is that should you require the CPAP pressure test, it would need to be adjusted to the medications you'll be taking to sleep at home.

Sometimes simply doing a screening test by videotaping yourself while sleeping can be helpful. Although you cannot see UARS on videotape, most people with this problem do snore. Because of this, if the videotape (or audiotape) shows that you do not snore, and the videotape does not show your legs jumping around or that you stop breathing during sleep, looking for sleep-disordered breathing or restless leg syndrome becomes less important.

TREATING SLEEP APNEA

There are several treatments for sleep apnea, and they fall into three main treatment categories: behavioral, pharmacologic, and mechanical. Let us consider each in turn.

BEHAVIORAL TREATMENTS

As noted, being overweight is the main cause of OSA. Because of this, weight loss is one of the most effective ways to treat it. When you are treated for CFS/FMS, it often becomes easier to lose weight. In fact, it is not uncommon to lose twenty to thirty pounds. Markedly cutting back on your carbohydrate intake and increasing your protein intake can help as well. I often prescribe medications that help treat CFIDS/FMS and that also assist with weight loss, among them dextroamphetamine (Adderall, Dexedrine), thyroid hormone, and certain antidepressants. As we discuss later, although I think Dexedrine is overused in hyperactive children, these medications actually help restore balance in CFS/FMS and can be beneficial in this setting.

Avoid sleeping in positions that the videotape shows cause you to snore and have sleep apnea, especially lying on your back. Sleep apnea can often be decreased by taking a tennis ball, putting it into a cloth pocket, and then sewing it into the mid-back of your pajama shirt. The tennis ball makes lying on your back uncomfortable, forcing you to roll onto your side or stomach without waking you. Finally, avoid bedtime alcohol, which can aggravate sleep apnea.

PHARMACOLOGIC TREATMENTS

Several drugs have been used for OSA, but with limited success. A few patients have also been helped by supplemental oxygen. This is especially helpful if you live at a high altitude.

Drugs that contribute to weight loss (including the ones noted above), as well as antidepressants that help weight loss, such as Prozac, can also be useful. It is important, though, not to take these drugs later in the day if they interrupt sleep.

MECHANICAL TREATMENTS

There are several mechanical devices that change the shape of the upper airway and help prevent the throat from collapsing. Orthodontic devices can help keep the lower jaw and tongue forward. These are most likely to be help-ful for mild cases of sleep apnea, UARS, and people who cannot tolerate the CPAP machine. Many people are not willing to continue with the CPAP treatment because of the noise of the machine, the discomfort of wearing the mask, and the cost. However, patients who are able to tolerate the CPAP for at least three to six months become adapted to the treatment. Fortunately, the newer CPAP machines have become much more user-friendly.

Another possibility is surgery to reshape the throat so it stays open dur-ing sleep. Removing the tonsils, nasal surgery, and surgically trimming back the soft palate and the uvula (the tiny thing that hangs down in the back of your throat) are the most common treatments performed. Although these surgeries can be helpful for snoring, they are less likely to help resolve sleep apnea.

It is controversial whether using more aggressive treatments for sleep apnea are worthwhile for people who have fewer than fifteen episodes of apnea per hour. The more conservative approaches (for example, weight loss and avoiding sleeping on your back) are more reasonable ways for those with mild apnea to begin treatment.

NARCOLEPSY

Narcolepsy is a sleep disorder characterized by excessive sleepiness during the day and a condition called cataplexy, a sudden temporary loss in muscle strength. It is often triggered by strong emotions, such as anger or happiness, and can last for seconds or minutes. In severe cases, the person may collapse to the floor. More commonly, the head may sag and the mouth may droop, with only a momentary feeling of weakness. During cataplexy episodes, the person is fully conscious and can see and hear but may not be able to speak. Some people with narcolepsy also have sleep paralysis, an inability to move any muscles when initially falling asleep or waking. This can be frightening, but it is not dangerous. About 70 percent of patients with narcolepsy have only daytime sleepiness, with no cataplexy or sleep paralysis. Narcolepsy is be-lieved to affect one in every thousand people. A study done in New Zealand suggests that narcolepsy is fairly common in CFIDS/FMS.

DIAGNOSING NARCOLEPSY

A diagnosis of narcolepsy can be made with multiple sleep latency testing (MSLT) done in combination with sleep apnea testing. A person with narcolepsy often falls asleep repeatedly in less than five minutes if put in a quiet environment. If REM (dream) sleep occurs in two or more of four or five naps, a diagnosis of narcolepsy is confirmed.

TREATING NARCOLEPSY

Stimulants (specifically Dexedrine, Ritalin, or Adderall, which are amphetamines commonly used in patients with hyperactivity) can be very helpful for many people with CFIDS. The amount needed to maintain adequate alertness varies from person to person. Once the proper dose is found, it does not need to be, and should not be, raised. The maximum dose is 10 to 30 milligrams of any of these three medications taken three times a day, up to 60 milligrams a day. Most CFIDS patients with narcolepsy find 5 to 7.5 milligrams in the morning and 0 to 5 milligrams at noon to be optimal. I become more concerned about addiction if a patient needs more than 30 milligrams a day, and I rarely prescribe these higher doses.

A newer drug, modafanil (Provigil), has also been found to have a beneficial stimulant effect in chronic fatigue syndrome and in narcolepsy as well. The usual dosage is 200 to 600 milligrams a day. Provigil is not considered an amphetamine, like Dexedrine, Ritalin and Adderall, and there are fewer legal restrictions concerning its use. It is also unlikely to cause addiction, which I see in rare cases with high-dose amphetamine. However, I am still more comfortable with recommending Dexedrine, as it is more effective, and we do not know the long-term risks of taking Provigil.

Some patients find that their cataplexy and narcolepsy also improve with 20 to 60 milligrams of Prozac a day. Xyrem, which we discussed earlier under medications for sleep (page 65), can also be helpful for narcolepsy. Frankly, Xyrem is also likely to help your sleep, growth-hormone deficiency, and pain—and having narcolepsy "benefits" you by giving you a diagnosis that will make it easier for you to get insurance coverage for Xyrem, which costs approximately five hundred dollars a month.

RESTLESS LEG SYNDROME AND
PERIODIC LEG MOVEMENT DISORDER

People with restless leg syndrome (RLS) have the sensation that they need to continually move their legs while sleeping. Occasionally, RLS also occurs during the day. Limb movements tend to be repetitive and most frequently involve the legs. A person will often extend his or her big toe while flexing the ankle, the knee, and sometimes even the hip. This can occur with the arms as well, and sometimes even with the whole body.

Another pattern consists of a disagreeable leg sensation and sense of restlessness that is brought on by rest and often relieved by movement. It is not uncommon for your bed partner to be aware that your legs are kicking much of the night or are constantly moving. You may or may not be aware of your own movements. It has been estimated that as many as one-third or more of fibromyalgia patients have RLS. Although the cause of RLS is not clear, experts suspect it comes from a deficiency of the neurotransmitter dopamine. RLS can also be aggravated by iron deficiency (having blood ferritin levels less than 50), nerve injuries, vitamin B_{12} and folic acid deficiency, hypothyroidism, and other problems. In some people, RLS may be associated with hypoglycemia. Some medications, especially Elavil and perhaps lithium, can aggravate RLS.

DIAGNOSING RLS

If you tend to scatter your sheets and blankets, and especially if you tend to kick your bed partner or if you note that your legs tend to feel jumpy and uncomfortable at rest at night, you probably have RLS. You can also have a sleep study done to look for leg muscle contractions. If contractions occur every twenty to forty seconds and last for about one half to five seconds each, you have RLS. The sleep study will determine whether these leg movements are associated with waking from deep sleep into light sleep to a degree that would be expected to cause daytime fatigue. Leg movements are not considered significant unless one has associated daytime sleepiness—for example, CFS/FMS.

TREATING RLS

There are both natural and prescription approaches to treating RLS. Following are summaries of those that have been found to be most successful.

NATURAL TREATMENTS

Natural remedies for RLS focus on diet and nutritional supplementation. Avoiding caffeine is important.[34] Because RLS may be associated with hypoglycemia, eating a sugar-free, high-protein diet with a protein snack at night may decrease episodes of cramping and RLS at night.[35]

An estimated 25 percent of RLS patients have low serum iron levels.[36] As noted in Chapter 6, if your serum ferritin level is under 50, your doctor should prescribe an iron supplement. I recommend Chelated iron by Ultraceuticals or the prescription iron supplement Chromagen Forte because they also contain vitamin C, which helps the iron to be absorbed. Take iron supplements on an empty stomach. Iron can be toxic if too much builds up in the bloodstream, so be sure that your doctor continues to monitor your serum ferritin level while you are taking one of these supplements.

Vitamin E can also be very helpful, although it takes six to ten weeks of treatment to help.[37] Take 400 international units a day. If you have RLS in which pain, numbness, and lightning stabs of pain are relieved by movement or local massage, taking 5 milligrams of folic acid three times a day (available by prescription) is helpful. However, folic acid does not help cases of RLS where there is no discomfort.[38]

Finally, a few case reports have suggested that taking the amino acid L-tryptophan can be effective. Because it is hard to get this without a prescription, I recommend using the related compound 5-HTP (see page 58, "Natural Sleep Remedies").

PRESCRIPTION TREATMENTS

Ambien, Klonopin, and Neurontin or Gabitril are the medications I use to treat sleep disorders in patients whom I suspect have RLS. These medicines usually do a superb job in suppressing RLS. Although it is heavily marketed, I rarely use Requip. I tell patients to adjust the dose to not only get adequate sleep, but also to keep the bedcovers in place and to avoid kicking their partners.

Important Points

- Getting eight to nine hours of solid, deep sleep a night without premature waking or having a hangover is critical to getting well.
- Begin with natural sleep aids. I recommend Suntheanine, wild lettuce, Jamaican dogwood, hops, passionflower, and valerian. These can be found in combination in the Revitalizing Sleep Formula by Enzymatic Therapy.
- Because of the severity of the sleep disorder in CFS and fibromyalgia, most patients will need to add prescription medications for at least six to

eighteen months. A low dose of several medications is more likely to be effective without next-day sedation than a high dose of one medication. Ambien, Desyrel, and Klonopin are the three best prescription sleep medications. Most regular sleeping pills make you feel worse by keeping you in light sleep.

- Take whatever combination of treatments you need to get your eight hours of solid sleep a night.
- Treat sleep disorders such as upper airway resistance syndrome (UARS), sleep apnea, narcolepsy, and/or restless leg syndrome (RLS), if they are present.

Questionnaire (see Appendix B for treatments to check off)

Disordered Sleep

_____ 1. Trouble falling and/or staying asleep? If yes, is it

_____ A. Mild (If yes, check #11 and 12.)

_____ B. Moderate (If yes, check #11, 12, and 13.)

_____ C. Severe (If yes, check #11, 12, 13, and 14.)

_____ 1A. Do you only have trouble falling asleep? If yes, check #12 and 19.

For any of the medications above, natural remedies #12, 15, 16, and 23 can be tried first. Also read and follow the directions at the top of the "Sleeping Aids for Fibromyalgia" section in Appendix B.

Restless Leg Syndrome

_____ 2. Do your legs jump a lot at night or are your blankets (or bed partner) kicked around a lot at night? If yes, add #11, 12, 14, and/or 17 till legs are still at night. Also check off #78, and if your iron blood tests show a ferritin level under 50 or an iron percent saturation under 22 percent, check off #5.

Sleep-Disordered Breathing

_____ 3. Do you snore?

If yes: Sleep Apnea

_____ A. Are you more than twenty pounds overweight?

_____ B. Do you have periods where you stop breathing?

_____ C. Do you have high blood pressure?

_____ D. Do you fall asleep easily during the day?

If yes to A, B, C, or D, check off #78. If no, answer question #4.

UARS

_____ 4. Do you have nasal congestion or low blood pressure? If yes, check off #79.

H—Hormonal Support: Optimizing Adrenal, Thyroid, Testosterone, and Estrogen Function

4

*Y*our body's metabolism is controlled by a series of glands that create messengers called hormones. These hormones are controlled by feedback mechanisms that are constantly interacting with one another in an elaborate dance that is initiated by the hypothalamus, which is the body's master gland. It sends hormones to its next-door neighbor, the pituitary gland, which in turn controls the thyroid gland, the adrenal glands, and the ovaries in females and testicles in males. The hypothalamus monitors the levels of the hormones that all these glands make, and tells the glands whether to make more or less. Other hormones regulated by the hypothalamus include oxytocin, growth hormone, and prolactin.

Many factors determine how much hormone the hypothalamus directs each gland to make. A mysterious gland in the brain called the pineal gland makes melatonin and possibly also other hormones, as yet unknown. This gland also likely regulates your body's circadian rhythm—that is, your day/night cycles. Many functions in the body are rhythmic. The adrenal gland, for example, makes most of its cortisol hormones during the day. If it makes too much at night, the person has trouble sleeping. Evidence suggests that in people with chronic fatigue, the day/night cycles are off, and adrenal glands make too much cortisol at night and not enough during the day. Stress, such as having an infection, also causes the hypothalamus to direct the adrenals to make more cortisol. These are just a few of the many factors that regulate hormone production.

Functions of the Different Glands

As just noted, the pineal, hypothalamus, and pituitary glands, located deep within the brain, work together to direct and balance the metabolic system (the body's energy) and the immune system (the body's defense systems), as well as the autonomic nervous system (the part of the nervous system that controls blood pressure, pulse, sweating, and blood flow to the skin, muscles, and organs). We already know that current evidence suggests that a major portion of the symptoms of CFS and fibromyalgia are manifestations of a poorly functioning hypothalamus, but what roles do the other glands play?

- The adrenal glands are really several glands in one. They help direct the body's defense systems and fluid regulation while also making it possible for your body to deal with stressful situations. If they are underactive, the result is fatigue, recurrent or persistent infections, hypoglycemia with sugar craving, allergies or environmental sensitivities, low blood pressure, dizziness, and poor ability to cope with stress.
- The thyroid gland is the body's gas pedal. It slows or speeds up the metabolism. If it is underactive (that is, if it produces too little thyroid hormone, as is common in CFS/FMS), you can have fatigue, achiness, weight gain, poor mental functioning, and intolerance to cold.
- The reproductive glands support and cycle the reproductive system. The ovaries regulate menstruation in women, and both the ovaries and testicles contribute to libido (sexual desire). The male and female states of mind are powerfully influenced by the hormones produced in these glands. Although testosterone is known as a "male hormone," it is also important in females, as estrogen, the "female hormone," is important in men. If either testosterone or estrogen is low, the person may feel tired, achy, depressed, weak, or moody. He or she may also feel a loss of libido and suffer from disordered sexual function and hot flashes.

Suppression of the hormonal system plays a dramatic role in CFS and fibromyalgia. This often occurs despite your hormonal blood tests being normal. This chapter will present an overview of how to handle this problem.

The Problem with Blood Testing

Before we begin discussing each of the individual hormones, it is important to understand why we cannot rely on blood tests to tell us if there is a hormone-function problem. Many, if not most of you, have had the experience of going to the doctor convinced that your thyroid was low, only to experience the frustration of having the tests come back normal. This was probably not because you do not need supplementation with thyroid hormone. Rather, it is most likely because the testing is not reliable.

By definition, the normal range for most blood tests is created by doing a number of tests and defining only the highest and lowest 2.5 percent of the population as being abnormal (called "two standard deviations"). This does not work well if more than 2.5 percent of the population has a problem. To show how absurd it is to use a 2 percent cutoff, research shows that despite "normal" thyroid hormone levels, antibodies attacking the thyroid gland were present in 34 percent of FMS patients and in 19 percent of "healthy" controls.[1]

One way to understand the difference between the "normal" range, based on two standard deviations (e.g., your not being in the lowest 2 percent of the population), and the optimal range, which you would maintain if you did not have CFS/FMS, is as follows:

> Pretend your lab test uses two standard deviations to diagnose a "shoe problem." One hundred people go to the mall and their shoe sizes are measured. From these one hundred people, a normal shoe size range is established of 4 to 13. If you picked up a pair of shoes from a pile of shoes in this normal range that happened to be a size 12, they might—or might not—fit your foot. If your feet measure a size 12, for example, they fit just perfect.[14] However, if your feet measure a size 5, you are in trouble—even though the normal range derived from the standard deviation would not indicate so. Of course, you would insist that the shoes did not fit because they didn't feel right on your feet.

Like shoes, hormone levels are not "one size fits all." Because of this, treatment needs to be based predominantly on symptoms, using the blood tests only as one more piece of information. The goal in CFS/FMS management is to restore *optimal* function while keeping labs in the normal range for safety. Using this information, let's look at each gland, how to tell if there is a malfunction, and how to optimize function. Let's begin with the adrenal gland—your "stress handler."

The Adrenal Glands

The adrenal glands, which sit on top of the kidneys, are actually two different glands in one. The center of the gland makes epinephrine (also known as adrenaline—for the adrenaline "junkies" out there) and is under the control of the autonomic nervous system. Although it is known that this part of the nervous system is also on the fritz in chronic fatigue patients—contributing to such symptoms as hot and cold sweats, neurally mediated hypotension, and panic attacks—it is not understood whether or how this ties into the adrenals' ability to make adrenaline in CFS/FMS. More likely, adrenaline deficiency is a central brain problem.

The outer part of the adrenal gland, the cortex, also makes many important hormones. These include:

- *Cortisol.* The adrenal glands increase their production of cortisol in response to stress. Cortisol raises blood sugar and blood pressure levels, and moderates immune function, in addition to playing numerous other roles. If the cortisol level is low, the person has fatigue, low blood pressure, hypoglycemia, poor immune function, an increased tendency to allergies and environmental sensitivity, and an inability to deal with stress.
- *Dehydroepiandrosterone sulfate (DHEA-S).* Although its mechanism of action is not clear, DHEA is the most abundant hormone produced by the adrenal cortex. If it is low, you will feel poorly. DHEA-S levels normally decline with age, but appear to drop prematurely in chronic fatigue patients. Patients often feel much better when their DHEA-S levels are brought to the mid-normal range for a twenty-nine-year-old.
- *Aldosterone.* This hormone helps to keep salt and water balanced in the body.
- *Estrogen and testosterone.* These hormones are produced in small but significant amounts by the adrenals as well as by the ovaries and testicles.

Symptoms of Adrenal Insufficiency

If your adrenal glands are underactive, what might you be experiencing? Low adrenal function can cause, among other symptoms:

- Fatigue
- Recurrent infections
- Difficulty shaking off infections
- Poor response and "crashing" during stress
- Achiness
- Hypoglycemia (low blood sugar with irritability when hungry)
- Low blood pressure and dizziness upon first standing

Hypoglycemia deserves special mention. Many people with CFS/FMS sometimes become shaky and nervous, then dizzy, irritable, and fatigued. These people often feel better after they eat sweets, which improves their energy and mood for a short period of time. Because of this, these people often crave sugar, not realizing that it makes their blood sugar level initially shoot back up to normal, which is what makes them feel better, but then makes it continue shooting up beyond normal. The body responds to this by driving the sugar level back down below normal again. The effect, energy-wise, is like a roller coaster.

Dr. Jefferies has noted—and again, my experience confirms his finding—that most people with hypoglycemia have underactive adrenal glands. This makes sense because the adrenal glands' responsibilities include maintaining blood sugar at an adequate level during stress. Sugar is the only fuel that the brain can use. When a person's blood sugar level drops, he or she feels anxious, irritable, and then tired.

Causes of Adrenal Insufficiency

About two-thirds of chronic fatigue patients appear to have underactive adrenal glands.[1] One reason may be that the hypothalamus does not make enough corticotrophin-releasing hormone (CRH), which is the brain's way of telling the adrenals that more cortisol is needed. I suspect that many people also have adrenal exhaustion. Hans Selye, one of the first doctors to research stress reactions, found that if an animal becomes severely overstressed, its adrenal glands bleed and develop signs of adrenal destruction before the animal finally dies from the stress.

If you think back to your biology classes in high school, you may remember something called the fight-or-flight response. This is a physical reaction that occurs during times of stress. During the Stone Age, when a caveman met an animal that wanted to eat him, the caveman's adrenal glands activated multiple systems in his body that prompted him to either fight or run. This reaction helped the caveman survive. In those days, however, people probably had a couple of weeks or months to recover before facing the next major stress.

In today's society, people often experience stress reactions every few minutes. For example, when driving to work, a woman is delayed because of heavy traffic. While sitting behind the wheel, she frets about the consequences of her walking into the office late. Every time she hits a red light or pulls up behind a car that has slowed down, her adrenal glands' fight-or-flight reaction goes off again. When she finally arrives at work, she finds her boss waiting for her, which triggers the reaction once more. During the day, the woman may also have to deal with stresses such as angry customers or difficult coworkers. Her husband or children may phone, forcing her to deal with family stresses. If the woman is ill—suffering from CFS, for example—she has another major stress. The different problems associated with CFS, such as poor sleep, infections, and pain, put more stress on her adrenal glands.

I suspect that many people suffer adrenal exhaustion, but without the destruction that Dr. Selye saw in his experimental animals. With the kinds of stresses common in modern society, a person's adrenal test may initially show hormonal levels that are actually higher than usual (but possibly still inadequate to deal with the degree of stress), since the adrenal glands increase hormonal output to deal with the many burdens placed on your body. Over time, this may exhaust the adrenal reserve—that is, the adrenals' ability to increase hormone production in response to stress. At this point the hormone levels may then drop to overtly deficient levels. This is why some studies show low adrenal hormone levels and others show normal levels.[2]

Treating inadequate adrenal function when it is present is critical if your CFS/fibromyalgia is to resolve. A study published in the *Annals of the New York Academy of Sciences* discussed the evidence for hypothalamic-pituitary-adrenal (HPA) axis insufficiency in CFS and FMS. The study concluded: "Our group has established [that] the impaired activation of the hypothalamic-pituitary-adrenal axis is an essential neuroendocrine feature of this condition."[3] In addition, in endocrinologist William Jefferies's experience (and in mine as well), people with either low hormone production or a low reserve often respond dramatically to treatment with a low dose of adrenal hormone.[4, 5]

Dr. Jefferies's opinion is that everyone who has unexplained, disabling chronic fatigue should be given a low-dose trial of adrenal hormone.[5] Although Dr. Jefferies may well be on the mark, I tend to use this treatment first only on patients whose symptoms, in combination with lab tests, are suggestive of inadequate adrenal function. Most people are able to improve their adrenal function using the natural remedies that I discuss on pages 90–91, especially when used in combination with very low doses of natural prescription hydrocortisone.

PROBLEMS WITH ADRENAL TESTING

Although the adrenal glands make several kinds of hormones, the lab tests for these glands use the production of cortisol as their marker. However, unlike other lab tests, which measure against the two standard deviations we discussed, cortisol levels are only considered low in approximately one out of a hundred thousand people. Most people show morning cortisol levels of approximately 18 to 20 mcg/dl. However, a cortisol level of 10, half of what most people run, 8, or even 6.1 is considered totally normal. To technically have adrenal insufficiency, your morning cortisol needs to be less than six. Shockingly, insufficiency at a level of 5.9 is considered life-threatening. The method of evaluation goes from "normal" to deadly in just .01 mcg/dl. Unfortunately, the lab machine is only accurate within 3 to 4 mcg/dl. In fact, I've seen a 4 mcg/dl variation on two cortisol levels accidentally done on the same tube of blood. This rigid interpretation of test results doesn't make sense to me, and it certainly does not make sense when it comes to taking care of patients.

Not all blood tests are created equal, however, and the HPA axis has a sluggish response to stimulation as well. It has been shown that even the test considered to be more sensitive—the ACTH (cortrosyn) stimulation test—misses the majority of CFS/FMS patients that have adrenal deficiency. When a combination of stimulation tests is used, however, close to 100 percent of these individuals need adrenal support.

FURTHER EVIDENCE SUPPORTING THE NEED TO TREAT ADRENAL PROBLEMS DESPITE NORMAL BLOOD TESTS

For those of you who have a bit more of a technical bent, let's discuss some of the evidence that:

- adrenal axis dysfunction is shown to be present in many CFS/fibromyalgia patients[6–34, 48] despite normal cortisol levels
- when a combination of stimulation tests is used, such as the metyrapone test, or when more sophisticated analysis is used, close to 100 percent of these individuals have documented adrenocortical dysfunction[38–44] and
- treatment with low-dose cortisol has been shown to be safe, appropriate, and effective in these patients.[4, 5, 11, 15, 16, 30, 35]

A study in the *American Journal of Psychiatry* measuring urine hormone levels in 121 consecutive patients with CFS found low twenty-four-hour cortisol levels in all of the CFS patients. The authors conclude: "Urinary free cortisol was significantly lower in the subjects with chronic fatigue syndrome regardless of the presence or absence of current or past comorbid psychiatric illness. . . . From whatever cause, low-circulating cortisol is associated with fatigue; furthermore, raising cortisol levels can reduce fatigue in chronic fatigue syndrome. Thus, this study provides further evidence that adrenocortical dysfunction in chronic fatigue syndrome, whatever the etiology and whether primary or secondary, may be one piece of the multifactorial jigsaw underlying the production of symptoms in chronic fatigue syndrome."[37]

Another study, published in the *Journal of Endocrinological Investigation*, performed a combination of stimulation tests on FMS patients. The researchers found that more than 95 percent of these patients had hypothalamic-pituitary-adrenal (HPA) axis dysfunction.[9] They state: "The etiology and pathophysiology of this disease [are] not fully understood but the current data [suggest] that the PFS [primary fibromyalgia syndrome] is not a primary disease of muscle. In contrast, an increasing amount of evidence suggests that the central stress axis, the HPA axis, seems to play an important role in the development of PFS [fibromyalgia]."[9]

The inability of the adrenal glands to respond adequately to stress is important. For example, cortisol levels normally increase with pain, but it has been shown that patients with CFS/FMS either cannot appropriately increase cortisol production in response to pain or that the patients' inability to increase cortisol causes the increased pain. A study published in the journal *Arthritis and Rheumatism* showed a strong relationship between cortisol levels and pain in individuals with CFS and FMS, and that low cortisol levels alone explained 38 percent of the variation in pain upon waking. The authors conclude: "The results of this study indicate that pain symptoms in women with FMS are associated with low cortisol concentrations during the early part of the day. . . . These data support the hypothesis that HPA axis function is associated with symptoms in FMS and accounts for the substantial percentage of pain symptom variance during the early part of the day."[45]

In addition to what was found in Professor Jefferies's decades of experience and in my studies, a placebo-controlled study was published in *The Lancet* in which patients with chronic fatigue syndrome were treated with low-dose hydrocortisone (5 to 10 milligrams/day), thus increasing their cortisol levels, or placebo. The study found significant improvements in those treated with low-dose hydrocortisone versus those treated with placebo, and 28 percent improved to normal levels. The authors concluded: "This study shows that low-dose hydrocortisone results in significant reduction in self-rated fatigue and disability in patients with chronic fatigue syndrome. . . . The degree of disability was reduced with hydrocortisone treatment, but not with placebo."[16] This also supports the effectiveness and appropriateness of raising cortisol levels through supplementation.

Another study, published in *JAMA*, also found significant improvement in fatigue scores with hydrocortisone replacement, but these researchers used excessive dosing of 25 to 35 milligrams of cortisol, which resulted in mild adrenal suppression and marked worsening of sleep.[51] Therefore, I limit patients to a maximum of 20 milligrams/day, as this dose has been shown to be quite safe.[11, 17, 46, 47]

TREATING ADRENAL INSUFFICIENCY

People with hypoglycemia, which in CFS/FMS is most often caused by inadequate adrenal function, can treat low-blood-sugar symptoms by cutting sugar and caffeine out of their diets; having frequent, small meals; and increasing their intake of protein while decreasing carbohydrates. It's best to avoid white flour and sugar and to substitute complex carbohydrates such as whole grains and vegetables. Fruit—not fruit juices, which contain concentrated sugar—can be eaten in moderation, about one to two pieces a day, depending on the type of fruit. If you get irritable, eat something with protein. For quick relief, put a quarter to half a teaspoon of sugar (or even just one or two Tic Tacs) under your tongue at the same time. This is enough to quickly raise your blood sugar level but not enough to put you on a sugar "roller-coaster ride."

More directly, treating the underactive adrenal problem with low doses of adrenal hormone usually quickly banishes the symptoms of low blood sugar. I like to begin with natural hydrocortisone such as Cortef (by prescription at most pharmacies) or, better yet, sustained-release hydrocortisone from a compounding pharmacy. This immediately gives your body the support that your adrenal glands are unable to give, and may help you feel much better quickly. The added cortisol also takes some of the strain off your adrenals so that they can heal.

If you and your doctor decide that treating the problem with natural hydrocortisone is not in your best interest, there are also many natural things you can take that can both help to support your adrenal glands and naturally raise your body's cortisol level.

NATURAL ADRENAL SUPPORT

Below are several things that can help your adrenal glands heal:

1. Adrenal glandulars supply the raw materials that your adrenal glands need to heal. It is critical, however, that you get them from reputable companies (I recommend Enzymatic Therapy) so that the purity and potency are guaranteed and so that you can be sure they come from cows that are not at risk of transmitting infections.
2. Vitamin C is crucial for adrenal function. Your body's highest levels of vitamin C are found in the adrenal glands and brain tissues, and the urinary excretion of vitamin C is increased during stress. Optimizing vitamin C intake by taking 500 to 1,000 milligrams a day also helps immune function.
3. Pantothenic acid, a B vitamin, also supports adrenal function, and pantothenic acid deficiency causes shrinking of your adrenal glands. Optimal levels are approximately 100 to 150 milligrams daily, although some physicians use even higher levels for adrenal support.

4. Licorice slows the breakdown of adrenal hormones in your body, helping to maintain optimal levels. There is no licorice in licorice candies in the United States because of this, as too much licorice can raise cortisol levels too high. Another beneficial effect of the licorice is that it helps in the treatment of indigestion, and it is even as effective as the prescription heartburn medication Tagamet. Do not take licorice if you have high blood pressure, as too much licorice can cause excess adrenal function and worsen high blood pressure. You can safely take 200 to 400 milligrams a day of a licorice extract standardized to contain 5 percent glycyrrhizic acid.

5. Chromium also helps decrease the symptoms of low blood sugar. Take 200 micrograms a day.[49]

If you'd rather not take these natural remedies separately, or just to simplify the supplementation, you can take Adrenal Stress End, which I helped the Enzymatic Therapy Company develop. Take one to two capsules in the morning. If symptoms recur in the afternoon, add another capsule at lunch. Adrenal Stress End, combined with the Energy Revitalization System vitamin powder, supplies everything noted above, as well as many other nutrients that will help support adrenal function. You can also put together your own supplement program using these and any of the other supplementation recommendations in this book.

Toxicity of Cortisone

Adrenal hormones are essential for life. Without them, a person dies. But, as with any hormone, too much can be dangerous, and any cortisol supplementation should be closely monitored by your CFS/FMS specialist. In the early studies using adrenal hormones, the researchers had no idea what dose was normal and what was toxic. When they gave injections of the hormone to arthritis patients, the patients' arthritis went away, and they felt better. However, they gave patients many times more than the normal amount, and many patients became toxic and died. Because of this, the researchers became frightened and avoided using adrenal hormones whenever possible. Medical students were taught to avoid adrenal hormones unless no other treatment choices existed.

The use of adrenal hormones needs to be put into perspective, however. Imagine if early thyroid researchers had given their patients fifty times the usual dose of thyroid hormone. Thyroid patients would have routinely died of heart attacks. The thyroid researchers, though, were fortunate enough to stumble upon the healthy dose early on and to skip negative outcomes (likely because too high a dose of thyroid caused immediate side effects). If they had not, people today would not be treated for an underactive thyroid until they displayed symptoms of advanced thyroid disease (myxedema) and were nearly comatose. Medical science is just beginning to learn that a person can feel horrible and function poorly even with a minimal to moderate hormone deficiency. Waiting for the person to "go off the deep end" of the test's normal scale is simply not healthy.

Dr. Jefferies has found that as long as the adrenal hormone level does not exceed the normal range, the main toxicity that a patient might experience is a slight upset stomach, as the body is not used to absorbing the hormone through the stomach.[11, 50] If this occurs, taking the hormone with food usually helps. In addition, some patients gain a few pounds. This is because a low adrenal level can cause a person's weight to drop below the body's normal set point, even if that set point is high because of CFS/FMS. However, any weight gain usually is more than offset by the eventual weight loss resulting from being able to exercise and function once again.

As discussed, many physicians do not like to prescribe even low doses of adrenal hormones. If your doctor is uncomfortable with hydrocortisone (Cortef, the natural and safer form of the adrenal hormone), and natural remedies do not provide sufficient relief, invite him or her to read Dr. Jefferies's material on the safety of low-dose cortisone as well as our study, which is available on my Web site (www.vitality101.com).[11, 50]

Additionally, the NIH Institute of Allergy and Infectious Diseases showed that what they called "low-dose" Cortef (25 to 35 milligrams a day) moderately helped CFS patients but caused some patients' adrenal glands to "go to sleep."[51] This is a concern, but as noted in my letter to the editor printed in the *Journal of the American Medical Association*, the dose used in the NIH study was two to three times as high as most CFS patients need and therefore dramatically worsened the sleep disorder.[52] Another study (using 10 milligrams of Cortef a day in CFIDS) and studies of CFS/FMS patients show significant benefit using lower doses without significant toxicity.[4, 11, 53] Indeed, most patients only need 5 to 12.5 milligrams a day—a dose lower than most doctors have ever prescribed. This dosage is equivalent to 1 to 3 milligrams a day of prednisone, which is the more toxic synthetic adrenal hormone used by most physicians. However, Cortef is better than prednisone for people with CFS/FMS, as it is bioidentical and more closely mimics your body's own hormonal activity. After feeling well for six to eighteen months, most people are able to begin slowly decreasing their adrenal hormone dosage, eventually discontinuing the treatment entirely as their adrenal glands resume normal function.

Our studies and clinical experience show that ultra-low-dose cortisol is unlikely to cause adrenal suppression, and this conclusion has been supported by other research. In a study published in 2001 in *Journal of Clinical Endocrinology & Metabolism*, the authors checked adrenal function in thirty-seven patients with CFS and then treated these patients with low-dose cortisol. They found that the treatment resulted in significant improvement and not only was there no adrenal suppression, but rather there was an improvement in the HPA axis function. They concluded: "In this group, there was a significant increase in the cortisol response to human CRH, which reversed the previously observed blunted responses seen in these patients. We conclude that the improvement in fatigue seen in some patients with chronic fatigue syndrome during hydrocortisone (cortisol) treatment is accompanied by a reversal of the blunted cortisol responses to human CRH."[54]

The safety of low-dose cortisol was also addressed in a forty-eight-page review article published in the *Annals of Rheumatic Diseases*. This extensive review assessed the safety of long-term low-dose glucocorticoid (cortisol) therapy in rheumatoid arthritis, considering "low dose" to be 40 milligrams hydrocortisone (much higher than the 10 to 20 milligrams we recommend). The researchers concluded: "Adverse effects of glucocorticoids are abundantly referred to in literature. However, in the available literature on low-dose glucocorticoid therapy very little of the commonly held beliefs about the incidence, prevalence, and impact of GC [glucocorticoids] proved to be supported by clear scientific evidence. Additional data from the randomized controlled clinical trials reviewed showed that the incidence, severity, and impact of adverse effects of low-dose glucocorticoid therapy in rheumatoid arthritis trials are modest, and often not statistically different to those of placebo."[55] This considerable safety and negligible risk is also confirmed in endocrinology texts.[56]

Recently, studies have been published about bone loss with the use of low-dose adrenal hormones, but even these studies do not use the very low doses that we use.[57] Nonetheless, it is reasonable to take bioidentical estrogen (that is, estrogen identical to what our bodies make) if you are a menopausal or estrogen-deficient female. If you have low bone density, also take 600 to 1,500 milligrams of calcium a day, 340 milligrams of strontium (more effective than Fosamax), and 600 to 4,000 units of vitamin D daily (see Chapter 8). You can also get your calcium by adding two cups of yogurt with live and active yogurt cultures to your daily diet. Your doctor can guide you further on your calcium needs.

ADRENAL FUNCTION AND BLOOD PRESSURE

Another important function of the adrenal glands is maintaining blood volume and pressure by keeping salt in your body. Low blood pressure, low blood volume, and dehydration are common in CFS patients. In adults with CFS/FMS, I have found dextroamphetamine (Dexedrine) and the antidepressant fluoxetine (Prozac) to reverse the dizziness and low blood pressure of neurally mediated hypotension (NMH).[58–61] In fact, antidepressants have actually been proven to increase exercise performance in CFS/FMS.[62] I would also note that Dexedrine and Ritalin, which I believe are overused in ADHD and underused in CFS/FMS, are helpful in CFS/FMS and have been shown in a placebo-controlled study to also help both fatigue and concentration in these syndromes.[63] A medication called ProAmatine (midodrine) may also be helpful occasionally. It is critical to begin with the basics, however, which includes drinking plenty of water and getting enough salt and potassium.

Though not helpful in adults, a salt- and water-retaining adrenal hormone called Florinef can be of benefit for those under age twenty-two. Young people can take one-quarter of a 0.1-milligram tablet per day and increase by a quarter tablet every four to seven days until they reach one whole tablet. Effects may not be evident for three to six weeks. An even simpler treatment may be to simply increase the intake of salt. In fact, Dr. David Bell, a physician specializing in pediatric CFS, found that nineteen of his twenty-five CFS patients felt much better when they received a quart of salt water (normal saline) intravenously each day.

To summarize, if your symptoms started suddenly after a viral infection, if you suffer from hypoglycemia (and irritability when hungry), or if

Getting Kids and Young Adults Well—
Information for Patients Under Age Sixteen

If you're under age sixteen, you most likely have neurally mediated hypotension (NMH)—sort of like low blood pressure—and an allergy to milk proteins. Some doctors do a type of test called the tilt-table test to diagnose NMH, but I treat NMH without doing the test first. It's not a bad idea to have it done, but it is expensive and uncomfortable.

To treat NMH, your doctor can prescribe the medications fluoxetine (Prozac), midodrine (ProAmatine), fludrocortisone (Florinef, which is modestly effective), and/or methylphenidate (Ritalin) or dextroamphetamine (Dexedrine). Of all of these, Dexedrine and Ritalin are most helpful for those under twenty years of age. In addition, the following things can be helpful:

- Avoid sugar. Stevia is a healthy sweetener you can use instead.
- Take the Energy Revitalization System vitamin powder or a similar multivitamin supplement.
- Dramatically increase your intake of salt and water. Aim for 8 to 15 grams of salt and one gallon of water each day.
- If you have stomach or bowel symptoms, cut out all milk products and any foods containing casein or caseinate (milk protein) for two to three weeks to see if this helps.
- If you have taken a lot of antibiotics and/or steroid medications (cortisone, prednisone, or others), ask your doctor to consider treating you with natural antifungals for five months and fluconazole (Diflucan) for six to twelve weeks to get rid of possible yeast overgrowth (see Chapter 5).
- If you run frequent fevers (temperatures over 98.8°F), you likely have a hidden infection. A three-to-six month trial of antibiotics should be considered (see Chapter 5). In addition, get a parasite test done by a laboratory that specializes in this type of testing, such as the Parasitology Center or the Genova/Great Smokies Diagnostic Laboratory (see Appendix E: Resources).
- Consider thyroid treatment with Cytomel (see page 101).

If you're not better, then refer to the rest of the program outlined in this book. Chapter 5 offers more detailed information on treating infections.

Fortunately, these simple suggestions help most kids get better.

you have recurrent infections that take a long time to resolve, you probably have underactive adrenal glands. About two-thirds of my severe chronic
fatigue patients have underactive or marginally functioning adrenal glands
or a decreased adrenal reserve.

Although I prefer natural products to pharmaceuticals, in this
situation I am comfortable adding standardized bioidentical hormones to
the natural therapies. By using these natural remedies in conjunction
with Cortef, you may need a lower dose of the bioidentical hormone than
you would otherwise. And you may be able to stop the cortisol supplementation sooner by helping your adrenal glands and hypothalamus heal. If
the amount of hormone given is within the body's normal range, the body
can decide for itself how much of the hormone it wants to use, making
these treatments very safe.

Dehydroepiandrosterone (DHEA)

The adrenal glands make many hormones in addition to cortisol. One of
these is DHEA, which is often low in CFIDS patients. Although DHEA's
function is not yet fully understood, it appears to be important for good
health, which makes a low DHEA level worth treating.[64-66] For many
CFS/FMS patients, when a low DHEA level is treated, the result is a dramatic boost in energy. Some studies suggest that the higher a person's
DHEA level is, the longer that person will live and the healthier he or she
will be. However, I'm concerned that pushing the blood level above the
upper limit of normal may increase the risk of breast cancer, so you should
work with your doctor to be sure blood DHEA-S levels do not exceed a
safe limit.

If your DHEA sulfate (DHEA-S, not DHEA) level is low (under 120
micrograms per deciliter [mcg/dL] of blood for females or 325 mcg/dL for
males), I recommend beginning treatment with 5–25 milligrams of DHEA
per day and slowly working up to what feels like an optimal level to you.
For women, I suggest keeping the DHEA-S level at around 150–180 mcg/
dL, which is the middle of the normal range for a twenty-nine-year-old
female. For men, I keep the DHEA-S level between 350 and 500 mcg/dL,
which is the normal range for a twenty-nine-year-old male. The low ends of
the normal ranges are normal only for people over eighty. If you have side
effects, such as facial hair or acne, which are uncommon, check your blood
level of DHEA-S and decrease your dose. A good form of DHEA (some are

not) is available without a prescription at compounding pharmacies, my Web site, and the General Nutrition Centers.

We have found that roughly 10 percent of women with CFS/FMS actually have an elevated DHEA-S level. This is often associated with an elevated testosterone level as well. When I see this, I suspect and look for polycystic ovarian syndrome (PCOS) and insulin resistance. If a fasting morning insulin level is higher than 10 (suggestive of insulin resistance), especially if ovarian cysts or infertility are also present, these patients often improve significantly with a diabetes medication called metformin, 500 to 1,000 milligrams one to two times a day, which improves insulin sensitivity. This can also assist with restoring fertility, as well as helping the patient lose excess weight. As metformin can cause vitamin B_{12} deficiency, it is critical that a high-dose B_{12} supplement be taken with it. Polycystic ovarian syndrome may also improve with low-dose hydrocortisone and with chromium supplementation of 1,000 micrograms daily.[67]

The Thyroid Gland

The thyroid gland, located in the neck area, is the body's gas pedal. It regulates the body's metabolic speed. If the thyroid gland produces insufficient amounts of thyroid hormones, the metabolism decreases and the person gains weight. Other symptoms of hypothyroidism include intolerance to cold, fatigue, achiness, confusion, and constipation (though diarrhea from bowel infections is common in CFS/FMS).

The thyroid makes two primary hormones. They are:

- *Thyroxine (T_4)*. T_4 is the storage form of thyroid hormone. The body uses it to make triiodothyronine (T_3), the active form of thyroid hormone. Most synthetic thyroid medications, such as Synthroid and Levothroid, are pure T_4. These synthetics are fine if your body has the ability to properly turn them into T_3. Unfortunately, many people with CFS/FMS find that their bodies do not have this ability.
- *Triiodothyronine (T_3)*. T_3 is the active form of thyroid hormone. Although in some life-threatening illnesses the body appropriately makes less T_3, research suggests that when CFS/FMS occurs, the body may not be able to adequately turn T_4 into T_3, or it may need much higher levels of T_3.

THE PROBLEM WITH THYROID TESTS

Many years ago, while I was in medical school, physicians were taught to diagnose hypothyroidism, or low thyroid function, by using the newly discovered method of measuring the metabolic rate while the patient ran on a treadmill. We doctors thought that this was a wonderful new test and that we finally had a way to identify patients with underactive thyroids. We congratulated ourselves on being so clever. But then a new test came out. The new test measured protein-bound iodide (PBI). When we began using the PBI test, we realized that we had missed diagnosing many people with a low thyroid, but thought that this new test would pick up everybody who had a problem. We patted ourselves on the back and told all our newly discovered thyroid patients that it turned out that they were not crazy—they just had a low thyroid. We were comfortable that we could now determine with certainty when someone had a thyroid problem.

Then the T_4-level thyroid test was developed, and we thought that the old PBI test had missed many people with a low thyroid, but this new test would find everyone. Then the T_7 test, which adjusts for protein binding of thyroid hormone, came out, and then the thyroid-stimulating hormone (TSH) test. Modern medicine is now beyond the fifth generation of TSH tests, and this is the only test that many doctors use to monitor thyroid function. With each new test, doctors realize that they missed many people with underactive thyroid function. In 2002, the American Academy of Clinical Endocrinologists noted that anybody with a TSH under 3 should be treated for hypothyroidism, and that 13 million Americans had an underactive thyroid that was not being treated because labs were being misinterpreted. Despite this, most labs still have a normal range for TSH that goes up to 5.5. To make matters more difficult, if the thyroid is underactive because the hypothalamus is suppressed, the TSH test, which depends on normal hypothalamic function to be at all reliable, may appear to be normal, or may even suggest an overactive thyroid. In fact, when lecturing at a fibromyalgia conference in Italy, I spoke with Professor Gunther Neeck—the world's foremost expert on hypothalamic-thyroid axis dysfunction in fibromyalgia.[8] I asked him a simple question: "Is the TSH test reliable in fibromyalgia?" He gave a very simple answer: "Absolutely not!" Fortunately some doctors are finally starting to catch on.

In two studies done by Dr. G. R. Skinner and his associates in the United

Kingdom, patients who were felt to have hypothyroidism (an underactive thyroid) because of their symptoms had their blood levels of thyroid hormone checked. The vast majority of them had technically normal thyroid blood tests. These data were published in the *British Medical Journal*.[68] He then did another study in which the patients with normal blood tests who had symptoms of an underactive thyroid—those whose doctors would likely say had a normal thyroid and would not need treatment—were treated with thyroid hormone. A remarkable thing happened when this was done (well, maybe we're not surprised). The large majority of patients, despite being considered to have a normal thyroid, had their symptoms improve upon taking thyroid hormone (Synthroid), at an average dosage of 100 to 120 micrograms a day.[69]

These two studies, plus another one showing that thyroid blood tests are only low in about 3 percent of patients whose doctors sent blood tests in, confirm what we have been saying all along.[70] Our current thyroid testing will miss most patients with an underactive thyroid. Doctors of decades ago were on target when they believed that one has to treat the patient and not the blood test. Most blood tests cannot accurately measure T_3 thyroid deficiency because readings measure only the level of T_3 in the blood, and it's the level inside your cells that is important. Nonetheless, it may still be worthwhile to check total or free T_3 levels if you and your doctor suspect T_3 deficiency. Testing should occur before beginning T_3 therapy, as the tests become unreliable once you begin taking hormones that contain T_3. (For a more complete discussion of the interpretation of thyroid tests, see Appendix G: For Physicians.)

TREATING AN UNDERACTIVE THYROID

We are constantly learning powerful new tricks for treating hypothyroidism, and there are many reasonable treatment approaches. Our treatment protocol information checklist (see Appendix B) gives the "nuts and bolts" of some approaches.

What treatment will work best often depends on what is causing your thyroid levels to be inadequate. Common causes of underactive thyroid hormone in CFS/fibromyalgia include:

1. *Hypothalamic dysfunction.* Your thyroid gland may be fine, but it is not getting adequate stimulation from the hypothalamus and is basically "asleep." In this situation, simply taking a mix of T_4 and T_3 (see below)

at the dose that feels best may be adequate. As the CFS resolves and hypothalamic function recovers, it is often possible to wean oneself off the thyroid hormone.

2. *Hashimoto's thyroiditis.* In this autoimmune process, your body's immune system attacks and damages the thyroid. This can be diagnosed by a blood test called an "anti-TPO antibody." If the anti-TPO antibody is elevated, you likely have Hashimoto's thyroiditis and may need to take thyroid supplementation for the rest of your life.

3. *Inadequate conversion of the T_4 thyroid hormone to active T_3.* In this situation, which is common in fibromyalgia, patients often respond best to treatment with pure T_3 hormone.

4. *Receptor resistance.* In this situation, your body is making adequate amounts of thyroid hormone but the areas that it stimulates are very slow to recognize the thyroid hormone's presence. Because of this, it takes a very high level of pure T_3 hormone to get a normal response. This problem often resolves over one to two years on the high-dose T_3 treatment as the body heals from fibromyalgia and/or chronic fatigue syndrome.

Given the multiple causes of thyroid insufficiency in CFS and fibromyalgia, let's discuss how to best treat these problems.

THYROID HORMONE

Most doctors prescribe T_4 (Synthroid) to treat an underactive thyroid. T_4, though, is fairly inactive until the body converts it into T_3, or activated thyroid hormone. If the problem is only with the thyroid gland itself, prescribing Synthroid will work just fine. However, during periods when the body wants to conserve energy (for example, during times of infection or with CFS/FMS), the body slows down its metabolism. It does this by decreasing the production of active T_3 from T_4, which is turned into inactive "reverse T_3" instead. In some cases, the body may get "stuck" and become unable to make adequate T_3. Because of this problem, many physicians prefer to use compounded or Armour Thyroid, which contains a mix of T_4 and T_3.

If you suffer from chronic fatigue and have achy muscles and joints, heavy periods, constipation, easy weight gain, cold intolerance, dry skin, thin hair, a change in your ankle reflexes called a delayed relaxation of the deep tendon reflex (DTR), or a body temperature that tends to be on the low side of normal, you should consider asking your doctor to prescribe a low dose of Armour Thyroid. As long as you do not have underlying heart disease and you follow up with a blood test to make sure that your free T_4 thyroid levels are in a safe range (going above the upper limit of normal may aggravate osteoporosis, a problem already common in CFS/FMS), a trial of low-dose thyroid hormone treatment is usually quite safe and may be dramatically beneficial.

I prefer to start with a trial of compounded T_3 plus T_4 or with Armour Thyroid, in which both T_3 and T_4 are already present. I begin with ¼ grain (15 milligrams) a day and increase it to ½ grain (30 milligrams) a day in one week. Then, I increase it by ½ grain each one to six weeks until the patient finds a dose that feels best. If this treatment does not bring about relief, a trial of Synthroid, which contains only T_4, may help. One hundred micrograms (0.1 milligrams) of Synthroid "equals" ¾–1 grain of Armour Thyroid. Often, one hormone treatment works when the other does not. Adjust the dose as above. You will know if the treatment is working within one to six weeks on a given dose.

If you are shaky or hyper, or have a racing heart (for example, a pulse over ninety beats per minute), lower the dose. In addition, try taking the full dose of thyroid in the morning on an empty stomach or half the dose twice a day to see which feels best. Do not take thyroid hormone within several hours of taking iron or calcium supplements, or you won't absorb the thyroid.[70A]

Once you have found a dose that feels best, or once the 2- and 3-grain levels are reached, your doctor should check the free T_4 blood levels. The first test should be administered about one month after you've reached the optimum level described above and then once every six to twelve months. You may need to slowly adjust the thyroid supplementation so that you remain within normal range for blood free T_4 thyroid hormone levels.[71] Do not allow your doctor to do a TSH test. It will be low (because of the hypothalamic dysfunction) and your doctor will incorrectly think you're on too much thyroid—even if your blood T_4 hormone levels are low normal. This will make you and your doctor crazy. Although many patients can stop taking thyroid hormone after twelve to twenty-four months, you can stay on Armour Thyroid or Synthroid for as long as it is needed.

Another approach, used by John Lowe, DC, a researcher in Boulder, Colorado, is to use pure T_3 hormone (Cytomel). He feels that FMS patients have "thyroid resistance"—that is, it takes a much higher level of thyroid to obtain the normal effect. Even though the body may only make about 25 to 30 micrograms of T_3 a day, his studies found it took an average of

120 micrograms a day to make his FMS patients feel healthy.[72, 73] We have found this approach to be helpful in many patients. For more information, see www.drlowe.com.

All thyroid treatments must be prescribed and monitored by a physician. Holistic physicians are more likely to be familiar with and open to trying these new treatment approaches. Unfortunately, many doctors are (incorrectly) trained to stop increasing the dosage of thyroid hormone once an individual's thyroid tests are in the "normal" range—even if the dose is inadequate for that person. Synthetic T_4 (Synthroid) and pure T_3 (Cytomel) are available at any pharmacy. Sustained-release T_3, which works better for many patients, can be obtained from compounding pharmacies. There has been a significant problem with quality control for T_3 hormone, so I recommend that you use ITC Pharmacy (see Appendix E: Resources). When you settle on an optimal dose, the compounding pharmacy can then make a single capsule of that dosage to be taken one or two times a day. This is less expensive because the cost tends to be based more on the number of capsules than the actual amount of T_3 in them.

POTENTIAL SIDE EFFECTS

If someone has blockages in the arteries that feed the heart and is on the verge of a heart attack, taking thyroid hormone can trigger a heart attack or angina, just as exercise can. Thyroid treatment can trigger heart palpitations as well. These are usually benign, but if chest pain or increasing palpitations occur, stop the thyroid supplementation and call your doctor at once. Because of this concern, I often recommend that patients at significant risks of angina—people who smoke, have high blood pressure, are over age forty-five, have cholesterol levels over 260, or have a family history of heart attacks in individuals under sixty-five years old—have an exercise treadmill test done before treatment, even if they can't complete the test.

To put the risk in perspective, in the many thousands of my patients on a thyroid supplement, none experienced heart attacks or other major health issues from taking it. In the long run, I suspect that thyroid treatment is much more likely to decrease one's risk of heart disease by lowering cholesterol.

The other main concern is that excess thyroid hormone can cause osteoporosis. In my research, I have seen no studies showing any increase in osteoporosis in premenopausal women, or even in postmenopausal women if they are on estrogen, if one keeps the T_4 thyroid blood level in the normal range. As noted earlier, TSH is simply not a reliable monitor of thyroid levels in CFS/FMS because of hypothalamic dysfunction. We don't know for sure if keeping the T_3 level above normal in FMS patients with thyroid resistance worsens the osteoporosis already commonly seen in CFS/FMS, but this has not been a problem in Dr. Lowe's experience with thousands of patients. If you need to keep the T_3 or T_4 above the upper limit of normal, you should have a DEXA (osteoporosis) scan every six to twenty-four months. If this scan shows osteoporosis, lower the thyroid dose. If this is not possible, consider other osteoporosis-prevention measures we discuss in this book (see page 225) with your physician.

The Reproductive Glands

Many people going through midlife develop fatigue, poor libido, or depression.[74] This includes men and women alike. Researchers have found that if the estrogen and testosterone levels in females or the testosterone level in males is low, a trial replacement of these hormones can bring about dramatic improvement and is therefore worth considering. Underactive adrenal glands can aggravate this problem.

LOW TESTOSTERONE—NOT ONLY A MALE PROBLEM

Low testosterone is associated with many problems, including fatigue, depression, poor stamina, osteoporosis, muscle wasting, diabetes, high cholesterol, weight gain, and poor libido. Low testosterone, classified as being in the lowest 20 percent of the normal range, is a major problem in 70 percent of my male patients with CFS/FMS. The severity of the problem has worsened, as men's average testosterone levels have dropped by 16 percent over the last fifteen years.[75] Although testosterone levels are normally much lower in females, deficiencies in women cause similar problems. Testosterone is critical in females as well as males, and I find low free testosterone levels in most female CFS/FMS patients as well. It is important, then, to check the free, or unbound, blood testosterone level in both men and women. This measures the active form of the hormone. A serum (or total) testosterone level measures mostly the inactive storage form of the hormone. Inactive (total) testosterone levels are often normal despite an inadequate level of the critical active (free) testosterone.

Optimizing testosterone levels can result in many benefits in people with CFS and fibromyalgia. After six to eight weeks, the effect of treatment is often marked. Benefits include:

1. In women with fibromyalgia, a study done by Professor Hilary White of Dartmouth University showed that giving natural testosterone decreased fatigue and pain.[76]
2. Fibromyalgia and CFS are associated with decreased red blood cell levels. Testosterone supplementation is a highly effective way of increasing the red blood cell levels.
3. Testosterone can improve libido, which is low in 73 percent of CFS and fibromyalgia patients.[77–79]
4. Testosterone increases bone density, therefore decreasing the risk of osteoporosis.[80]
5. Testosterone improves mood and decreases depression.[81]
6. Testosterone increases muscle strength and decreases fat levels.
7. Research has shown that men who have low testosterone are at greater risk of premature death. For example, one study that followed men over forty years old for five years found that the men with low testosterone levels were 88 percent more likely to die during that period.[82, 83]
8. Low testosterone is associated with an increased risk of high cholesterol, angina[84, 85] and diabetes.[86]
9. Chronic fatigue syndrome has been associated with a possible decrease in the heart's ability to pump blood, and testosterone improves heart function.[87]

As is the case with most hormones, keeping testosterone levels optimal using bioidentical hormones seems to be very helpful in CFS and fibromyalgia and also appears to be associated with increased health and longevity. However, it is important that we not confuse giving safe levels of bioidentical natural testosterone with the high-dose, synthetic, and toxic testosterone that bodybuilders sometimes use.

TESTING FOR LOW TESTOSTERONE

Again, it is important to check the free (not just total) testosterone. Most laboratories can test free testosterone only if they also measure the total testosterone—this is a normal procedure.

Be sure that the normal ranges for the lab results are broken down by ten-year age groups—thirty-one to forty years old, forty-one to fifty years old, and so on. It is meaningless to have a normal range that includes eighty-year-olds if you're twenty-eight.

Also, bizarrely, some labs even have a normal range for women's testosterone levels that begins at zero. This would be like having a normal range for women's heights that goes from 0 to 72 inches. If your result is below normal, or even in the lowest 25 percent of the normal range, I would consider a trial of natural, bioidentical testosterone therapy.

TREATING LOW TESTOSTERONE

For men, I recommend using topical testosterone creams or gels, applying 25 to 100 milligrams to the skin each day. This is available from regular pharmacies (Testim 1 percent gel), but the form made by compounding pharmacies is much less expensive for those without prescription insurance. Be aware that if the skin where it is applied comes in contact with a woman's skin (e.g., after a hug or if you do not wash your hands after applying the cream), this can result in very high, undesirable, and unsafe levels in that woman's body. Always be sure to wash your hands after applying the cream.

I do not recommend taking testosterone by mouth in males, as it can dramatically worsen cholesterol levels since testosterone goes to the liver first when taken by mouth, which is where cholesterol is made. I also do not recommend injections because this results in very high levels for the first few days afterward and in very low levels a week later. Testosterone pellets that are injected under the abdominal fat each four to six months may well be the best approach, but it is difficult to find physicians trained in this technique.

For women, testosterone treatment is easier. I recommend the natural testosterone creams made by compounding pharmacies. The usual dose is 2 to 5 milligrams a day. If you also need estrogen or progesterone (see page 107), all three of the hormones can be combined in the same cream, resulting in increased simplicity and a lower cost. With this dosing, most women have more energy, thicker hair, younger skin, and improved libido.

Adjust the testosterone level to the dose that feels best, checking blood levels to make sure they do not go above the upper limit of normal. Most people feel best with a blood level around the 70th percentile of the normal range.

POTENTIAL SIDE EFFECTS

In men, acne suggests the dose is too high. It is important to monitor levels because, as in bodybuilders who abuse testosterone by taking many times the recommended dose, elevated levels can cause elevated blood counts, liver inflammation, a decreased sperm count with resulting infertility (usually reversible), and elevated cholesterol with increased risk of heart disease. Because of this, in men, a testosterone level, PSA, complete blood count (CBC), cholesterol test, and liver enzyme test should be done occasionally. Testosterone supplementation can also cause elevated thyroid hormone levels in men taking thyroid supplements. In men who are on thyroid supplements, consider rechecking thyroid hormone levels after six weeks if you get a racing heart or anxious/hyper feelings.

It is important to note that testosterone can be converted to two other hormones: estrogen and DHT (dihydrotestosterone). If the estrogen level rises too high in males, breast size may increase and erections may decrease. Because of this, it may be reasonable to also check total estrogen levels while on testosterone and, if they are elevated, to add a medication called Arimidex (0.5 milligrams every other day), which blocks the conversion to estrogen. DHT level can also become elevated, resulting in a higher risk of prostate enlargement.[88]

As noted above, in men, most studies show that bringing low testosterone up to the normal level decreases angina and leg artery blockages, and decreases diabetes. If DHT goes too high, however, it can cause prostate enlargement and a worsening of male pattern baldness. If this occurs, these side effects can usually be blocked by taking the herb saw palmetto (160 milligrams twice daily) along with the testosterone. Fortunately, both of these problems have been fairly uncommon.

Treatment with testosterone in men has not been shown to increase prostate size (if DHT is normal) or the blood test marker for prostate cancer (PSA).[89] In addition, there is currently no evidence from studies of natural testosterone treatment showing that it increases the risk of prostate cancer.

If acne, intense dreams, or darkening of facial hair occurs in women taking testosterone, the dose is too high and should be decreased. These effects, which can also occur with DHEA supplementation, are usually reversible. These side effects can also be caused by an estrogen level that is too low relative to testosterone, and may be avoided by supplementing both together.

If you choose to take testosterone and estrogen separately, it may be best to use estrogen for four to eight weeks before starting testosterone. This often decreases side effects.

For many patients with CFS and fibromyalgia, treating low testosterone levels has been critical in leading to dramatic improvements in stamina, energy, and overall sense of wellness.

LOW ESTROGEN AND PROGESTERONE

Although not likely to be a problem with men, deficiencies of estrogen and/or progesterone can be major problems in women with CFS/FMS. A book by Dr. Elizabeth Lee Vliet, *Screaming to Be Heard: Hormonal Connections Women Suspect . . . and Doctors Still Ignore*, reviews the role of estrogen deficiency in causing fatigue, brain fog, disordered sleep, fibromyalgia, poor libido, PMS, low levels of serotonin and other neurotransmitters, interstitial cystitis, and other problems. She notes that the perimenopausal period (the period as you approach menopause) has a gradual onset, and symptoms of estrogen deficiency can occur five to twelve years before your blood tests and periods become abnormal. As previously noted, hypothalamic dysfunction can also cause estrogen deficiency.

Although checking blood levels gives some information, these levels do not register as abnormal until you have been estrogen-deficient for many years. In addition, levels vary dramatically throughout the month. I have found that the best way to tell if a trial of natural estrogen is needed is to ask the simple question: "Are your CFS or fibromyalgia (not PMS) symptoms worse around your period?" If the answer is yes, that is, your fatigue, pain, and brain fog are worse around your period, when estrogen and progesterone levels are lowest, this suggests that estrogen and progesterone deficiency are contributing to your symptoms. In addition, hormone levels drop at midcycle around ovulation. For example, panic attacks, migraines, and palpitations that occur for one to two days around ovulation or around your period are often triggered by dropping estrogen levels. Because of this, it can be helpful to keep a symptom log relative to your periods.

One other point is critical to note. If you have had a hysterectomy, even if your ovaries were not removed, you will likely become estrogen deficient within two years. Though this research was done at Yale, most physicians are not aware of this fact and presume that as long as the ovaries remain, estrogen deficiency will not occur. This is why so many women, even in their twenties, develop CFS/FMS after a hysterectomy. Although it has not been researched, I suspect this may also occur after tubal ligations.

The importance of estrogen deficiency is reflected in research, which shows that 25 percent of women said that their FMS symptoms started with the onset of menopause and 26.4 percent said that the severity of their previous symptoms increased after menopause. Of all the premenopausal females, 45 percent admitted to higher pain severity and 57.5 percent to a higher fatigue severity during their menses, when estrogen levels are the lowest.[90]

TREATING LOW ESTROGEN AND PROGESTERONE

I strongly recommend that bioidentical hormones be taken in a balance that mimics that found in a thirty-year-old woman. These are made by compounding pharmacies. The form of estrogen that I use in my practice is called BiEst, and 2.5 milligrams daily (containing 0.5 milligram of estradiol and 2 milligrams of estriol) is a good dose for most women.

If you take supplemental estrogen, you must also take natural progesterone to prevent uterine cancer. I usually add natural progesterone even in women who have had a hysterectomy, because progesterone also improves sleep and decreases anxiety. You'll probably find that a dose between 30 and 100 milligrams a day, taken at bedtime, is best. Higher doses can aggravate the depression that often accompanies CFS/FMS, so it's important to pay attention to how you feel when you start taking these medications. Taking both estrogen and progesterone every day (instead of cycling hormones by only taking them for the first twenty-five days of each month) will often result in your periods going away after six to nine months, and most women over forty-eight prefer this approach.

The discussion of estrogen and progesterone supplementation is an important one. Although many women are concerned with studies showing an increased risk of breast cancer associated with the use of synthetic estrogen and progesterone, the data suggest that this risk is predominantly associated with the use of Premarin and synthetic progesterones, and perhaps estradiol. Premarin is the brand of estrogen most commonly prescribed for menopausal women. It contains a form of the hormone that comes from pregnant horse urine (pre = "pregnant," mar = "mare," in = "urine"). I think it's medically absurd to prescribe this for human females. There is not likely to be an increased risk with the bioidentical hormones we are recommending (see below). In fact, estriol, the estrogen that goes up most during pregnancy, is likely to actually decrease breast cancer risk. This is reflected in many studies, including those showing that multiple pregnancies are associated with less breast cancer risk. In addition, estriol has dramatic immune-altering effects, which cause multiple sclerosis to improve and which are also likely to help CFS/FMS. Estriol is likely one of several reasons that CFS/FMS improves during pregnancy.

Research and clinical experience show that bioidentical hormones are safer than their synthetic counterparts and leave women feeling better. It is my impression that nonbioidentical hormones have been used mainly because they are patentable and therefore more profitable for drug companies. However, the tide looks to be turning as more and more well-informed doctors are speaking out on the safety and efficacy of natural, bioidentical hormone supplementation.

For more information on the safety of bioidentical hormone replacement, see the article by Dr. Kent Holtorf on the *From Fatigued to Fantastic!* notes section at www.vitality101.com. Dr. Holtorf is the medical director of the Holtorf Medical Group, Inc, Center for Hormone Imbalance and Fatiguing Conditions, in Los Angeles (310–375–2701). Although highly technical, it will likely leave you comfortable with the safety of bioidentical hormone replacement therapies.

The Women's Health Initiative Study and the HRT Controversy

Natural bioidentical hormones for hormone replacement therapy (HRT) are unlike their synthetic versions, often having completely different effects. Thus, it is critical that women be given the information that these natural hormones do not have the negative side effects of the synthetic hormones and in no way pertain to the conclusions reached by the Women's Health Initiative (WHI) study. Natural hormones are a safe and more conservative approach to hormone replacement therapy and without the risks associated with Premarin and Provera.

Clinically, patients feel much better on the natural hormones, while synthetic hormones do not work as well and cause severe side effects. Medical research confirms our clinical experience[2,50] and shows that HRT with bioidentical hormones is also safer.[1–79]

HRT and the Risk of Heart Disease and Stroke

The WHI study demonstrated that when synthetic progesterone (Provera) was added to Premarin, there was a substantial increase in the risk of heart attack and stroke.[12–17,34–36,49–51,53,54,65,70–73]

Natural bioidentical estrogen and progesterone, on the other hand, have an opposite effect, decreasing the risk of heart attack and stroke.[49,50,61,67,70,71,72,76,77]

One of the causes of heart attack and stroke is blood vessel spasm, which is decreased by natural estrogen and progesterone.[13–15, 68, 69] Unfortunately, synthetic progesterone actually increases spasm and heart attack risk,[13–15,69] to the degree that researchers noted the following:"We conclude that medroxyprogesterone (Provera) in *contrast to progesterone* increases the risk of coronary vasospasm[13] [emphasis mine]." In women who already had chest pain (angina) with exercise, natural progesterone increased how much exercise the women could do versus how much they could do when taking Provera. This was marked enough that the researchers found that "these results imply that the choice of progestin in women at higher cardiovascular risk requires careful consideration. Provera is expected to increase the risk of heart attack and stroke, while progesterone is not."[14]

For many years, doctors believed that estrogen protected the heart. This is indeed the case, as natural HRT decreases blocked arteries by half.[61] However, when Provera is used, this benefit is negated and diabetes risk is increased.[49,51,52,62,73,75] Natural progesterone by itself[76,77] or in combination with estrogen[15,51,61,66,67,70–72] will protect the heart, while Provera reverses estrogen's heart-protective benefits.[15,51,53,54,63–65,70,72] In fact, a major review article found that the scientific research "taken together, provide[s] a basis for concern, not about all progestogens, but specifically about MPA [Provera]."[15] Natural progesterone is also more effective than Provera in improving good cholesterol (HDL) levels.[12,34] This effect was so marked that Elizabeth Connor, a cardiologist and researcher on the major PEPI (Postmenopausal Estrogen/Progestin Interventions) study stated: "If I were treating a woman primarily because she was worried about heart disease or . . . HDL cholesterol, I would probably see if she wanted to take micronized [natural] progesterone. I was quite impressed with the better effect."[12] In addition, the president of the American Heart Association stated that a woman who changes her medication from Provera to natural progesterone would significantly lower her risk for heart disease.[35] Finally, Premarin, an oral estrogen, will increase clotting factors and inflammatory proteins, increasing the risk of blood clots.[16,18] This does not occur with natural transdermal estrogens.[18] Given all this, it is no surprise that the WHI study showed an increased risk of heart attacks and strokes using synthetic hormones. The good news is that bioidentical hormones have actually been proven to protect your heart.

HRT and the Risk of Breast Cancer

The synthetic estrogen Premarin increases breast cancer risk by 23 percent, and adding the synthetic progesterone Provera to the mix increases that risk by 38 percent to 67 percent.[9, 10, 78] This is in contrast to natural estrogens and progesterones, which reduce the risk of breast cancer.

Premarin is made from pregnant horses' urine, hence its name Pre (pregnant)-mar (horse)-in (urine). It consists of a combination of conjugated equine (horse) estrogens that are much more potent and cancer-causing than bioidentical estrogens.[20–22,80]

Most compounded bioidentical hormones are a mix of estriol, which is normally present but rises during pregnancy, and estradiol, which is the hormone used in estrogen patches. Estriol is shown to cause much less breast cell proliferation and is felt to be even safer than estradiol[40–48] and much safer than Premarin.[23–27, 39] Estriol appears to inhibit breast cancer,[24, 26, 39] and the higher your estriol level, the lower your risk of breast cancer.[25,26,56,57,59,60] In fact, an analysis of six studies found that there are higher estriol levels in populations with lower risks for breast cancer.[26] The protective effects of estriol against breast cancer are so pronounced that a study in the *Journal of the American Medical Association* found that 37 percent of women with breast cancer who were given estriol actually had remission, or arrest, of their cancer. The author of the accompanying editorial notes, "Enough presumptive and scientific evidence has been accumulated that we may say that orally administered estriol is safer than estrone or estradiol. . . . Let us have the estrogen that causes the least risk."[27] Premarin, on the contrary, increases the risk of breast cancer.[20–22,80]

As one more added benefit, estriol improves multiple sclerosis while other estrogens make it worse, another indication of its profoundly different effects.[28, 29] Because of this, the bioidentical estrogen I recommend is called BiEst, a mix of estriol 2 milligrams and estradiol 0.5 milligram a day.

Several studies also show that synthetic progesterones, such as Provera, also increase breast cancer risk,[4–10, 19,33,55,78,79,81] while natural progesterone is breast-protective.[1,8,30,31] In fact, a Johns Hopkins study found that the risk of breast cancer was 5.4 times higher in women with a low progesterone level when compared to those with a normal level.[30]

Numerous studies indicate that with respect to the risk of breast cancer, heart disease, heart attacks, and stroke, natural hormones offer a safe and more conservative approach to HRT. In fact, a large amount of scientific evidence overwhelmingly demonstrates that natural hormones are safer than the study drugs of the WHI, Premarin, and Provera. Unfortunately, the overwhelming majority of women, and their physicians, do not know that there are safe alternatives to their current HRT or to the one they stopped once the results of the WHI were released. The good news is that bioidentical estrogen (especially estriol) and progesterone decrease your breast cancer risk and protect you from heart attacks and stroke.

Notes for this article follow those for Chapter 4.

POTENTIAL SIDE EFFECTS

It is important to be aware that using the SHIN protocol will routinely result in your periods becoming irregular for six to twelve months—whether or not you take estrogen. This occurs in part because your hypothalamus cycles back to its normal rhythm as it starts to heal—and this controls the timing of your cycle. The more common side effects of bioidentical estrogen and progesterone (not synthetic, as discussed above) are fluid retention, moodiness, spotting, breast tenderness, and depression resulting from the progesterone supplementation.

Pregnancy and CFS/FMS

Women often worry about getting pregnant with CFS/FMS. The good news is that most people with CFS/FMS do very well with pregnancy—and even after the pregnancy, given the proper support.

Most of you will actually feel much better during your pregnancy. It is after the pregnancy that you'll need both nutritional and hormonal support to prevent the CFS/FMS from recurring. I do recommend that, if possible, you follow the treatment protocol discussed in this book for a year before getting pregnant, so you can stop the medications and other treatments that would not be appropriate during pregnancy, without losing the benefits. Although most people with CFS/FMS do not have problems with infertility, it is more common in this population. The good news is that there are many effective natural treatments for infertility. Because they are not expensive, however, they do not get the attention that in vitro fertilization gets. I have created a section in my Web site notes using a question-and-answer format (adapted from an interview that I'd done) to answer some of the most common concerns. This is followed by general advice for a healthy pregnancy and how to deal with infertility naturally if you are having trouble conceiving. (Visit www.vitality101.com.)

Here's wishing you a happy and healthy pregnancy, baby, and life.

Other Hormones

In addition to the more publicized hormones above, others are also important in CFS/FMS.

Low Oxytocin

Research has shown that oxytocin, a neurotransmitter/hormone produced by the hypothalamus, is also low in fibromyalgia sufferers. Oxytocin is recognized primarily for its function in labor and lactation (milk production), but it also appears to play a major role in the day-to-day performance of the hypothalamus, and is an important neurotransmitter in the brain.[91] Fortunately, it's easy to tell if oxytocin will help you feel better by simply taking one injection. People who are pale and have cold extremities seem most likely to benefit from oxytocin treatment. Your doctor may choose to prescribe this injection, and will teach you how to administer the daily dose of 10 international units (1 cc by intramuscular injection). If the oxytocin treatment is going to help, it should do so in thirty to sixty minutes, resulting in increased energy and mental clarity with decreased pain. Oxytocin may cause transient anxiety.

GROWTH HORMONE

Current research suggests that inadequate levels of growth hormone (GH) may be an important factor for some patients with CFS/FMS who do not respond to adrenal hormone, thyroid hormone, oxytocin, estrogen, and testosterone treatment.[92] Growth hormone, sometimes called the "fountain of youth hormone," is synthesized and stored in the pituitary gland, and assists in protein synthesis and bone growth. It is also responsible for stimulating DHEA production, which as we know may be inadequate in those with CFS/FMS. In addition, this important hormone decreases pain and weight and increases stamina. For those who are unable to find relief with other hormonal treatments, suboptimal levels of growth hormone should be tested for with a blood test called an IGF-1 level.

Research studies by Dr. Robert Bennett and others show that people with CFS/FMS have significantly diminished GH levels. Other studies have shown that low GH levels can be associated with significant fatigue and CFS-like symptoms. Getting deep, restorative stage 3 and 4 sleep may well be the best way to raise growth hormone without supplementation; however, these stages of sleep are often missing in CFS/FMS.[93] In addition, growth-hormone release during exercise is blocked in fibromyalgia. Dr. Bennett found, however, that growth-hormone release could be restored by prescribing a medication called Mestinon at a dosage of 30 to 60 milligrams, three to four times a day. It may take three to five months to see the full effect of this treatment.

Over the years, I've also become much more comfortable with recommending injections of growth hormone for patients with low levels. Unfortunately, it requires expensive daily insulin-like injections, and insurance companies are often unwilling to cover the cost. Nonetheless, for those who are willing and can afford them, the shots can be helpful.

VASOPRESSIN

Vasopressin, which is also known as the antidiuretic hormone (ADH), is secreted by the pituitary gland, and keeps the body from losing too much water by increasing the amount that is reabsorbed by the kidneys. People who are light-headed or drink more water than normal—that is, most CFS/FMS patients—may be low in vasopressin.[94] This can cause low blood pressure, dehydration, and secondary fatigue. The simplest treatment to compensate for a low vasopressin level is to increase your salt intake and to drink enough water to keep your mouth and lips moist.

PROLACTIN

Prolactin is synthesized and stored in the pituitary gland, and is best known for stimulating milk production after childbirth. Unlike other hormones, which are usually low in people with CFS/FMS, prolactin levels are sometimes mildly elevated. The hypothalamus normally suppresses, instead of stimulates, prolactin production, but the hypothalamus is often dysfunctional in people with CFS/FMS. To make sure that no (benign) pituitary tumor exists, however, I may order a magnetic resonance imaging (MRI) scan in patients who still have elevated prolactin levels after four months of treatment with the SHIN protocol. The MRI generally shows that everything is normal. Some medications, such as risperidone (Risperdal), can also elevate prolactin levels, as can high-dose melatonin. Taking vitamin B_6 at a dose of 200 milligrams a day can lower an elevated prolactin level, and this can be helpful, as excess prolactin can cause both a drop in the neurotransmitter dopamine and infertility.

As you can see, many problems can occur when the body's glands do not function properly. The good news is that most can be effectively treated. In my experience, this often results in dramatic improvement. It is important, though, to treat the whole person, not simply the hormonal problems.

Important Points

- Because the hypothalamus controls many hormones, CFS/FMS patients often need supplementation with adrenal, thyroid, and reproductive hormones.

- Blood testing is not a reliable way to tell if you need hormonal support. The normal range for most blood tests does not tell you whether your hormone levels are adequate; rather, it measures only whether you are in the lowest 2.5 percent of the population.
- Underactive adrenals are common in CFS. Treat low or borderline adrenal function with very low-dose hydrocortisone (e.g., Cortef at under 20 milligrams daily) and natural adrenal support (e.g., Adrenal Stress End). If DHEA-S blood levels are suboptimal, add DHEA supplementation.
- Hypothyroidism is also common in CFS. Treat symptoms of low or borderline thyroid function with a thyroid product that contains a mix of T_4 and T_3 hormones or high-dose pure T_3—even if your blood tests are normal.
- If your blood pressure is low, you get dizzy upon standing, and you crash after exercising, you might have NMH (neurally mediated hypotension). If so, increase your water intake and make sure you consume a high-salt diet; Dexedrine and Prozac can also be helpful. If you are twenty-two years of age or younger, consider a therapeutic trial of Florinef.
- For both men and women, if the testosterone blood level is in the lowest quarter to third of the normal range, consider treatment with natural testosterone.
- If you are menopausal or if your CFS/FMS symptoms are worse around your period, consider a trial of the bioidentical estrogen and progesterone.
- If other hormone treatments do not work for you, you may have growth-hormone deficiency. Growth hormone can be raised by deep sleep, exercise, sex, growth-hormone injections, or the medication Mestinon.

Questionnaire (See Appendix B for treatments to check off.)

Adrenal Checklist

_____ 1. Hypoglycemia

_____ 2. Shakiness relieved with eating or irritability when hungry

_____ 3. Recurrent sore throats/infections that take a long time to go away

_____ 4. Low blood pressure or frequent dizziness on first standing

_____ 5. Long-term prednisone (cortisone) usage since illness began, and feeling better when you took it

If the answer to any of these (1 through 5) is yes, check off #28, 29, and 30.

Thyroid Checklist

_____   6.   Weight gain of more than ten pounds

_____   7.   Low body temperature (under 98 degrees F)

_____   8.   Achiness

_____   9.   Cold intolerance

_____   10.   Dry skin or thin hair

_____   11.   Females only: heavy periods

If the answer to any of these (6 through 11) is yes, check off # 25 (unless your free T_4 blood test is elevated).

Iodine deficiency

_____   12.   Breast cysts or tenderness

If yes and your physician has ruled out breast cancer, check off #26.

Estrogen

_____   13.   Decreased vaginal lubrication

_____   14.   Did your CFS/FMS begin within three years after you had a hysterectomy, ovaries removed, or a tubal ligation?

_____   15.   Are your symptoms worse the week before your period?

If the answer to any of these (13 through 15) is yes, check off #31 (unless you have a history of breast cancer or blood clots).

Vasodepressor Syncope (NMH)

_____   16.   Frequent dizziness on standing or low blood pressure (under 100/60)?

_____   17.   Did you ever have a positive tilt-table test?

If the answer to either of these (16 and 17) is yes, check off #30 and 57.

I—Infections: Destroy Your Body's Hidden Invaders

5

Medical science has known for quite some time that chronic fatigue syndrome is associated with changes in the body's immune system. In fact, the acronym CFIDS stands for chronic fatigue and immune dysfunction syndrome. People with CFIDS (which can be used interchangeably with CFS) usually have many different and unusual infections at the same time. Some of these infections need to be treated directly. Others will go away on their own as your immune (defense) system comes back "online" as a result of using the effective treatment protocol detailed in this book. In this chapter, we will look at some of the more common, yet often missed, infections.

What kinds of infections are people with CFIDS/fibromyalgia most at risk for? Although there are literally dozens of infections implicated in CFS, the most important ones to deal with fall under four categories:

1. Yeast or fungal infections
2. Parasites
3. Antibiotic-sensitive infections
4. Viral-infections

In some cases, it is not the infection itself but your body's reaction to it that causes your symptoms. For example, the body produces interferon to fight viral infections. When a person with cancer or hepatitis is injected with interferon, he or she becomes achy, fatigued, and brain-fogged—all symptoms of CFS/FMS.[1] Underactive adrenal glands, commonly associated with CFS/FMS, can also cause interferon levels to become elevated.[2] Because of this elevation, it is more accurate to say that the body's immune system is not functioning properly than to say that it is underactive. Indeed, in many ways, the immune system may be in overdrive early in the illness and then exhaust itself. The immune system malfunctions in many other ways as well, decreasing the effectiveness of the body's natural killer cells, which are an important defense mechanism.[3, 4]

Many recurrent or unusual infections can occur when one has a malfunctioning immune system. Chronic sinus, bladder, prostate, and respiratory infections are common, and are often treated with repeated courses of antibiotics. The large amount of antibiotics introduced into the system can then lead to a secondary yeast overgrowth, as the antibiotics change the natural balance between the bowel's healthy bacteria and yeast. The original immune dysfunction combined with a high sugar intake (which feeds the yeast) also contributes to the yeast overgrowth. Although the theory is controversial, many physicians believe that chronic yeast overgrowth due to overuse of antibiotics and sugar is a potential and strong trigger for chronic fatigue, fibromyalgia, and further immune dysfunction. What makes the theory controversial is that no definitive tests exist to distinguish fungal overgrowth from normal fungal levels. Nonetheless, a recent study showed that bowel candida levels are much higher in CFS patients when their illness is flaring,[5] and most doctors who try treating yeast in at least three or four CFIDS patients see how well this treatment works and continue to utilize it.

There are also other bowel infections. One-sixth of those with CFS/FMS have bowel parasite infections.[6] Bowel parasites can cause severe allergic or sensitivity reactions, which in turn can trigger fibromyalgia and fatigue. Often, a patient will finally recover from long-standing and disabling fatigue within a week or two after beginning treatment for bowel parasites.

CFS that begins suddenly often seems to be triggered by viral infections—for example, infection with the Epstein-Barr virus (EBV), human herpesvirus 6 (HHV-6—*not* the same as genital herpes or cold sores), or cytomegalovirus (CMV). In some cases, CFS occurs when you first get the infection. In others, these infections occurred years before and are still present but no longer active (latent). When your immune system becomes weakened, however, they are able to resurface. This is fairly common. For example, most people still have chicken pox virus in their body from when they had it as a child. Shingles occur if that virus resurfaces when your immune system is suppressed. In the same way, old Epstein-Barr (mono), HHV-6, or CMV infections can reactivate during chronic fatigue syndrome. More than 90 percent of healthy adults have had these infections in the past, usually without even knowing it. In many cases, the fatigue caused by viral infections responds to the treatments discussed in this book. A subset of people will, however, need antiviral treatments for their immune system to recover and their CFS to resolve (see p. 138).

Antibiotic-sensitive infections with unusual organisms such as rickettsia, chlamydia, and mycoplasma may also be problematic. Unfortunately, there is also no effective test available for physicians to confirm these infections, so it is often necessary to rely on symptoms to determine the appropriate treatment. Let's review each category of infection in more depth, beginning with the most important—yeast/fungal overgrowth.

Yeast/Fungal Overgrowth

Everyone's immune system has strengths and weaknesses. For example, some people never get colds but have frequent bouts of athlete's foot or other skin fungal infections. Others never get fungal infections but tend to get colds. However, many people seem to have a diminished ability to fight off fungal infections.

I use the terms yeast, fungi, and candida interchangeably for this discussion. Fungal overgrowth may suppress the body's immune system. It is suspected that this occurs in part because the bowel yeast infections cause what is called leaky gut syndrome. This means that food proteins get absorbed into the blood system before they are fully digested. Because of this, the immune system has to complete the digestion process, which often overtaxes it. Many physicians feel that yeast overgrowth causes a generalized suppression of the immune system. In other words, once the yeast gets the upper hand, it sets up a cycle that further suppresses the body's defenses.[7]

Yeast is a normal member of the body's "zoo." It lives in balance with bacteria—some of which are helpful and healthy, and others that are detrimental and unhealthy. The problems begin when this harmonious balance shifts and the yeast begins to overgrow.

Many things can prompt yeast overgrowth. One of the most common causes is frequent antibiotic use. Antibiotics kill off the good bacteria in the bowel along with the bad bacteria. When this happens, the yeast no longer has competition and begins to overgrow. The body is often able to rebalance itself after one or several courses of antibiotics, but after repeated or long-term courses—and especially if the body has an underlying immune dysfunction—the yeast can get the upper hand.

The body may also develop allergic reactions to components of the yeast. This allergic reaction was suggested in a study that connected the fungal organism Candida albicans with allergic skin dermatitis (eczema).[8] It found that there is a significant correlation between the body having antibodies to Candida albicans and eczema. In addition, we have found that unexplained rashes that have lasted for many years often clear up with antifungal treatment.

Other factors are also important. Studies have shown that animals that are sleep-deprived and/or have increased sugar intake develop immune suppression and bowel yeast overgrowth. Many physicians feel that eating sugar stimulates yeast overgrowth in people as well, so as you prepare your meals, remember—sugar is food for yeast.

Diagnosing Yeast Overgrowth

There are no definitive tests for yeast overgrowth that will distinguish yeast overgrowth from normal yeast growth in the body. In my experience, using Dr. William Crook's yeast questionnaire is still the most reliable way to tell if a person is at risk of yeast overgrowth. (I've placed a modified one at the end of this chapter.)

In addition, anyone with CFS/FMS meeting the following criteria should be treated with antifungals:

- Has chronic nasal congestion or sinusitis or
- Has spastic colon (gas, bloating, diarrhea, and/or constipation) or
- Has been on recurrent or long-term antibiotics (especially tetracycline for acne), or
- Who intermittently has painful sores in the mouth (not cold sores on the outer lips) that last for about ten days at a time and who has CFS/FMS.

Sinusitis and bowel symptoms are some of the more overt symptoms that are caused by yeast—and both of these usually resolve with antifungal treatments. Since so many people suffer from these symptoms and there is no test available to determine yeast overgrowth, it is reasonable for everyone with CFS/FMS to be treated with an empiric trial of antifungal therapies.

TREATING YEAST OVERGROWTH

A number of effective treatments can be used to eliminate yeast overgrowth. I find that the best approach is to combine dietary changes, natural remedies, and prescription medications.

DIETARY CHANGES AND NATURAL REMEDIES

The most important part of treating yeast overgrowth is avoiding sugar and other sweets, although I will add the three magic words, "except for chocolate." You can also enjoy one or two pieces of fruit a day, but don't consume concentrated sugars like fruit juices, corn syrup, jellies, pastry, candy, or honey. Stay far away from soft drinks, which have ten to twelve teaspoons of sugar in every twelve ounces. This amount of sugar has been shown to markedly suppress immune function for several hours. Be prepared to have your CFS/FMS symptoms flare for about one week when you cut sugar out of your diet.

Using stevia as a sweetener is a wonderful substitute for sugar. Despite some misconceptions, stevia is safe and natural, and you can use all you want. There are even cookbooks available for using stevia. The brand of stevia that you choose is important, however. Most brands of stevia are not filtered and therefore are bitter. The two that won the taste test in our office are made by Body Ecology (see Appendix E: Resources) and Stevita.

Several books have been written on the yeast controversy and offer additional dietary methods to try. One of the best is *The Yeast Connection and Woman's Health* by the late Dr. William Crook, a physician who advanced our understanding of CFIDS/FMS considerably.

One of those dietary methods that can help restore balance in the bowel is the intake of acidophilus—that is, milk bacteria, a healthy type of bacteria. Acidophilus is found in yogurt that has live and active yogurt cultures. Indeed, eating one cup of yogurt a day can markedly diminish the frequency of recurrent vaginal yeast infections.[9] Acidophilus is also available in supplement form, but the brand you use is important because many brands do not actually contain the amount that the label claims or contain dead bacteria— which do not put up much of a fight against yeast. I like to use Acidophilus Pearls by Enzymatic Therapy. The pearls act like little tanks that protect the milk bacteria while they pass through the acidic environment of the stomach. Once the pearls hit the alkaline environment of the small intestine, they dissolve and release the bacteria to fight the yeast. I recommend that you take two pearls twice a day for five months, after which time many people choose to continue taking one a day for prevention. Although the box claims 1 billion bacteria per pearl, the laboratory assays actually show that each of these pearls contains 2.4 billion bacteria. If you are on antibiotics (not antifungals), take acidophilus at least three to six hours before or after the antibiotic dose.

In addition to using acidophilus against the yeast, chemical weapons can also be helpful, and I recommend that they be taken with the acidophilus. I find that grapefruit seed extract, such as Citricidal, is helpful. I recommend the capsule or tablet form, taking 200 milligrams twice a day for five months. Use less if it upsets your stomach.

Many other natural antifungals may be helpful, but when used individually in a high enough dose to kill the yeast they also irritate the stomach. Because of this I like to combine multiple antifungal herbs. My favorite combination is Anti-Yeast by Ultraceuticals, which contains 240 milligrams of coconut oil powder (50 percent caprylic acid), 200 milligrams of oregano powder extract, 120 milligrams of uva ursi extract, 240 milligrams of garlic powder (deodorized), 160 milligrams of grapefruit seed extract, 80 milligrams of berberine sulfate, 200 milligrams of olive leaf extract, 50 milligrams of alpha lipoic acid, 50 milligrams of milk thistle extract, and 50 milligrams of N-Acetyl-L-Cysteine. Another antifungal supplement product that I recommend is Phytostan, by Integrative Therapeutics (see Appendix E: Resources).

PRESCRIPTION TREATMENTS FOR YEAST OVERGROWTH

It is critical to add a prescription antifungal, because the natural products only kill yeast in the gut and are not as strong. I recommend that almost all of my CFS/FMS patients use Diflucan 200 milligrams a day for six to twelve weeks. If stool cultures (which are negative even in most people who need yeast treatment) show the yeast to be resistant to Diflucan, then your doctor may choose to substitute Nizoral at 200 milligrams a day for six weeks. Nizoral can lower adrenal hormone levels, so if your cortisol is low your doctor should consider adding adrenal support when prescribing Nizoral.

Nystatin, an antifungal medication, has been helpful in treating yeast overgrowth in the past. Unfortunately, more and more fungi seem to be developing nystatin resistance. In addition, nystatin is poorly absorbed, which means that it has little impact on the yeast outside of the bowel. Because of this, I am now using the herbals listed on page 122 instead.

Any effective antifungal can initially make the symptoms of yeast infection worse. In addition, Diflucan can cause liver inflammation, although this is uncommon, and I have not seen it to be a significant problem in the more than three thousand patients I've treated. Nonetheless, if you are taking Diflucan or Nizoral for more than six to twelve weeks, blood tests should be performed to check liver function—specifically checking blood levels of alanine aminotransferase (ALT) and aspartate transaminase (AST), two compounds that are good indicators of injury to the liver. If you have preexisting active liver disease, you should be cautious about using Diflucan—or not use it at all. The Anti-Yeast herbal on page 122 contains lipoic acid, milk thistle extract, and N-Acetyl-L-Cysteine, natural supplements that help protect and heal the liver. For that matter, I strongly recommend lipoic acid for anyone with severe active liver disease (for example, hepatitis), at a dose up to 1,000 to 3,000 milligrams a day, as it may prevent and/or help treat cirrhosis.

If symptoms of yeast overgrowth are caused by an allergic or sensitivity reaction to the yeast body parts, symptoms may flare up when mass quantities of the yeast are suddenly killed off. This is called a die-off (Herxheimer) reaction and can occur with the treatment of any chronic infection. To decrease the risk of this reaction, start your treatment with acidophilus and a sugar-free diet for one to two weeks, followed by the herbals for two weeks before beginning the Diflucan. If symptoms flare up, take just 25 to 100 milligrams of Diflucan each morning for the first three to fourteen days. If symptoms recur after you stop the Diflucan, I recommend continuing the medication for an additional six weeks at 200 milligrams a day.

As your doctor will inform you, when taking Diflucan, do not use the heart medicine quinidine or cholesterol-lowering medications in the statin family, which includes Mevacor, Baycol, Lescol, Lipitor, Pravachol, and Zocor, as these combinations can be deadly. In addition, these cholesterol-lowering medications can actually trigger fibromyalgia, and I almost never use them in my CFS/FMS patients. Cholesterol can usually be effectively lowered naturally using herbal treatments such as garlic, berberine, inositol hexaniacinate, and oats (as found in Life cereal or Cheerios). For more information on natural ways to lower cholesterol, see Chapter 8. I would note that the cholesterol medications also deplete coenzyme Q_{10}, so I recommend that anyone taking cholesterol-lowering medications take coenzyme Q_{10} (Vitaline form) at a dose of 200 milligrams a day. Your holistic doctor can guide you on how best to safely treat high cholesterol.

Once the yeast symptoms of sinusitis and spastic colon have been effectively decreased and kept that way for six to twelve months, you can try adding small amounts of sugar back into your diet. If symptoms recur, however, stop the sugar again. Continuing either to eat yogurt with live and active acidophilus cultures or to take Acidophilus Pearls is very helpful.

Many books on yeast overgrowth advise readers to avoid all yeast. This information is based on the theory that an allergic reaction to yeast is the cause of the problem. However, the yeast that is found in most foods (except beer and cheese) is not closely related to candida, which is the predominant yeast that seems to be involved in yeast overgrowth.

In my experience, trying to avoid all yeast in foods results in a nutritionally inadequate diet and does not substantially help most people. Although a few people do appear to have true allergies to the yeast in their food, they account for fewer than 10 percent of my patients with suspected yeast overgrowth. These people may benefit from the stricter diet recommended in Dr. Crook's books. Interestingly, once adrenal insufficiency and yeast overgrowth are treated, most people find that their allergies and sensitivities to yeast and other food products seem to improve or disappear.

Nutritional deficiencies such as low zinc or low selenium may also decrease resistance to yeast overgrowth.[10] A good multivitamin supplement (see Chapter 6) should take care of these deficiencies. This is simply another example of how all the factors involved in CFIDS are closely interrelated.

The best thing you can do to combat yeast overgrowth is to try to avoid it in the first place. When you get an infection, immediately begin treating it naturally (see "Treating Infections Without Antibiotics," on page 126). Hopefully, you will be able to prevent it from turning into a bacterial infection that might require an antibiotic. Ask your doctor what measures you can take before resorting to antibiotics. Many good over-the-counter remedies are available. A knowledgeable compounding pharmacist can also be a wealth of information. Your local bookstore or health food store also has books on natural infection-fighting measures.

If you find, however, that you must take an antibiotic, all is not lost. You can still lessen the severity of yeast overgrowth by avoiding sweets and by taking the Anti-Yeast herbal plus either taking acidophilus (again, not within three to six hours of an antibiotic) or by eating one cup of yogurt with live and active acidophilus cultures daily. Don't eat yogurt or drink milk, however, if you have sinusitis or pneumonia, because the milk protein causes mucus to thicken and makes it hard for the body to fight these infections.

WHAT IF THE YEAST COMES BACK?

It is normal for yeast symptoms to resolve after treatment. After six weeks on Diflucan, most people feel a lot better. If not, you may have Diflucan-resistant candida, and a trial of Nizoral may be helpful. However, symptoms may recur soon after you stop taking the antifungal. If this happens, I recommend that you take Diflucan or Nizoral for another six weeks or for as long as is needed to keep the symptoms at bay. More frequently, people feel better after treatment and stay feeling fairly well. Although many people never need to be treated again for yeast, others need to repeat a course of antifungals after six to twenty-four months, especially after eating too much sugar or taking antibiotics.

The best marker that I have found for recurrent yeast overgrowth is a return of bowel symptoms, with gas, bloating, and/or diarrhea or constipation; vaginal yeast; mouth sores; and/or recurring nasal congestion or sinusitis. If these symptoms persist for more than two weeks, especially if there is also even a mild worsening of the CFIDS/FMS symptoms, it is reasonable to re-treat yourself with six weeks of Anti-Yeast and Diflucan. If a second round of treatment resolves the symptoms, you may opt to repeat this regimen as often as is needed, usually every six to twenty-four months. By using some of the natural remedies listed earlier in this chapter, however, you may be able to avoid repeated use of antifungals and the possible risk of becoming resistant to them.

Some people find that they need to stay on the antifungals for extended periods of time—years, in some cases—or the symptoms recur. If this is necessary, I recommend using the natural remedies. I do, however, also prescribe prescription medications when needed. The main risk of long-term use of the antifungals Nizoral and Diflucan is liver inflammation, and if these medications are used for extended periods, liver function should be monitored. Consider checking the ALT and AST liver tests (also called SGOT and SGPT tests) every three to six months and anytime a severe flu-like feeling or worsening of fatigue or pain occurs. As an alternative, instead of taking the antifungals every day, many people find they can get long-term suppression of the yeast by taking 200 milligrams of Diflucan twice a day, one day each week (for example, each Sunday). As HHV–6 viral infections can suppress immune function and your resistance to yeast, it is worth looking for an HHV–6 infection if you need long-term antifungals.

Treating Infections Without Antibiotics

Many people do not realize how many things they can do before resorting to using an antibiotic to clear an infection. If you feel you are coming down with a respiratory infection such as a cold or the flu, I recommend that you try the following:

- *Take natural thymic hormone.* This is available as a product called Pro Boost (see p. 142), and it is an outstanding immune stimulant. Dissolve the contents of one packet under your tongue three times a day and let them absorb there (any that is swallowed will be destroyed by your stomach acid). A study in CFIDS patients with markedly elevated Epstein-Barr antibody levels showed a dramatic drop in the antibody levels after twelve weeks of treatment with thymic hormone. Many physicians are finding that thymic hormone has been helpful for CFIDS/FMS patients with persistent viral, yeast, bowel, or other infections. I have found that using it for two or three days at the onset of an infection can shorten the length of the infection dramatically, and often stops it on the first day. It should be in everyone's medicine cabinet and should be begun immediately at the start of any infection.
- *Take herbal immune stimulants.* An excellent immune stimulant is Leuko-Stim by Ultra-ceuticals, which contains olive leaf extract, Beta 1,3, glucan, maitake mushroom, Arabino-galactan (larch), and aloe vera powder extract.
- *Take 1,000 to 8,000 milligrams of vitamin C a day*—enough to stimulate diarrhea. Then cut back to a comfortable level.
- *Suck on a zinc lozenge five to eight times a day.* Make sure that the lozenges have 10 to 20 milligrams of zinc per lozenge. Less than this will not be effective. Zinc lozenges have been known to speed the time it takes to recover from a sore throat by about 40 percent. The brands of zinc sold by General Nutrition Centers and the Vitamin Shoppe are the brands I recommend.
- *Drink plenty of water and hot caffeine-free tea* (or hot water with lemon) and rest!

- *Take Oscillococcinum,* a homeopathic remedy available at most health food stores and some supermarkets, if you have flu-like symptoms such as chills, fever, achiness, and/or malaise. It speeds healing and eases discomfort. It is best taken early in the infection—as soon as you have any symptoms.
- *If you have a sinus infection, try nasal rinses.* Dissolve $\frac{1}{4}$ teaspoon of salt in a cup of lukewarm water. Inhale some of the solution about one inch up into your nose, one nostril at a time. Do this either by using a baby nose bulb or an eyedropper while lying down, or by sniffing the solution out of the palm of your hand while standing by a sink. Then gently blow your nose, being careful not to hurt your ears. Repeat the same process with the other nostril. Continue to repeat with each nostril until the nose is clear. Rinse your nasal passages at least twice a day until the infection improves. Each rinsing will wash away about 90 percent of the infection and make it much easier for your body to heal.
- *Gargle* with salt water, mixed as described above for the nasal rinse, to help a sore throat.
- *If you use acetaminophen frequently,* you should also take 500 milligrams of supplemental N-Acety-L-Cysteine (NAC) each day so you don't deplete your glutathione levels.
- *Try using a humidifier or vaporizer in your bedroom.* You can also make a steam room by running a hot shower in your bathroom and then breathing in the steam. Or try using a steam inhaler, such as the one available from Sinus Survival (see Appendix E: Resources). This also helps alleviate chronic and acute sinusitis.
- *Take at least 500 milligrams of vitamin C a day for prevention.*

There is a point where it is important to seek medical advice. If nasal and lung mucus is yellow after seven to fourteen days, or if you are feeling worse after three to four days, you may have to consider taking a course of antibiotics. If you do, you should take the Anti-Yeast formula or Diflucan while on the antibiotic. Erythromycin antibiotics such as azithromycin (Zithromax) and clarithromycin (Biaxin) are usually preferable to penicillin antibiotics. Interestingly, my patients have sometimes found that all their CFIDS symptoms (not just the cold) improve while they are taking an erythromycin or tetracycline antibiotic. If that happens, I recommend a twelve-week course of Zithromax 250 to 600 milligrams a day or 500 milligrams of Biaxin or 100 milligrams of doxycycline twice a day. If you feel better on the antibiotic (take thymic hormone and the Anti-Yeast herbal in conjunction with it), keep repeating six-week courses until the symptoms stay gone. For most of my patients who repeatedly get respiratory infections that take forever to go away, I also consider an empiric trial of prescription hydrocortisone, as their adrenal function is probably impaired (see Chapter 4).

As a preventive for respiratory infections, the flu vaccine is a double-edged sword for people with CFS/FMS. In some patients, it can cause mild flu-like symptoms for a few days or, in rare cases, a severe flare-up of symptoms. Still, unless you are one of the 10 percent of CFS/FMS patients who feel worse after the flu shot or other vaccinations, I recommend that you get a flu shot each year. For most people, the benefit can significantly outweigh the risk. Taking at least 500 milligrams of vitamin C a day is also a good idea. It is also helpful to dress warmly during cold weather, as a cold breeze blowing across your muscles or neck can make fibromyalgia symptoms flare up.

CHRONIC SINUSITIS—THE YEASTY BEASTIES REVISITED!

Although we will be discussing some unusual infections, CFS/FMS patients also get more of the day-to-day variety of infections. These include chronic sinusitis, which in my experience is predominantly caused by the underlying yeast/fungal infection. The result is a stuffy nose, eventually leading to nasal passages swelling shut. In the body, any time something gets blocked (e.g., an appendix or gallbladder), it results in a secondary bacterial infection— and the sinuses are no exception. When this happens, your nasal mucus turns yellow-green, and you go to the doctor in pain. She or he then gives you an antibiotic, which knocks out the bacterial infection and leaves you feeling better. Unfortunately, the antibiotic worsens the underlying yeast infection in your nose, causing more swelling and blockages and therefore more attacks of bacterial infections. This is why sinusitis in the United States usually becomes chronic. An interesting study reported in the Mayo Clinic Proceedings supports this thought, noting that previously "fungus allergy was thought to be involved in less than 10 percent of cases . . . our studies indicate [that], in fact, fungus is likely the cause of nearly all of these problems and that it is not an allergic reaction but an immune reaction."[11] In the study, researchers found that most people with chronic sinus infections had fungal growth in their sinuses. This research is interesting because more and more studies are showing that treating chronic sinusitis with antibiotics doesn't really do much and that shorter courses of treatment work just as well as long courses. I find that conservative treatments (e.g., nasal rinses) are more effective than antibiotics for chronic sinusitis.

In my experience, sinusitis (even chronic) usually responds dramatically to yeast treatment with Diflucan and a compounded nose spray that my patients love. It contains Bactroban and xylitol, which kill the bacterial infections, low-dose cortisol to shrink the swelling, and an antifungal. I recommend patients use one to two sprays in each nostril twice a day while on the Diflucan. That is usually enough to knock out the sinusitis, although some patients like to stay on it long term or use it intermittently for recurrent infections. The spray is available by prescription and can be mailed from ITC Compounding Pharmacy (see Appendix E: Resources). Simply have your physician ask for the sinusitis nose spray. Another helpful over-the-counter treatment for sinusitis is silver nose spray (see Appendix E: Resources). In low doses, this mineral is an anti-infectious agent against both viral and bacterial infections, and liquid silver can even be used orally for many types of difficult-to-treat chronic infections (see Appendix B, items 33, 49, and 50). Silver also works well in combination with the prescription sinusitis nose spray.

Besides the annoyance of your nose constantly running, sinusitis causes other problems. Work by Dr. Alexander Chester has shown that chronic nasal congestion can actually trigger chronic fatigue. In addition, having a chronic bacterial infection in the nose can drag your energy down. A fringe benefit of treating yeast overgrowth with Diflucan is that, especially when combined with the nose spray mentioned above, it also frequently eliminates chronic sinusitis and spastic colon/irritable bowel syndrome.

For those few patients with persistent chronic sinusitis despite treatment, I recommend the book *Sinus Survival* by Robert S. Ivker, a physician whose heart embodies what it means to be a healer (see Appendix D: Recommended Reading). His Web site at www.sinussurvival.com has many helpful tools and resources.

Chronic Urinary Tract/Bladder Infections (UTIs)

The main symptoms of a UTI/bladder infection are dysuria (discomfort—for example, a burning sensation—when urinating), urgency (the feeling that you have to go very badly and right away when there is not much urine there), and frequent urination with low urine volume. This group of symptoms is also common in CFS/FMS patients in the absence of bladder infections and, when very severe, is called interstitial cystitis (IC). However, I would not say that a person has interstitial cystitis unless this is the major symptom of their CFS/FMS, because almost everyone with this illness has some urinary urgency and frequency. The few people who have IC need to be careful, as many vitamin supplements can cause bladder symptoms to flare up, and they should begin with very low doses to be sure they are tolerated. For more information on treating the disorder, see my book *Pain Free 1–2–3* and/or contact the Interstitial Cystitis Association (www.ichelp.org).

Taking antibiotics will kill a bladder infection but will also kill the healthy bacteria in the bowel. This sets you up for yeast overgrowth and other problems. So unless you have fever, blood in the urine, back pain over the kidneys, or a toxic feeling, it is reasonable to try natural remedies for one to two days before going with the antibiotics.

Because bladder symptoms can be seen in both UTIs and CFS/FMS, it is important to have a urine culture done before initiating treatment with antibiotics to make sure it is an infection, and not just muscle spasms in the bladder, that is causing these symptoms. If there is an infection, more than 90 percent of the time it will involve *Escherichia coli* (*E. coli*), a bacterium normally found in the intestines and, with the exception of a few rare, dangerous forms, a healthy part of normal bowel bacteria. The problem occurs when the E. coli gets out of the bowel, where it belongs, and into the bladder. Unlike most other infectious organisms, E. coli have little Velcro-like projections that stick to the bladder wall, so they cannot be washed out by urination.

There are two natural remedies that can keep the E. coli from sticking to the bladder wall—cranberries and D-mannose. In addition, taking high doses of vitamin C (500 to 5,000 milligrams a day) can acidify the urine, making it inhospitable to the bacteria. Drinking a lot of water also helps wash out the infection.

CRANBERRIES

Because approximately 20 percent of the female population suffers from UTIs, several studies have been done to find a remedy.[12] They showed significant benefits to drinking six to sixteen ounces of cranberry juice a day. Because most cranberry juice products have a lot of sugar, which can promote yeast overgrowth and aggravate other symptoms in CFIDS/FMS, I think it is much better to use pure cranberry juice powder in capsule or tablet form. Choose a cranberry product that is standardized to contain 11 to 12 percent quinic acid. The therapeutic dose is one to two capsules a day. You can also use unsweetened cranberry juice and add stevia as a natural sweetener if needed.

D-MANNOSE

D-mannose is even more effective for bladder infections than cranberry juice and is what I most strongly recommend. Mannose is a natural sugar (not the kind that causes symptoms or yeast overgrowth) that is excreted promptly into the urine. Unfortunately for the E. coli bacteria, the "fingers" that stick to the bladder wall stick to the D-mannose even better. When you ingest a large amount of D-mannose, it spills into the urine, coating all the E. coli so that the E. coli are literally washed away with the next urination.[13–15]

The nice thing about the natural approach, as opposed to antibiotics, is that cranberries and D-mannose do not kill healthy bacteria, and therefore do not disturb the normal balance of bacteria in the bowel. In addition, D-mannose is absorbed in the upper gut before it gets to the friendly E. coli that are normally present in the colon. Because of this, it helps clear the bladder without causing any other problems.

D-mannose is quite safe, even for long-term use, although most people need it for only a few days. People who have frequent recurrent bladder infections may, however, choose to take it every day to suppress the infections. The usual dose of D-mannose is ½ to 1 teaspoon every two to three waking hours to treat an acute bladder infection or ½ to 1 teaspoon a day to prevent chronic bladder infections. It is best taken dissolved in water. If you get bladder infections associated with sexual intercourse, you can take a teaspoon of D-mannose one hour before and/or just after intercourse to prevent an infection. If you cannot find the D-mannose at your local health food store, it is available at www.vitality101.com.

You should feel much better within twenty-four to forty-eight hours on D-mannose. If you don't, see a doctor for a urine culture (you may want to get the culture at the first sign of infection) and consider antibiotic treatment after two days if the culture is positive. Some evidence exists that the antibiotic nitrofurantoin (also sold under the brand name Macrobid) causes less yeast overgrowth than do other antibiotics.[16] Even with other antibiotics, most bladder infections are knocked out by one to three days of antibiotic use, instead of the old seven-day regimen.

Prostatitis

Although women tend to be the ones plagued with bladder infections, men also have problems to deal with. It is very common for men with CFIDS/FMS to have prostatitis, an inflammation or infection of the prostate that is usually seen in men between the ages of twenty and fifty. There are three main types of prostatitis:

1. *Bacterial prostatitis.* This is an acute or chronic infection in the gland that causes prostate swelling and discomfort, and in which an infection can be found by doing a culture. Although normal bacteria are the most common causes, some bacteria transmitted through sexual contact can also cause prostatitis.

2. *Nonbacterial prostatitis.* This is a condition that causes you to feel swelling of the prostate with no detectable infection. My suspicion is that it is not uncommon for nonbacterial prostatitis to be associated with yeast overgrowth or other infections that cannot be cultured.

3. *Prostadynia.* This is a general irritation of the prostate that causes a burning sensation with urination, urinary urgency, and frequency, without any infection or swelling of the prostate. This can come from a number of causes including, I suspect, chronic spasm or tightening of the muscles of the pelvic floor. Although there are several causes of prostatitis, contributing factors include excessive consumption of caffeine, alcohol, and spicy foods. Sitting for long periods while traveling (for example, as a truck driver) can also cause irritation of the prostate.

The symptoms of chronic prostatitis can come and go and be mild or severe. They include:

- Pain or tenderness in the area of the prostate. It is also common to have burning on the tip of the penis.
- Discomfort in the groin and, occasionally, lower back pain.
- Urinary urgency and frequency with pain on urination.
- Pain with ejaculation.
- In some cases, a slight discharge from the penis. If the discharge is cloudy, it is most likely bacterial prostatitis and you'll need to go to your doctor for antibiotics. Your doctor will probably also check to make sure that the discharge is not indicative of a sexually transmitted disease before beginning treatment.

Severe symptoms accompanied by fever, chills, and extreme fatigue point to acute bacterial prostatitis, requiring treatment with antibiotics. The main medications used for bacterial prostatitis are tetracycline antibiotics (for example, doxycycline), ciprofloxacin (Cipro), or sulfa drugs (such as Bactrim or Septra DS). Unfortunately, since it is hard for antibiotics to be absorbed into the prostate, symptoms often recur, even after six weeks of treatment. I recommend that people with CFS/FMS ask their doctor to prescribe either doxycycline or Cipro because these may be effective against other hidden infections that contribute to their underlying disorders. In many cases of prostadynia, the cause is an underlying fungal infection. Diflucan can help, though it may require six to eighteen months of treatment. If symptoms persist, however, it is reasonable to consider a therapeutic trial of the antibiotics noted above.

To help relieve prostatitis and prostadynia symptoms while taking antibiotics, you may wish to take 500 milligrams a day of the bioflavonoid quercitin.[17]

Bowel Parasite Infections

Parasites should not be thought of as just a problem encountered when traveling. In some places throughout the United States, the water supply is contaminated with parasites—something we may never consider a problem here in our country. You may remember the news reports a number of years ago, when an infection by a bowel parasite called cryptosporidium killed scores of Milwaukeeans. Doctors in the United States also frequently see cases of infection by giardia, amoebae, and numerous other bowel parasites.[18] The symptoms of parasitic infections can mimic those of CFS, and, in immune-suppressing situations like CFIDS, all parasites should be treated.[19–21] Indeed, people with suppressed immune function are especially unable to combat parasitic attack.

DIAGNOSING BOWEL PARASITES

Most laboratories miss parasites when they do stool testing. I initially tested for bowel parasites by sending my patients' stool samples to a respected local lab. The tests kept coming back negative, so I eventually stopped testing. Finally, I started doing my own laboratory stool testing. Doing the testing properly was time-consuming, taking up to five hours per specimen. However, when the tests were processed properly, they frequently turned out positive. In my experience—and in that of other physicians as well—when you treat a patient for parasites, the person's fatigue, bowel symptoms, and achiness often improve dramatically.[20, 21]

If you would like your stool tested, make sure that the laboratory doing the test specializes in this area. The routine random tests performed in most standard laboratories are generally not adequate or reliable. In speaking with several lab technicians, I was told that they had less than one hour of training in looking for parasites—which they found to be useless. In fact, a gastroenterologist friend once noted that during a bowel exam he had performed, he saw a large number of parasites swimming in the patient's bowel. Yet when he sent a sample for confirmation and identification, it came back negative. This is why I stress that stool testing must be done at a lab that specializes in parasitology. I no longer have to do the testing in my office because I can mail specimens to two excellent labs: Parasitology Center and Genova Labs, previously called the Great Smokies Diagnostic Laboratory (see Appendix E: Resources).

TREATING BOWEL PARASITES

Common parasites include giardia, blastocystis, and amebic infections. The appropriate treatment for bowel parasites depends on which organism is causing the problem. For an updated list of treatments for some of the more common infections, see the "Treatment Protocol" link at www .vitality101.com. When a parasitic infection is suspected, but no parasites have been identified, it is reasonable to ask your doctor to consider treating you empirically with albendazole (Albenza).

NATURAL IMMUNE BOOSTERS AND ANTIVIRALS

There are several natural products that both stimulate immune function and have anti-infectious properties. I discussed Pro Boost (see pages 126, 142) and silver (page 129) earlier in this chapter. Some other excellent ones (from Ultracenticals) include:

1. *Leuko-Stim.* This mix mostly stimulates immune function, but the olive leaf may also have antiviral properties. It contains olive leaf extract, Beta 1,3, glucan, maitake mushroom extract, and arabinogalactan (larch).
2. *Maitake D-Fraction.* This contains 330 milligrams of maitake mushroom and extract (an immune stimulant).

3. *Antiviral.* This contains a mix of milk thistle extract (80 percent silymarin), phylanthus amarius, phylanthus uraria, monoammonium glycyrrhizinate, L-lysine, N-Acetyl-L-Cysteine, astragalus herb powder, lactoferin, olive leaf extract, dionea (Venus flytrap extract), and selenium (Selenomethionine).

If a chronic viral or bacterial infection is suspected, consider treating it with a three-month antiviral regimen, using Leuko-Stim or Maitake D-Fraction, plus Pro Boost. Adding the silver solution may also help. These natural supplements can be taken on their own or with antibiotics and antivirals. Though these are more expensive than many other natural supplements, they can be very helpful in fighting these infections and are well tolerated. You'll see effects from treatment in about three months.

Natural Antiviral Treatments Available by Prescription

Two treatments deserve special mention. The first is a natural antiviral derived from animal livers. Called Nexavir (formerly sold as Kutapressin), it is given by daily injection, either subcutaneously or intramuscularly. In my practice, I have seen dramatic improvement with regular use of the Nexavir. However, daily injections are a must, and the few patients who used it only three times a week did not get much, if any, benefit. The downside is that it costs about twenty dollars a day, and the symptoms may return when the injections are discontinued.

The second natural antiviral prescription treatment is gamma globulin. These are the actual antibody infection fighters derived from the serum of numerous blood donors. The serum is first treated to kill off any infections the donors may have had and then the antibodies are harvested. Although these antibodies can be helpful against both bacterial and viral infections, in patients with the latter we have seen a die-off reaction (initial flaring of symptoms) with the first few injections of gamma globulin. I am now advising patients to start with the Nexavir first and add the gamma globulin one to three weeks later. I recommend that 2 cc be given intramuscularly one to two times a week for six weeks, and then as needed. Although it can also be given through an IV, this delivery method is expensive and does not seem to bring any additional benefit.

Both Nexavir and gamma globulin are expensive treatments, and few people find them necessary. However, if you are unable to resolve your chronic infections using any of the other methods described in this chapter, you may wish to discuss these treatments with your CFS/FMS specialist.

THE IMPORTANCE OF FILTERING WATER

As demonstrated in the Milwaukee example, drinking water can be a major source of parasitic infection. As the American water supply becomes more contaminated, parasitic bowel infections will likely become more common. These infections, as well as the overgrowth of yeast or toxic bacteria caused by the use of antibiotics, contribute to the problems of people with CFS/FMS.

Water filters can be helpful in the fight against parasitic infection, and can help to improve health in general. However, not all units are designed to filter out parasites. For a water filter to remove parasites, it must be rated by the National Sanitation Foundation (NSF) for cyst removal. A good example is the Multi-Pure water filter (see Appendix E: Resources). Most filters on the market do not remove parasites and a wide range of contaminants. Solid carbon block filters and reverse-osmosis filters are the best types of units.

When shopping around for a water filter, request the NSF International Listing. The NSF is an independent, not-for-profit organization that tests and certifies drinking-water-treatment products. The unit you buy should meet both NSF Health Effects Standard 53 for cysts (giardia, cryptosporidium, entamoeba, toxoplasma), as well as their standards for the following contaminants: VOCs (pesticides, herbicides, and chemicals), endocrine disrupters (PCBs), trihalomethanes (cancer-causing disinfection by-products), heavy metals (lead, mercury), MBTE (a gasoline additive), chloramines, and asbestos. Solid carbon block filters can reduce chlorine, taste and odor problems, particulate matter, and a wide range of contaminants without removing healthful, naturally occurring minerals. They also require no electricity and add no salt to the water. Any unit that does not meet all of these standards, particularly the health standard, is inadequate.

In addition to verifying that a water filter meets the NSF standards, ask to see its Product Performance Data Sheet. Many states require that this sheet be given to all prospective customers of drinking-water-treatment devices. Also ask about the range of contaminants that the unit can reduce under NSF Health Effects Standard 53. Most units certified under Standard 53 list only turbidity and cyst reduction. The number of units that also reduce all of the contaminants listed above is very small. Make sure that the water filter you are considering can remove the specific contaminants that concern you without removing beneficial minerals. Beware of sales agents who tell you that NSF certification is not important.

Be sure to ask if the unit is licensed in such states as California, Colorado, and Wisconsin, which have some of the toughest certification procedures in the United States. Finally, ask about the unit's service cycle, which is stated in gallons of water treated. Find out how often you will need to change the filter and what the replacement filters cost. Proper investigation into these details will ensure that you find the water filter that is best for your needs. I recommend getting one from Pure Water (see Appendix E: Resources).

Antibiotic-Sensitive Infections

People with CFS/FMS are at high risk for multiple viral and antibiotic-sensitive infections because of their immune system dysfunction. That people usually have not just one but several infections simultaneously is significant. It suggests that although these infections may be a trigger for the illness in some cases, most of the infections occur because of the illness, setting you up for multiple and sometimes unusual infections that persist. These infections may then drag you down, further suppressing your immune system.

Fortunately, most people improve (and often get very healthy) by simply treating sleep, hormonal, nutritional, and yeast problems. Once these areas are treated, your body can often eliminate many persistent infections by itself. Some people, though, have infections that need treatment with antivirals and/or antibiotics.

How can you tell if you need such treatments? First, I would try the other approaches discussed in this book. I would consider drug treatments if the following symptoms persist:

- Predominantly flu-like symptoms, with debilitating fatigue and little or no pain or fever. People with these symptoms are more likely to have an underlying persistent viral infection, such as HHV–6, CMV, or EBV.
- A fever over 98.6°F—even 99°F—and/or lung congestion, sinusitis, a history of bad reactions to several different antibiotics (people misinterpret this die-off reaction as an allergic reaction), scabbing scalp sores,

or other chronic bacterial infections. People with these symptoms seem to be more likely to have bacterial, mycoplasma, or chlamydia infections that respond to special antibiotics.

Let's look at these two situations and how to approach them.

Viral Infections

Human herpesvirus 6 (HHV–6) is a virus that is related to the Epstein-Barr virus (EBV), cytomegalovirus (CMV), and the herpes viruses that cause cold sores and genital herpes. All of these are in the human herpesvirus family and stay in the body (usually in an inactive latent form for EBV, CMV, and HHV–6) for the rest of your life. Usually HHV–6 is transmitted like the common cold, and more than 90 percent of adults have had HHV–6, as well as EBV and the cold sore virus, by the time they are twenty years old.

THE PROBLEM WITH LAB TESTING FOR INFECTIONS IN CFS

Unfortunately, there is no test that clearly distinguishes old dormant infections from viral reactivation. When you first have an infection, antibodies in the IgM family (M antibodies are like your body's storm troopers) are elevated for six to twelve weeks, telling doctors that you have an active new infection. After that time, the IgM test will be negative. The IgG antibody levels then stay elevated (G antibodies are like regular troops, suppressing the latent infection) for the rest of our lives. Because of this, when you check the standard IgG antibody testing almost everybody (including healthy people) tests positive for EBV and HHV–6 and many will test positive for CMV. That the IgG test is elevated, however, does not tell you if you have an active infection because of viral reactivation or simply an inactive, dormant infection. Other tests available to your doctor, such as PCR testing, are also still unreliable for a number of reasons, and the IgM test will not be positive in the vast majority of those with reactivated viral infections.

Nonetheless, these infections are common in CFS, and the available IgG test may still offer useful information. Unfortunately, despite all of the data to the contrary, most doctors are not familiar with the research and still mistakenly think a negative IgM antibody test confirms that there is no active infection. Because most physicians are not aware of this research, and it may be important for your doctor to know about, I invite the more scientifically oriented reader to read the sidebar "Research on Viral and Antibiotic-Sensitive Infections in CFS/FMS." Getting past the miscon-

---

Research on Viral and Antibiotic-Sensitive Infections in CFS/FMS

- A study by Dylewski et al in the *New England Journal of Medicine* demonstrates that in immune-compromised patients, as occurs in CFS/FMS, active infections correlate with elevations in IgG antibodies without elevations of IgM antibodies and that a lack of elevation of IgM is not useful in these patients as a way to rule out active infection. A high clinical suspicion must be maintained, and implementation of anti-infective treatment should be based on elevated IgG levels.[22]

- In addition to mycoplasma, numerous studies have also demonstrated other bacterial and viral infections such as EBV, CMV, HHV–6, and enterovirus in CFS and FMS patients that cause or contribute to the symptoms. The research also demonstrates that these infections are present and that an active infection correlates with an elevated IgG antibody, despite the lack of IgM antibodies.[23–33] As with mycoplasma infections (see page 143), because these infections are generally not acute but rather reactivation of an old infection, an elevation of IgM antibodies is typically *not* seen with active infections of EBV, CMV, HHV–6, Borrelia (Lyme), and enterovirus.[23–33] Because of the immune dysfunction seen in CFS, there may even be a lack of IgG antibodies present despite the presence of an active infection.[30,34,35]

- Immune-suppressed patients have also been shown to be helped by antiviral therapy in a number of studies.[36–40]

- It is clear that multiple infections are present in CFS/FMS patients. For example, one study found that 52 percent of CFS patients had active mycoplasma infection, 30.5 percent had active HHV–6 infection, and 7.5 percent had chlamydia pneumonia infections versus only 6 percent, 9 percent, and 1 percent of healthy people, respectively. They conclude: "The results indicate that a large subset of CFS patients show evidence of bacterial and/or viral infection(s), and these infections may contribute to the severity of signs and symptoms found in these patients."[41]

---

ception that these infections are not active if the IgM test is negative is important, as we finally have treatments that are effective against many of these infections. Let's look at some of the more important infections.

HHV–6

A reactivated HHV–6 viral infection is present in many patients with CFS. A study in the *Annals of Internal Medicine* found that 70 percent of patients with CFS had active HHV–6 infection.[42] In another study of HHV–6 in CFS patients, 89 percent with very high HHV–6 IgG antibody levels of 1:320 and above were found to have active infections by cell culture. To compare, most healthy adults have levels of 1:40 to 1:160. Though not all of the studies were able to document the infections, as CFS expert and Harvard professor Anthony Komaroff notes in his recent review, "the great majority of studies have found evidence of active replication of HHV–6 more often in patients with CFS than in healthy control subjects."[43]

When HHV–6 is present, it seems to affect the immune system's natural killer cells, which are critical in fighting infections and are also often malfunctioning in CFS. Natural-killer-cell function is described in what is called lytic units—which means the ability of cells to lyse, or break down, foreign invaders. An average person has a lytic unit level of 20 to 250, with more than 80 percent of healthy people having more than 40 units. However, in people with CFIDS, the mean natural-killer lytic-unit level is just 12 units. With your immune system so low, the reactivated HHV–6 can then also cause reactivation of the Epstein-Barr virus. In addition, both HHV–6 and EBV can suppress immune function, and HHV–6 can also suppress your body's ability to fight fungal/yeast infections.

Until recently, there was no readily available treatment for HHV–6. Even though it is related to other herpes viruses, HHV–6 is resistant to acyclovir (Zovirax), valacyclovir (Valtrex), famciclovir (Famvir), and the other antivirals that are commonly used for herpes infections. Fortunately, there is a new and promising oral antiviral called Valcyte that has been shown in early studies to be beneficial in CFS patients who have both HHV–6 and EBV viruses. Unfortunately, this drug can have significant side effects, although it causes no problems in most CFS patients, and is expensive. If you have an open-minded doctor and are interested in exploring Valcyte treatment, the information in the sidebar on page 141 may be helpful to your physician.

Diagnosing and Treating Reactivated HHV–6 Infections in CFS

In a recent study by Professor Jose Montoya of Stanford University, CFS patients were treated with the new antiviral drug Valcyte if they had elevated IgG tests for HHV–6 and EBV and had at least four of the following symptoms—impaired cognitive functioning, slowed processing speed, sleep disturbance, short-term memory deficit, fatigue, and symptoms consistent with depression. In their first study of twelve patients, nine out of twelve (75 percent) patients "experienced near resolution of their symptoms, allowing them all to return to the workforce or full-time activities. In the nine patients with a symptomatic response to treatment, EBV VCA IgG titers dropped from 1:2560 to 1:640, and HHV–6 IgG titers dropped from a median value of 1:1280 to 1:320 . . . serious adverse events were not observed among the twelve patients."[44]

I had the pleasure of speaking with Professor Montoya in January 2007 to get further details on his treatment protocol. In CFS patients whose symptoms began with a flu-like illness and who have an EBV VCA IgG antibody level of at least 1:640 plus an HHV–6 IgG antibody of at least 1:640 (or 1:320 if the EBV is at least 1280), he treats as follows:

1. Valcyte 900 milligrams two times a day is given for three weeks, then
2. Valcyte 900 milligrams one time a day is given for twenty-three weeks.

To monitor for bone marrow, liver, and kidney toxicity (which he has not found to be a problem in CFS patients) he does the following testing:

CBC and chemistries (BUN, Cr, ALT, AST) twice a week for three weeks, then once a week for three weeks, then every other week for three weeks, and then monthly while on the treatment.

He avoids prescribing Valcyte for those with severe neuropathic (nerve) pain in their hands as well as in patients with inadequate kidney function or who have white blood cell counts of less than 3,500, as a potential toxicity is bone marrow suppression. He found that all patients who improved had an initial flare of their symptoms from about the second to the fourth weeks of treatment—often leaving them housebound for that two-week period. Most noticed significant improvement beginning at about three to four months into treatment. The patients I have spoken with who have taken it have been very pleased, but a few have developed recurrent symptoms when they stopped the medication after six months and are considering repeating the treatment. Though there is the potential for toxicity from this medication, current experience suggests that this has not been a major problem in the CFS population.

This treatment is promising, with the main limiting factor now being its cost. Sixty 450-milligram tablets (a one-month supply) costs about two thousand dollars from Consumers Discount Drugs (1-323-461-3606) and is available from Canada by mail for $1,500. This makes the six-month cost $10,000 to $13,000.

EBV AND CMV

The roles of EBV (Epstein-Barr virus) and CMV (cytomegalovirus) in CFIDS are not clear. It is not uncommon for antibody levels of these viruses to be elevated in people with chronic fatigue syndrome. However, we do not know if this elevation reflects an old inactive infection or an on-going infection with these viruses. Given the findings with HHV–6 and the drop in EBV antibody levels after treatment, I am inclined to believe that reactivation is occurring with these viruses as well. As discussed in reference to HHV–6 infection, I have not found the antiviral Valtrex to be helpful in treating CFS symptoms and no longer use it. Valcyte still holds much greater promise and is effective against HHV–6, CMV, and EBV. As the HHV–6 seems to trigger reactivation of EBV, it is possible that suppressing the HHV–6 infection is enough to allow the body to also overcome the EBV infection.

In addition to Valcyte, there are also several other treatments that may be helpful in fighting CMV and HHV–6.

- Thymic protein A, marketed under the brand name Pro Boost, is an excellent natural immune stimulant. Although not a hormone, thymic protein A mimics the natural hormone produced by the thymus, the gland that stimulates the immune system. I find it to be extraordinarily effective in fighting common acute infections of any kind that seem to pop up, and recommend that it be in everyone's medicine cabinet. In fact, whenever my kids get a cold, the first thing they say is, "Dad, where's the white powder?" (the Pro Boost).

   Although taking it for one to three days will quickly eliminate most acute infections, for the chronic infections of CFIDS, one packet three times a day for three months is needed. In one study, this dropped EBV IgG levels by 70 percent after three months in CFS patients.
- Extracts of maitake mushroom have also been shown to increase natural-killer-cell function.
- Lysine is an amino acid (one of the building blocks of protein) that inhibits oral and genital herpes viruses by depleting arginine, another amino acid that the virus needs to grow. It is not known whether lysine also inhibits EBV, HHV–6, or CMV, but these viruses are all

members of the herpes family. Lysine is safe and inexpensive. The recommended dosage is 1,000 milligrams three times a day. Arginine is used by the body to make both nitric oxide and growth hormone. Decreasing arginine may therefore also decrease excessive nitric oxide activity in CFS. The downside is that it may also decrease growth hormone—which is too low in CFS. Because of this, it may be reasonable to take lysine for six months, but I would not use it on a long-term basis in CFS.

- Another treatment that may be helpful is vitamin C. High doses of 15–50 grams of vitamin C, administered intravenously, are often dramatically helpful for CFS when given as part of intravenous nutritional therapy your doctor may administer (page 364).

- In addition, your clotting system may be activated by several infections, making it difficult to eliminate the viruses. Using the anticlotting treatment that we discuss later (see page 149) can also make it easier for your body to eradicate infections.

ANTIBIOTIC-SENSITIVE INFECTIONS
SUCH AS MYCOPLASMA, CHLAMYDIA, AND LYME DISEASE

Research by Dr. Garth Nicolson and his wife, Nancy L. Nicolson, has shown that other antibiotic-sensitive infections, including mycoplasma and chlamydia, can be important in CFIDS. These microorganisms can cause persistent infections, and have similar characteristics. Mycoplasma are a type of ancient bacteria that lack cell walls and are capable of invading a number of types of human cells. They can cause a wide variety of human diseases. These organisms can cause the types of symptoms seen in people with CFIDS and, according to Dr. Nicolson, tend to be immune-suppressing. Unfortunately, they cannot be readily cultured in a culture dish.

In medicine, we have a bad habit of focusing on things that are easy to test for and making believe that things that are hard to test for do not exist. Because of this, bacterial infections such as pneumonia, bladder infections, and skin infections—in which one bacterium on a cell dish will rapidly turn into millions by the next day and be visible to the human eye—get all our attention. Unfortunately, mycoplasma and chlamydia, which cannot be easily cultured, tend to be ignored.

Although mycoplasma and chlamydia are common in the environment, they usually are fairly noninvasive. It may simply be that once your immune system is weakened, these infections can get into cells where they don't belong. When that happens, even some of the common ones that are normally considered noninfectious can wreak havoc. When these infections reproduce slowly, they tend to be low-grade and chronic, as opposed to the acute and more prominent symptoms seen with bacterial and viral infections that multiply and divide rapidly.

Interestingly, the Nicolsons found that in patients with chronic fatigue syndrome or fibromyalgia, approximately 70 percent (144 out of 203 patients) had a positive PCR test for at least one—and usually several—species of mycoplasma or chlamydia. When the Nicolsons tested seventy healthy patients, only six (less than 9 percent) were positive for any of the mycoplasma species. This is a highly significant difference. Only two of these seventy healthy people were positive for mycoplasma fermentans. Similar results have been published by other doctors.

It is likely that there is a group of underlying problems and not a single one that triggers CFS/FMS. This applies to infections as well. This is why we see positive tests for both viral and mycoplasma/chlamydia infections in so many people with this disease. For mycoplasma alone, when the Nicolsons checked for four different types of mycoplasma, more than half of the ninety-three CFS patients who were positive had more than one type of infection. More than 20 percent of them tested positive for three out of the four mycoplasma infections. The more infections they tested positive for, the worse their symptoms were and the longer they had had CFS/FMS. Unfortunately, testing for these antibiotic-sensitive infections is not reliable in most people. Although in research settings one can quickly run a PCR (polymerase chain reaction), a test for the DNA of different organisms, my experience is that blood samples sent by mail are not fresh enough to be useful. In addition, there are many other antibiotic-sensitive infections for which we have no good testing. These include organisms such as Lyme and babesiosis. Because of this, I am starting to believe that it is better to simply treat with antibiotics based on symptoms, instead of using expensive lab tests that have limited reliability. The early data, however, suggest that finding an abnormally high elevation in the IgG antibody levels for these organisms may also suggest active infection. Hidden dental infections can also be problematic.

Lyme disease is especially problematic, as there is *no* gold standard test. I suspect that as many as half of the people who have Lyme infections have

Help for Dental Infections

People with CFS/FMS seem especially vulnerable to cavities. This usually comes from the dry mouth, which can be caused by CFS/FMS as well as medications (especially Elavil). To treat dry mouth, add fish oil and the vitamin powder to increase saliva production and eliminate medications that cause dry mouth. Some patients will get "cavitations" in their jaws, which can serve as hidden infections. Cavitations are poorly understood, so I asked Dr. Stephen Hubert, a Maui dentist specializing in dental infections, to give us more information about them.

Cavitations are groups of infections caused by remnants of roots of extracted teeth and the periodontal ligament. They are commonly associated with "wisdom tooth" extractions, infected "root canalled" teeth, and even apparently healthy teeth that have undergone root canals. These incomplete extractions may leave behind potent toxins such as hydrogen sulfide and methylthiol.

Cavitations can be diagnosed with a good panoramic X-ray, and treatment consists of surgical excision and removal of tooth fragments and the associated connective tissue. A hard tissue laser is often used in this surgery because of its ability to sterilize the surgical site as it "ablates," or destroys, the infected tissue.

A significant source of chronic dental inflammation is infection under the gum known as "periodontal disease." This disease is diagnosed by microscopic analysis of biofilm samples from tooth root surfaces under the gum, especially any inflamed bleeding pockets. Many biological dentists have a Phase Contrast Microscope that allows identification of potent pathogens and the accompanying high number of white blood cells that mark this condition. This infection can be eliminated with a series of antiseptic, under-the-gum irrigations using a Waterpik device fitted with a special connector. Ozone/oxygen can be applied directly to the anaerobic environment under the gum, which also helps kill the infections.

---

negative tests and, conversely, that if you randomly check Lyme tests, as many as half of the people who test positive do not have Lyme disease. This creates enormous confusion, as CFS/FMS symptoms are similar to those of Lyme disease. Because of this, many people desperately looking for an explanation for their symptoms who have found one of many Lyme tests to be positive cling to this diagnosis as they seek an explanation for their disability. Many of these patients feel better on antibiotics and take this as confirmation. Indeed, many excellent physicians feel that the large majority of CFS/FMS patients have Lyme disease. The majority of physicians only believe a Lyme infection is present if a test called the western blot is positive—ignoring that this test is negative in a large percent of those with Lyme disease.

To show how severe the lack of awareness of proper diagnosis is of these infections in the medical community, the U.S. legislature passed a resolution strongly recommending that physicians become aware of the lack of sensitivity of current tests for Lyme disease and consider appropriate treatment based on clinical grounds. It notes: "The committee is distressed in hearing of the widespread misuse of the current Lyme disease surveillance case definition. . . . The definition is reportedly misused as a standard of care for . . . medical licensing hearings." Sadly, even this law has been ignored by some physicians.

Given all of the above, we simply do not know for sure if many people with CFS also have Lyme disease. If you had a history of tick bite and a bull's-eye rash and have fatigue or pain, I consider it reasonable to treat for possible Lyme disease even if the tests are negative. The approach I currently recommend (until we have better testing) is to simply acknowledge that the testing used in CFS/FMS patients for antibiotic-sensitive infections in general is unreliable, that the research shows that these infections are common in CFS/FMS, and that the research also shows that many patients improve when given antibiotics such as azithromycin (Zithromax) or doxycycline—even if testing is negative. Given this situation, it is reasonable for physicians to use their clinical judgment and treat with antibiotics when appropriate, even if there is no test to confirm the type of infection.

Should your doctor also come to this conclusion, you should be informed of an approach to treating possible Lyme disease and other antibiotic-sensitive infections that has worked for many patients.

Treating the Hidden Antibiotic-Sensitive Infections

As we have discussed, testing for these infections is difficult and, therefore, it is often necessary to simply treat based on clinical symptoms. Because of this, I am more likely to treat with antibiotics if any of the following are present:

- A chronic or recurrent fever over 98.6°F—even 99°F
- Chronic lung congestion
- Recurrent scalp sores that scab

- A history of bad reactions to several different antibiotics (people mis-interpret the die-off reaction as being an allergic reaction)
- A history of CFS/FMS transiently improving in the past when given an antibiotic
- Severe vertigo (when you feel like you or the room is spinning in a cir-cle, which is not to be confused with the disequilibrium experienced by most of us with CFS)

People with these symptoms seem to be more likely to have infections that respond to special antibiotics. Fortunately, Lyme disease, mycoplasma, and chlamydia infections, and many other infections that are difficult to test for in CFS, are often sensitive to the right antibiotics. The antibiotics most likely to affect these organisms are the following:

- *Doxycycline or, preferably, minocycline, usually at dosages of 100 milligrams twice a day.* These two antibiotics are in the tetracycline family. They are effective against a number of unusual organisms (for example, Lyme disease). They sometimes cause some stomach upset, so if this occurs, either take the medicine with food and a full glass of water or lower the dose. These antibiotics should not be given to children under eight years old because they can cause permanent staining of the teeth.
- *Ciprofloxacin (Cipro), usually 500 to 750 milligrams twice a day.* Although expensive, this is usually a well-tolerated antibiotic. It has a wide range of effectiveness against a large number of organisms. Cipro has an additional benefit for men, as it also treats any hidden prostate infections, as does doxycycline. You should not take oral magnesium or any supplement containing magnesium within four to six hours of taking Cipro or you may not absorb the Cipro as completely. A small percentage of the population has a genetic defect that prevents them from breaking down Cipro. In this group, taking Cipro can actually trigger FMS, and this family of antibiotics should be avoided if you have a family member who developed fibromyalgia after taking Cipro.
- *Azithromycin (Zithromax), 250 to 600 milligrams a day taken with food, or clarithromycin (Biaxin), 500 milligrams twice a day, taken on an empty stomach.* These antibiotics are in the erythromycin family. Zithromax tends to be fairly well tolerated. Biaxin is more likely to cause a bit of nausea in some patients, but it is usually also well tolerated. These

two may work against infections missed by doxycycline and Cipro. Begin with this antibiotic if you have scalp or skin sores or scabs.

Although all of these antibiotics can be effective, it is not uncommon for infections that are sensitive to the erythromycin antibiotics (Zithromax and Biaxin) to be resistant to tetracycline antibiotics (doxycycline, minocycline) and Cipro, and vice versa. Therefore, it is best to try either doxycycline or Cipro first. If they are not effective, then try the Zithromax or Biaxin. The antibiotic should be taken for at least six months. If there is no improvement in four months, switch to the other antibiotic or simply stop the treatment.

As mentioned earlier, I am more likely to use antibiotics for CFS patients who have temperatures over 98.6°F, even if they are only 98.8°F (I consider 98.8°F a fever because CFS/FMS patients usually have low body temperatures). If you do have low-grade chronic temperature elevations, be sure that you monitor your temperature during treatment. If your temperature drops with the antibiotic, it suggests that you do have one of these nonviral infections and that the antibiotic is helping. This would encourage me to continue the antibiotic trial—even if it takes up to eighteen months to see an improvement in your symptoms.

If you are clearly better, you should probably take the antibiotic for at least six to twelve months. It can then be stopped. If symptoms recur, keep repeating six- to eight-week cycles until the symptoms stay gone. It may take several years of treatment for the infection to be totally eradicated. To put this in perspective, this is how long children often take antibiotics for acne—which, unfortunately, if not taken with antifungals, can lead to yeast overgrowth and possibly trigger CFS. You should therefore take two tablets of the herbal Anti-Yeast mix twice a day while on the antibiotic. It is a good idea to take an acidophilus supplement as well. Also, be aware that birth control pills may be ineffective while you are taking antibiotics, so be sure to use an alternative form of birth control.

It is very common to get what is called a die-off (Herxheimer) reaction that includes chills, fever, night sweats, and general worsening of CFS/FMS symptoms when the antibiotic first kills off the infection. Many people mistakenly confuse these with an allergic reaction. These symptoms can be severe and can last for weeks. Stop the antibiotic and let the die-off reaction subside. Then resume the antibiotic at a much lower dose (e.g.,

25 milligrams of minocycline every other day) and work the dose up slowly. The Nicholsons, who pioneered this treatment of antibiotic-sensitive infections, note that if you have been sick for years, it is unlikely that you will recover in less than one year of treatment, so you should not be alarmed by symptoms that return or worsen temporarily. In addition, some other unusual infections may require the simultaneous use of multiple antibiotics.

One more antibiotic-sensitive infection deserves mention. If spastic colon symptoms persist after treatment for yeast and parasites, consider treating for SIBO (small intestinal bacterial overgrowth), which is common in CFS/FMS and which is another key cause of bowel symptoms. Research has shown that treating empirically with the antibiotic Rifaximin for ten days can result in long-lasting improvement of the symptoms of irritable bowel syndrome/spastic colon.[45]

What to Do When All Else Fails—the Role of the Blood-Clotting System

Although more than 85 percent of CFS/FMS patients improve by using the SHIN protocol, we are constantly looking for new treatments. Using the blood thinner heparin has been able to help half of those who failed all other treatments. We do not begin with this treatment because it carries more risk. Fortunately, none of our patients have developed problems on it.

Work done by David E. Berg, director of Hemex Laboratories in Phoenix, has shown that a number of infections can trigger the blood-clotting system to become active, thus setting up a low-level chronic clotting cascade. Some of the infections that can do this are HHV–6, mycoplasma, CMV, and chlamydia, which can trigger production of antibodies against clot-protective proteins on the inner surfaces of blood vessels, called antiphospholipid antibodies. One of these is called beta-2-glycoprotein 1. This then triggers the clotting cascade. Once the clotting system is triggered, the body produces what are called soluble fibrin monomers (SFMs). The theory is that these SFMs are like long, thin sheets of a Teflon-like substance, similar to a scab that covers a cut, but microscopic in size, and that these sheets then coat the blood vessels. This makes it hard for nutrients and oxygen to get in and out of the blood vessels to the cells where they are needed.

Why Would an Infection Trigger the Clotting System?

Many infectious organisms do not survive well in the presence of oxygen. These are termed anaerobic. Mycoplasma (which can be anaerobic) and other organisms may trigger the clotting system to create a shell, which then acts like a suit of armor, protecting them from oxygen, your body's defense system, and antibiotics. This would explain why these infections may have evolved a way to trigger the clotting mechanism. The fibrin armor preventing antibiotics from getting to the infection could also explain why some people with these infections may not respond to antibiotics. Indeed, some physicians have found that the antibiotics work better once someone has been on a blood-thinning medication, which may dissolve the armor.

This Is an Interesting Theory, but How Do We Know This Is Going On?

Mr. Berg and others have done studies showing that the results of blood tests to look for these clotting changes are abnormal in CFS/FMS patients, whereas they are normal in most other people. Results of two of the tests in the panel must be abnormal for the result to be considered positive. When these tests were performed, fifty of fifty-four CFS/FMS patients had abnormal results (that is, only 7.4 percent of the patients had normal blood test results). In healthy people, twenty-two out of twenty-three (96 percent) had normal blood test results. This means the test is both sensitive and specific, picking up people with CFS and excluding healthy people. Almost everyone with CFS whom I have tested has turned out to have these clotting changes, although I personally have not tested healthy people to see if this also occurs with them. Interestingly, many people with unexplained infertility also test positive for these changes, as do many people with multiple sclerosis, Parkinson's disease, autism, inflammatory bowel disease, and some other illnesses.

These results suggest that these tests can be helpful in deciding whether to treat people with CFS/FMS with blood thinners. On the other hand, when a test is positive in 93 percent of patients and costs about three hundred fifty dollars, a good argument can also be made for simply treating without doing the test. Your doctor will determine whether he or she feels comfortable with empirical treatment.

Treating the Blood-Clotting System

First of all, it is important to note that using heparin injections as a treatment for CFIDS/FMS is still controversial and is considered by some to be experimental. I much prefer to use treatments that are as safe as possible. Although there are risks of potentially fatal bleeding or drops in platelet counts (the cells that cause your blood to clot), we have not seen or heard of any serious toxicity occurring in the thousands of CFS patients who have been treated with heparin. In addition, I find that about half of my patients with the most severe and refractory symptoms of CFS/FMS get better with this treatment.

While a patient is on heparin, I perform tests to measure blood thinning frequently during the first month of treatment. If the patient is not better and the partial thromboplastin time (PTT) test is still within the normal range, I will increase the prescribed heparin to as much as 8,000 units twice a day. To put this dosage in perspective, most hospital patients who require heparin receive 1,000 units per hour (a total of 24,000 units a day) intravenously. Those with chronic fatigue syndrome and fibromyalgia take heparin by subcutaneous injection using an insulin syringe for the first six weeks of treatment. Then, some patients can switch to a nose spray or sublingual form.

If the heparin is going to help, you'll start to feel better at about the ten- to fourteen-day point. I then consider adding doxycycline (a tetracycline) or antiviral therapies based on symptoms or lab results for six to twelve months. At the end of four to twelve months, if the heparin helps, we try to taper off the heparin because it is a powerful medicine, and its main risk is excessive bleeding. Although we are using very low doses that are usually well tolerated, life-threatening bleeding can rarely occur. In addition, if used for more than a year, a DEXA scan for bone density should be performed, as heparin could cause osteoporosis.

Most people tolerate these treatments quite well and many, many more people die from taking aspirin and Motrin family medications called NSAIDs (for example, for arthritis) than from taking heparin each year. Still, heparin is riskier than the other treatments I recommend, and I tend to use it as a last resort. As an aside, I would note that I am not convinced that this clotting theory is entirely accurate or the reason heparin works, because I have found other blood thinners like Coumadin and nattokinase to be useless for CFS. However, we know by clinical experience that heparin is helpful for many patients. I suspect that we'll find that this could be because heparin is also an antiviral.

The treatment approach I am recommending for infections in CFS/FMS patients is getting more and more support over time. For a more detailed discussion (and numerous references) about the lack of reliability of current testing and the proven benefits of treating infections in CFS empirically based on the symptoms and history, see the *From Fatigued to Fantastic!* notes at www.vitality101.com.

In summary, several infections can cause or be caused by CFS and FMS. These are usually associated with immune system malfunction. Testing for infections may be helpful but can be expensive. If you can afford the tests and/or your insurance will pay for them, they are worth checking and will make it easier to adjust therapy over time. Otherwise, it is reasonable to treat empirically—that is, without testing. If you have lung congestion and/or recurrent temperatures over 98.6°F, scalp scabs, vertigo, or a history of repeated "allergic" reactions to antibiotics, or if your CFS improved with antibiotics in the past, your doctor may be able to effectively treat you with antibiotics. If you have chronic flu-like symptoms or if your illness began with a flu-like infection, and your blood tests show EBV VCA and HHV–6 IgG antibodies elevated at 1:640 or higher, you should consider the antiviral regimen with Valcyte. I would usually only use the antibiotics, Valcyte, or heparin if symptoms persist after treating sleep, hormonal issues, infections, and nutritional deficiencies. Fortunately, there are now physicians around the country who can expertly guide you through these therapies (see Chapter 12, "Finding a Physician"). Our new understanding of how to diagnose and treat the infections offers exciting new hope.

Important Points

- An important component of CFIDS is disordered immune function, which opens the door to repeated infections, repeated treatment with antibiotics, and yeast overgrowth.
- Treat yeast overgrowth by avoiding antibiotics and sweets. Many patients have found herbal antifungals such as Anti-Yeast, probiotics such as Acidophilus Pearls, and other antifungal medications, such as Diflucan, 200 milligrams a day for six to twelve weeks, to be helpful.
- Bowel parasites are common in CFIDS patients, whose symptoms often improve with treatment. However, most laboratories do not adequately detect parasites through stool testing. To get an accurate test result, use a laboratory that specializes in stool testing (see Appendix E: Resources).
- Prevent parasitic infection by filtering your water with an effective filtration unit. I recommend the Multi-Pure water filter (see Pure Water in Appendix E: Resources).
- If you have lung congestion and/or recurrent temperatures over 98.6°F, scalp scabs, vertigo, or a history of repeated "allergic" reactions to antibiotics, or if your CFS improved with antibiotics in the past, I would treat with the antibiotics. Take antifungals while on the antibiotic to prevent yeast overgrowth.
- If you have chronic flu-like symptoms despite treatment for yeast and underactive adrenal glands, consider trying the antiviral, immune-stimulating protocol discussed in this chapter.
- If you feel chronically flu-like or if your illness began with a flu-like infection, and your blood tests show EBV VCA and HHV–6 IgG antibodies elevated at 1:640 or higher, you should consider the anti-

viral regimen with Valcyte combined with the natural antivirals and immune boosters.

Questionnaire (Items to be checked are in Appendix B.)

Parasites

_____ 1. Did your problems begin with a diarrhea attack?

_____ 2. Do you sometimes have diarrhea? If so, is it severe? _____

If you answered yes to either #1 or 2, check off #77.

_____ 3. Do you drink well water?

_____ 4. Have you had a parasite infection in the past?

If you answered yes to #3 or 4 and either #1 or 2, check off #45.

Antibiotic-Sensitive Infections

_____ 5. Has any antibiotic improved your CFS/FMS symptoms?

If yes, check off any of #46–48 that helped (or, if none of these, add the name of the antibiotic that was most effective).

_____ 6. Do you have scabbing scalp sores?

If yes, check off #48.

_____ 7. Do you have chronic respiratory infections/lung congestion?

_____ 8. Do you have chronic or intermittent low-grade fevers?

_____ 9. Do you have chronic vertigo (where it feels like you or the room is spinning in a circle)?

If yes to #7, 8, or 9, check off #47.

_____ 10. Have you had severe reactions (not including rash, itching, throat swelling, or trouble breathing) to two or more different antibiotics?

If yes, check off any of #46–48 that caused the reaction (or if none of these, add the name of the antibiotic that caused a die-off reaction) after discussion of the reaction with your CFS-expert physician.

_____ 11. Did your illness begin after a tick bite and a bull's-eye rash?

If yes, check off #47 and see a CFS or Lyme disease specialist.

Viral Infections

_____ 12. Did your CFS/FMS begin with a flu-like infection?

If yes, check off #80 and read the section on HHV–6 on page 140.

_____ 13. Do you have chronic flu-like symptoms despite being on Cortef/hydrocortisone?

If yes, check off #35, 44, and 44A.

Yeast/Candida Infections

_____ 14. Do you have sinusitis, nasal congestion, mouth sores, or spastic colon?

If yes to any of these, check off #36, 37, 38, 40, and 43 and skip question #15. If you get painful mouth sores, also check off #41.

_____ 15. Yeast Questionnaire

The total score for this section gives the probability of yeast overgrowth being a significant factor in your case.

Point Score (add up and put total below)

50 _____ Have you been treated for acne with tetracycline, erythromycin, or any other antibiotic for one month or longer?

50 _____ Have you taken antibiotics for any type of infection for more than two consecutive months, or shorter courses more than three times in a twelve-month period?

6 _____ Have you ever taken an antibiotic—even for a single course?

25 _____ Have you ever had prostatitis or vaginitis?

5 _____ Have you ever been pregnant?

15 _____ Have you taken birth control pills?

15 _____ Have you taken corticosteroids such as prednisone, Cortef, or Medrol?

15 _____ When you are exposed to perfumes, insecticides, or other odors or chemicals, do you develop wheezing, burning eyes, or any other distress?

20 _____ Are your symptoms worse on damp or humid days or in moldy places?

20 ____ Have you ever had a fungal infection such as jock itch, athlete's foot, or a nail or skin infection that was difficult to treat?

20 ____ Do you crave sugar or breads?

10 ____ Does tobacco smoke cause you discomfort (e.g., wheezing, burning eyes)?

Total:
If 70 or higher, check off #36, 37, 38, 40, and 43.

____ 16.   Do you get chronic bladder infections?

If yes, check off #51.

____ 17.   Do you get chronic sinus infections?

If yes, check off #49 and 50.

N—Nutrition: Optimizing Your Body's Ability to Heal

6

*F*or those of you who watch what you eat, here's the final word on nutrition and health. It's a relief to know the truth after all those conflicting medical studies:

1. The Japanese eat very little fat and drink very little red wine, and they suffer fewer heart attacks than the Americans.
2. The French eat lots of fatty cheese and rich food and drink lots of wine, and they suffer fewer heart attacks than the Americans.
3. The Italians drink a lot of red wine and eat lots of carbohydrate-rich pasta, and they suffer fewer heart attacks than the Americans.
4. The Germans drink a lot of beer and eat lots of sausages and fats, and they suffer fewer heart attacks than the Americans.

Conclusion: Eat and drink what you like. Speaking English is apparently what kills you.

This joke exemplifies the frustration many people feel toward the medical establishment. What is in vogue one day is forbidden the next. Nutrition and health recommendations seem to swing wildly from one extreme to the other for no apparent reason. Yet the truth is that there are some basic nutrition recommendations that can make a difference in health and quality of life.

Often, people come into my office complaining of long-standing fatigue that is not quite as disabling as the fatigue seen in chronic fatigue syndrome or fibromyalgia. I never cease to be amazed at how often these people improve dramatically by simply altering their diets—cutting down on sugar, caffeine, and alcohol intake; substituting whole grains for white flour; and adding simple yet powerful nutritional support to their daily regimens. So let us start with the easy things first.

Caffeine and Alcohol

I am constantly astonished at the number of people who drink more than three cups of coffee a day while complaining about being tired. Caffeine is a loan shark for energy, and also accentuates hypoglycemic symptoms. Many chronic fatigue patients fall into the trap of drinking ever-increasing amounts of coffee to boost their energy so that they can function. What these people do not realize is that as the day goes on, caffeine takes away more energy, than it gives. Coffee drinkers are often caught in a vicious cycle. I advise all such people to stop ingesting coffee completely for two to three months. After this initial period, I tell them that they can add back up to eight ounces of coffee a day if they are feeling better. However, black and green teas, in leaf and tea bag forms, are high in antioxidants, and are much more healthful than coffee. It is okay to drink one to two cups of brewed tea a day (not the sugar-loaded tea in bottles) to get your caffeine kick.

If you drink more than three cups of coffee a day, you should remove it from your diet gradually. To begin, cut your coffee consumption in half every week until you are down to about one cup a day. For example, if you generally drink four cups of coffee a day, cut your intake to two cups a day the first week, then to one cup a day the second week. The final week, continue with one cup a day or switch to caffeinated tea, which contains many antioxidants that improve your health.

Caffeine is an addictive drug, and removing it from the diet brings withdrawal symptoms—grouchiness, headache, and fatigue. Once the symptoms are gone, however, my patients usually feel much better and are happy that they went through the process. By tapering the coffee as just described, it takes a little longer to feel well, but the withdrawal symptoms are not as severe.

In addition to eliminating coffee from your diet, limit alcohol to one to three drinks a day. One drink equals six ounces of wine, twelve ounces of beer, or one and a half ounces of whiskey. If you drink more than these amounts, you should stop drinking alcohol completely for three months. If you decide to return alcohol to your diet at the end of that time, make three drinks a day your limit. Some people with yeast overgrowth find that even the smallest amount of alcohol makes them feel bad.

Sugar and White Flour

The average American's diet includes more than 140 pounds of added sugar per year.[1] This added sugar accounts for 18 percent of their caloric intake. The added sugar alone makes the typical American diet a disaster.

Sugar suppresses the immune system and stimulates yeast overgrowth in the intestines. Yeast grows by fermenting sugar, and the yeast say thankyou for eating sugar by making billions of baby yeasties. Physicians working in this field have found that although most sugar is usually absorbed before it gets to the intestines, excess sugar can still markedly aggravate yeast overgrowth.[2] Yeast can also aggravate sugar craving. This may mimic hypoglycemia, which is commonly found in people with underactive adrenal glands.

Another dietary disaster is white flour. In the United States, approximately 18 percent of the average person's calories come from white flour, which, just like white rice, has had the brown outer shell, or bran, removed. The bran, however, contains most of the vitamins and minerals that are present in rice.[3] Although some foods made of white flour are now fortified with vitamins and minerals to make up for this, most of the nutrients that were removed continue to be missing.

From just the use of white flour and added sugar, Americans often reduce their vitamin and mineral intake by around 35 percent. Add to this the nutrients that are lost in the canning of vegetables, which can cause vitamin losses of up to 80 percent, and in the processing of other foods, and you have a serious problem.[4, 5] As Dr. S. B. Eaton noted in his study in the *New England Journal of Medicine:* "Physicians and nutritionists are increasingly convinced that the dietary habits adopted by Western society over the past one hundred years make an important etiologic [causative] contribution to coronary heart diseases [angina], hypertension, diabetes, and some types of cancer."[6]

Vitamin and Mineral Supplements

The argument that the average modern American does not need vitamin tablets is simply not valid. One study that was reported in the *American Journal of Clinical Nutrition* showed that fewer than 5 percent of the study participants consumed the recommended daily amounts (RDAs) of all the needed vitamins and minerals.[7] What is frightening is that this study was conducted on U.S. Department of Agriculture (USDA) research center employees, people who would be especially aware of proper nutrition.

In the United States, nutritional deficiencies are a major problem and a key contributor to creating disabilities. A study out of Cornell University notes: "Low serum concentrations of vitamins B_6 and B_{12} and selenium predict subsequent disability . . . in older women living in the community. Nutritional status is one of the key factors to be considered in the development of strategies aimed at preventing or delaying the disablement process."[8] In addition, among overweight or obese men and women, long-term use of multivitamins, vitamin B_6, vitamin B_{12}, and chromium were significantly associated with lower levels of weight gain. Getting optimal nutrient levels can also even help you keep your teeth.[9]

Despite this, some physicians still like to say that vitamins are excreted in your urine, so all you're doing by taking vitamin supplements is making expensive urine. Using this line of reasoning, these cynics can stop drinking water (it just goes out in their urine). That way, they'll soon stop annoying people who are in the process of getting themselves well. The truth is, nutritional support is critical, even if the nutrients are excreted after they've done their job.

Patients often ask me what vitamins or minerals they need. The answer is that all of them are critical. The body depends on receiving vitamins and minerals from the diet because it cannot make them itself. If you are low in vitamins and minerals—whether it is because you are not taking in the required nutrients or because you are consuming the proper foods but your body is unable to metabolize them correctly—your CFS and fibromyalgia simply will not subside. In addition, higher levels than normal are often needed to compensate for the poor absorption of nutrients caused by the bowel infections, as well as the increased needs that result from the illness. For example, as discussed on page 178, optimal zinc levels are critical for proper immune function, and zinc deficiency contributes to the immune dysfunction in CFS/FMS. Chronic infections (due to immune dysfunction) result in large zinc losses, which then further suppress immune function, resulting in more infections and zinc losses. An excellent multivitamin supplement is therefore critical to your improvement.

Why are vitamins and minerals so important? Janet Travell, White House physician for Presidents John F. Kennedy and Lyndon B. Johnson and professor emeritus of internal medicine at George Washington University, cowrote *Myofascial Pain and Dysfunction: The Trigger Point Manual*, which is acknowledged as the authoritative work on muscle pain. In one chapter alone, coauthors Dr. Travell and Dr. David Simons reference 317 studies showing that problems such as hormonal, vitamin, and mineral deficiencies can contribute to muscle pain.[10]

Because each nutrient is critical to health, it is helpful to understand the roles that they play. In this chapter, I give you a nutrition primer, which reviews the key nutrients you should be getting from your diet and their optimal amounts. Don't panic! As you read this, realize that almost all of the nutrients can be obtained in one drink and one capsule daily. The exceptions include iron, which is toxic if you are not deficient; calcium, which blocks thyroid absorption and which most people do not need; and fish oil, which cannot be mixed with water. This one-drink, one-capsule regimen has been formulated to keep it inexpensive and easy so that you can get all of these, without being part of the "handful club" (where you take handfuls of supplements all day). You're probably already taking ribose supplementation to stimulate your energy production, and you may find that other natural supplements recommended throughout this book should also be added. To keep your daily supplement regimen as simple as possible, I suggest that you follow the nutritional supplement recommendations in this chapter first (plus ribose), then add other supplements as necessary during treatment for CFS/FMS.

In addition, for credibility's sake, I have a policy of not taking money from any supplement or pharmaceutical companies, and 100 percent of the royalties from my products (including this one) go to charity.

For simplicity, I do recommend the Energy Revitalization System vitamin powder and B complex capsule made by Enzymatic Therapy and also by ITI (Integrative Therapeutics, which sells through health practitioners), as this single drink and capsule replaces more than thirty-five supplement pills. I did help create this product; however, as noted above, my royalties are donated to charity.

In fact, I lecture frequently to more than four hundred of the world's leading nutritional experts at the International and American Association of Clinical Nutritionists (IAACN) annual conference, and I put out the challenge that if any of them can get what's in the one drink and capsule in less than thirty-five capsules, I'd give them fifty dollars (multiplied by four hundred attendees, my risk was twenty thousand dollars). No one has managed to do it yet, and these are experts. Try it yourself. It usually takes fifty-plus capsules (see Appendix E: Resources for further information).

Because the Energy Revitalization System is a powder, it can be taken many ways. Some like to add it to yogurt. Others add the orange-flavored form (my wife's favorite) to four ounces of orange juice and four ounces of milk so that it tastes like an orange smoothie. Others like the berry flavor (my favorite) and simply stir it in water to avoid the sugar in fruit juices. If hand mixing it instead of using a blender, know that the best way to mix powders is to put the powder in a dry glass, add two to three ounces of whatever liquid you're using, give it a few stirs till any lumps are gone, and then add the rest of the liquid. It's the most worthwhile ten seconds you'll spend each day.

The main side effects caused by multivitamins that give optimal nutritional support are gas, diarrhea, or an upset stomach, which occur in a small percentage of people. If this is a problem for you, try taking the vitamin powder or any other multivitamin that you take with a meal or at bedtime, or split it and take a quarter to half of the dose two times a day. If using the powder, half a scoop daily is plenty for most people for maintenance (even though the box says one scoop daily), so adjust it to the dose that feels best to you. The other side effect you may notice is that any supplement containing B vitamins will turn your urine bright yellow. This is normal and not something to worry about. The vitamin powder is safe for long-term use and is recommended for those with or without CFS/FMS. If, however, you have kidney failure or are on dialysis, any supplementation that includes magnesium should only be used under the careful supervision of your doctor. The Energy Revitalization System vitamin powder is available in most health food stores and at www.vitality101.com.

In addition, Chapter 2, "Create Your Individual Treatment Protocol—Beginning with Ribose for Energy Production," discussed other key, specialized nutrients that can powerfully boost energy production. These often can be stopped after four to nine months, although many people choose to take some of them long term as well.

Whether you choose to use the Energy Revitalization System vitamin powder or wish to develop your own supplement regimen, it's important to recognize which nutrients are critical to your health and why you should take them.

ANTIOXIDANTS

Although necessary for life, oxygen can be incredibly toxic. In fact, the greatest mass extinction in the history of the planet occurred when algae began to grow in the seas, generating large amounts of oxygen. This oxygen production led to high amounts of "free radicals" in the atmosphere, which set up ongoing, self-sustaining chain reactions of molecular damage. It is estimated that this overabundance of oxygen and the subsequent production of oxygen free radicals drove more than 95 percent of animal species then living into extinction. Antioxidants end these chain reactions and are critical to life. Species that developed antioxidant defense systems actually learned to thrive on oxygen. These same antioxidants are critical to your health today, and have been shown to be deficient in CFS/FMS patients.

Research has shown that people with CFS/FMS are under severely increased oxidative stress.[11] In fact, noted CFS expert Dr. Paul Cheney believes that a major component of chronic fatigue syndrome stems from the heart muscle working poorly because of inadequate energy production. He theorizes that this occurs because the body's mitochondrial energy furnaces (see Chapter 2) are unable to adequately handle oxygen free radicals and therefore shut down energy production. One antioxidant, called glutathione, is especially critical. This has also been supported by the work of Rich Van Konynenburg, Ph.D., who proposes a number of triggers for glutathione depletion. I have long respected Rich as being a leading thinker in CFS, and have added more-detailed information on his theories and the importance of antioxidants in the *From Fatigued to Fantastic!* notes at www.vitality101.com.

Although supplementation can be critical, there are even more fun ways to get your antioxidants. This is why when I recommend avoiding sugar to inhibit yeast overgrowth, I also add the three magic words "except for chocolate!" Chocolate, especially dark chocolate, contains high levels of antioxidants, as well as a natural mood enhancer. According to the results of a study conducted at Cornell University, the concentration of cancer-fighting antioxidants in hot cocoa was significantly higher than those in red wine, green tea, or black tea.

Chocolate's Sweet-Natured Side Effect

Chocolate has other benefits that go beyond its antioxidant power. According to a study at the University of Helsinki, in Finland, children born to women who regularly ate chocolate during their pregnancies were more likely to be "sweet natured." Researchers asked three hundred pregnant women to track their stress levels and chocolate consumption. When their children were six months old, their moms were surveyed on their babies' behaviors. The results showed that babies born to stressed women who ate chocolate daily smiled more frequently, laughed more often, and showed less fear of new situations than babies of stressed women who did not indulge in chocolate. Taking high levels of antioxidants during pregnancy also decreases the risk of the baby having asthma.[12] I guess that eating chocolate is simply a sacrifice that we need to make for our children.

In addition to being critical for the production of energy, antioxidants also seem to be very important for maintaining health and youth. In fact, doctors who specialize in "antiaging medicine" use antioxidants as key tools. In men, taking even low-dose antioxidants (120 milligrams ascorbic acid, 30 units vitamin E, 6 milligrams beta-carotene, 100 micrograms selenium, and 20 milligrams zinc versus a placebo daily for an average of 7.5 years) prolonged life dramatically.[13] Antioxidants protect against stomach cancer,[14] help in the treatment of liver disease,[15] are associated with a decreased risk of hip fractures,[16] and may protect against strokes.

VITAMIN C (500 MILLIGRAMS A DAY)

The antioxidant vitamin C is well known as a critical nutrient, being important for proper immune, adrenal, and antioxidant function. In addition, the antioxidant vitamin C can decrease hearing loss,[17] and it is estimated that three hundred thousand cases of macular degeneration (35 percent of cases), a leading cause of blindness, could be prevented simply by supplementation with antioxidants and zinc.[18,19] Vitamins C and E also help prevent osteoporosis,[21] and vitamin C may protect against developing angina or strokes[22] while also making it easier to lose weight.[23] Vitamin C also helps improve sperm count and motility, and can be helpful in treating infertility[24] (see the Web site notes on pregnancy and infertility at www.vitality101.com). With sperm counts dropping dramatically around the planet, it could be that natural selection will mean that only those taking their supplements will eventually be able to reproduce.

And, proving conventional wisdom right once again, vitamin C actually does make you less likely to catch a cold. In one study, people taking 500 milligrams of vitamin C daily had 18 percent fewer colds than those in the 50-milligrams-a-day group.[25] To protect against illness and optimize your health as discussed above, I recommend that you get at least 500 milligrams of vitamin C per day.

VITAMIN E (100 UNITS A DAY)

This critical antioxidant serves many functions, but taking more of any one antioxidant is not always better. Many nutrients, such as beta-carotene, are part of a larger "family," so taking very high doses of only one type can actually suppress the others and become problematic. This is also the case with vitamin E, as there are many types of vitamin E in the tocopherol family. Research suggests that taking more than 150 units a day can cause this suppression,[26] so I recommend taking 100 units a day as the optimal level in multivitamins. If you are taking higher levels to treat a specific problem, take it for only a few months and use natural vitamin E (mixed tocopherols), which contains all of the different types of vitamin E. Although more is not better, deficiency is a significant problem.[27]

Vitamin E in optimal doses (about 100 units a day) may also be cancer protective. Two studies presented at the 2004 annual meeting of the American Association of Cancer Research found that people who had a high intake of dietary vitamin E or who had high levels in their bloodstream were the least likely to have cancer. In one of the studies, vitamin E supplements in addition to a vitamin E–rich diet lowered the risk of bladder cancer. In the other, men with the most vitamin E in their systems had the lowest risk of prostate cancer. This was also discussed in another study, published in the *Journal of the National Cancer Institute*, where high blood levels of vitamin E cut the risk of prostate cancer by about 50 percent,[28] and a third study that showed that vitamin E caused prostate cancer cells to "self-destruct."[29] Adequate intake of vitamin E may also decrease the risk of breast cancer.[30]

The cancer-protection benefit is not the only reason to take vitamin E, and it's important to maintain optimal antioxidant support as you age. In a study on 1,033 people sixty-five and older, low plasma levels of vitamin E were found to be associated with a more than doubled risk of dementia and of suffering from cognitive impairment.[31]

Although there are many other antioxidants (and I discuss them in the following sections), simply looking at vitamins C and E gives us an idea of their importance. Each of the nutrients below is very important and the *From Fatigued to Fantastic!* notes at www.vitality101.com discusses each of them in depth. I invite you to read that information as well. In the sections below, I focus on the nutrients' importance in CFS/FMS, while briefly listing some of their other benefits and noting the recommended daily amount after each nutrient.

Other Vitamins

VITAMIN A (3,500 IU A DAY)

Vitamin A is critical for mucosal immunity and zinc function, but be careful not to get too much. The risk of fetal birth defects can increase in pregnant women taking more than 8,000 units a day, and higher dosing of vitamin A can also aggravate osteoporosis. At doses of more than 50,000 units a day, vitamin A can even cause liver injury, so I would only use doses higher than 8,000 units daily under the supervision of a holistic practitioner. Higher doses may be used by your practitioner to treat two problems often seen in CFS/FMS: acne, which is associated with low vitamin A levels[32] and which improves with high-dose vitamin A plus zinc (which augments vitamin A activity), and heavy menstrual periods during perimenopause. Called dysfunctional uterine bleeding (DUB), this bleeding often resolves without the need for a hysterectomy when patients take 50,000 units of vitamin A (with 25 milligrams of zinc) daily for three months. It is, of course, important to also treat low thyroid and iron levels, which are two other and more common causes of heavy periods.

BETA-CAROTENE (3,500 IU A DAY)

One of a large family of carotenoids (found in carrots), beta-carotene is the main one added to supplements. In proper dosing it can be helpful, and higher doses (to a point) are associated with increased longevity.[33] However, like vitamin E, beta-carotene is part of a larger "family," and taking very high doses of only one type can suppress the others and become problematic. For example, taking 25,000 units a day was associated with an increased risk of lung cancer. So more is not always better. Taking 3,500 units a day can keep you healthy—without this increased risk.

BIOFLAVONOIDS (500 MILLIGRAMS A DAY)

There are many members of this family, which can be found in the white part of citrus fruits just below the peel. They are important for blood vessel integrity and immune function. A high intake of flavonoids has been shown to lower heart attack risk,[34] and 500 milligrams a day of the quercitin form decreases the symptoms of prostatitis.

B Vitamins

These are especially critical for energy production, and the RDAs are inadequate for those with CFS/FMS. B vitamins are also important for immunity, nerve and brain function, and much more. Using high but safe doses is important.

B₁ (75 MILLIGRAMS A DAY)—THIAMINE

Vitamin B₁ is critical for proper brain functioning, making it especially important for those with brain fog. It is also critical for heart function, which in CFS patients suffers because of decreased energy production. In fact, a major cause of death in the United States is congestive heart failure, which is one symptom of vitamin B₁ deficiency. Although 33 percent of people with congestive heart failure are low in thiamine,[35] this easy treatment aid is often ignored. Thiamine is also used therapeutically in dementia, anxiety, neuropathy, fatigue, alcoholism, confusion, depression, pain, memory loss, and disequilibrium.

In a double-blind study by Dr. David Benton, an expert on thiamine, supplementation with vitamin B_1 improved mood, possibly by increasing synthesis of acetylcholine, a neurotransmitter that is associated with memory.[36] Deficiency of this neurotransmitter has also been suspected to occur in CFS, and supplementation with choline (see page 180) can also be helpful. Dr. Benton also found that giving 50 milligrams a day of thiamine (versus placebo) was associated with reports of being more clearheaded, composed, and energetic. These influences took place in subjects whose thiamine status, according to traditional criteria, was adequate.[37] Interestingly, symptoms of thiamine deficiency can mimic symptoms often seen in CFS/FMS, including:

- Increased auditory, tactile, or visual perceptions, which are acute enough to be unpleasant
- Rapid pulse, unusual sweating, and abdominal pain with or without diarrhea
- Sense of panic/anxiety and fear
- Mitral valve prolapse, premenstrual syndrome, temporomandibular syndrome, and irritable bowel syndrome[38]

Thiamine may also have antiviral effects in addition to improving cognitive function.[39]

B_2—RIBOFLAVIN (75 MILLIGRAMS A DAY)

This B vitamin is especially critical for energy production. In higher doses of 75 to 400 milligrams a day, it has been repeatedly shown to decrease migraine frequency (a common problem in CFS/FMS) by 67 percent after six to twelve weeks. Vitamin B_2 even helps decrease the risk of postpartum depression.[40]

B_3—NIACIN (50 MILLIGRAMS A DAY)

Niacin is also critical for energy production, being a key part of the energy molecule NADH, which also helps make the neurotransmitter dopamine. Niacin may also prevent Alzheimer's. A five-year study of more than 3,700 people published in the *Journal of Neurology, Neurosurgery, and Psychiatry* showed an inverse relationship between niacin intake and both Alzheimer's disease and age-related mental decline. While some benefits were noted to begin at 17 milligrams per day, a daily niacin intake of 45 milligrams offered the most protection from Alzheimer's disease and other causes of cognitive decline.[41] High doses over decades also seem to decrease the progression of arthritis.

PANTOTHENIC ACID (50 MILLIGRAMS A DAY)

Pantothenic acid and its cousin pantethine play many key roles in the body. Most importantly in CFS and fibromyalgia, pantothenic acid is critical for proper adrenal gland function. In addition, pantethine is also critical for proper handling of fats.[42]

B_6—PYRIDOXINE (85 MILLIGRAMS A DAY)

Vitamin B_6 (pyridoxine) serves many critical functions, including enhancing immune function[43] and decreasing the risk of heart disease[44] and colon cancer.[45]

I have also found that the fluid retention seen in CFS/FMS often improves with vitamin B_6 at a dose of about 200 to 250 milligrams a day—especially if you also optimize thyroid hormone levels. This has implications way beyond the rings on your fingers being too tight. For example, B_6 at a dose of 250 milligrams a day is very helpful in alleviating carpal tunnel syndrome (CTS), a common condition in CFS/FMS that is linked with fluid retention. The book *Pain Free 1–2–3* gives information on how to treat carpal tunnel syndrome simply and without surgery.

B_{12} (500 TO 1000 MICROGRAMS A DAY)

Vitamin B_{12} is another key nutrient in CFIDS. Technically, the B_{12} level is considered normal if it is over 208 picograms per deciliter (pg/dL) of blood. However, studies have shown that this "normal" level may be much, much too low. People can suffer severe and sometimes long-term nerve and brain damage from B_{12} deficiency even if their levels are 300 pg/dL[46] and signs of B_{12} deficiency sometimes occur with levels higher than 500 pg/dL.[47]

Why are the "normal" levels set so low? In part because the normal values were initially set according to what prevents anemia. But the brain's and nervous system's needs for vitamin B_{12} are often much higher than the levels needed to prevent anemia. Also, as much as I hate to admit it, the medical establishment has greatly enjoyed poking fun at the old-time doctors who gave vitamin B_{12} shots for fatigue. The use of B_{12} shots despite "normal" levels is considered almost a symbol of unscientific, archaic medicine. As noted in an editorial in the *New England Journal of Medicine*, however, current findings suggest that those old-time doctors might have been right.[48]

Other studies suggest that many people need significantly higher B_{12} levels than what is currently considered normal.[49] More importantly, recent research shows that despite their having normal B_{12} levels in the blood, CFIDS patients often have very low and sometimes absent B_{12} levels in their brains.[50] This suggests that because of the metabolic problems present in CFIDS/FMS, you may need quite high B_{12} levels in your blood to get adequate levels past the blood-brain barrier (the membrane that separates the brain from the blood to protect the brain from circulating toxins) and into the brain, where B_{12} is needed.

One benefit of vitamin B_{12} is that it helps reduce excessive levels of nitric oxide, a neurotransmitter that can be too high in people with CFIDS/ FMS and that can easily contribute to symptoms. More and more, research studies are supporting what doctors who effectively treat CFIDS/ FMS using B_{12} shots have said for years. Whatever the cause, I have found that treating patients with vitamin B_{12}, even if their levels are technically normal, often results in marked improvement in both energy and mental clarity. This is good, as vitamin B_{12} is both very safe and cheap, and using high doses can be critical in CFS/FMS.

The Importance of Vitamin B_{12}

Why is a low B_{12} level such a common problem in CFIDS patients? Several possibilities exist. Among them are the following:

- Vitamin B_{12} has trouble getting across the blood-brain barrier.[50]
- Nitric oxide excess is suspected in CFS, and B_{12} is a nitric oxide scavenger. For more information on this, see the article by Professor Martin Pall in the Web site notes section.
- Vitamin B_{12} is important for the repair of nerve injuries. Evidence suggests that brain dysfunction occurs in CFIDS. In repairing this injury, the body may overutilize vitamin B_{12} and deplete its stores.
- If an autoimmune process impairs the thyroid or adrenal glands, it may also attack the area responsible for our ability to absorb vitamin B_{12}.

- Overgrowth of yeast, bacterial infections, or parasites in the bowel causing problems with absorption may prevent the proper absorption of vitamin B_{12}.
- Vitamin B_{12} may be important for, and used up in, detoxification.

It is no surprise then, when their other problems are also treated, that many people respond dramatically to B_{12} injections. If your B_{12} level is under 540 pg/ml, your doctor may want to start treatment with a 1-cc (1,000- to 3,000-microgram) injection one to five times a week, giving at least fifteen total injections. These shots are safe and fairly inexpensive. Although most regular pharmacies carry only the 1,000-microgram-per-cc strength, holistic pharmacies (see Appendix E: Resources) can make up injectable vitamin B_{12} that contains 3,000 micrograms per cc. The methylcobalamin form of B_{12} is best (or if cost is an issue, hydroxycobalamin) when taking high-dose injections. If you are going to benefit from the shots, you'll see improvement by ten weeks. If you feel worse when the injections are stopped, your doctor may resume the shots, usually every one to five weeks (but as often as daily in some cases) for an extended period of time. Most people, however, can maintain their B_{12} level after fifteen injections by taking the Energy Revitalization System or by supplementing with 500 micrograms B_{12} per day.

In addition to directly addressing CFS/FMS, vitamin B_{12} helps other problems such as:

- Depression
- Neuropsychiatric disorders such as mental confusion, memory changes, cognitive slowing, mood disorders, violent behavior, fatigue, delirium, and paranoid psychosis[51]
- Osteoporosis[52]
- The risk of stroke[53]
- Increased blood clotting[54]—a problem that is common in CFS (see Chapter 5)
- Breast cancer risk[55]

FOLIC ACID (800 MICROGRAMS A DAY)

The dosage recommended here is the highest that can legally be added to a vitamin, as there is a concern that folate could mask vitamin B_{12} deficiency—which is not a problem if the supplement also has high levels of

B_{12}. Optimal levels of folic acid (folate) are critical in CFS/FMS because of its role in immune function, and it can also improve memory. In fact, it may be critical in preventing Alzheimer's dementia.[56, 57] In addition, it is critical in methylation reactions, which are impaired in CFS/FMS.

The benefits of folate begin early in life. Folic acid is known to protect against serious neural tube birth defects that develop in the earliest weeks of pregnancy, such as spina bifida, in which parts of the brain or spinal cord don't develop properly. For this reason, doctors recommend that women who are pregnant or trying to get pregnant take a vitamin supplement that includes folic acid. Interestingly, since food makers began adding extra folate to flour in 1998 to prevent birth defects, the rates of heart disease, stroke, blood pressure, colon cancer, and osteoporosis have all fallen, suggesting that the general public may have been folate deficient. Folate may also decrease the risk of ovarian cancer.[58]

BIOTIN (200 MICROGRAMS A DAY)

Biotin is a cofactor for a number of enzyme reactions, but seems especially important for healthy hair, skin, and nails. People with CFS/FMS often suffer from hair loss, dull skin tone, and brittle nails. It may take a year for improvement in these areas, but many people are thrilled when their nails and hair have become strong and healthy along with the rest of their body.

VITAMIN D (600 TO 4,000 IU A DAY)

The importance of vitamin D deficiency is finally gaining increasing attention. This nutrient deficiency is critical, causing tens of thousands of unnecessary deaths in the United States each year. Because of this, and the deadly recommendation to avoid being out in the sun without sunscreen, I am going to cover the importance of this nutrient in depth.

Vitamin D deficiency is common. In fact, a review in the *Mayo Clinic Journal* showed that approximately 36 percent of healthy young adults and 57 percent of general medicine inpatients in the United States have inadequate levels of the vitamin,[59] and deficiency is even more common in people with chronic pain.

This problem has increased ever since skin cancer awareness prompted many to forgo sunshine. The misguided advice from well-meaning doctors and media outlets was given to decrease the number of dangerous skin cancers called melanomas—a worthy goal. However, 90 percent of our vitamin D comes from the sun, and the skin cancers usually caused by sunshine (e.g., basal cell cancers) are usually benign and easy to treat. In fact, most melanomas are not in sun-exposed areas; they develop on skin covered by clothing. It is likely that the increase in melanomas is mostly occurring because of changes in diet, environment, and sleep, which are resulting in weakened immune systems. A good rule to remember is to avoid sunburn, not sunshine.

Many other cancers increase in the face of vitamin D deficiency. It is currently estimated that the advice to avoid sunshine is resulting in as many as eighty-five thousand unnecessary cancer deaths each year.[60] To give a few examples, increasing vitamin D levels is associated with:

- A decrease in lymphomas and leukemia (malignant white blood cell cancers)[61–64]
- A fifty percent decrease in breast and colon cancer risk[65–67]
- A lower prostate cancer risk[68]
- Lung cancer protection[69]
- A thirty percent drop in ovarian cancer[70]

In addition to causing upward of eighty-five thousand unnecessary cancer deaths each year, vitamin D deficiency contributes to weak bones and osteoporosis. Vitamin D is low in 98 percent of the elderly who break a hip, a major cause of these people losing mobility and therefore being in nursing homes.[71, 72] Vitamin D deficiency in pregnant women actually increases the risk of their children developing osteoporosis.[73, 74]

Vitamin D deficiency is also wreaking havoc in many other ways. Vitamin D is critical in regulating immune function, and a deficiency is implicated in multiple sclerosis, rheumatoid arthritis,[75] inflammatory bowel disease,[76] and diabetes.[77–81] Treatment with vitamin D can also improve lung function and help people with asthma,[82–85] while also decreasing the risk of heart disease[86] and stroke.[87]

This leaves the question of what level of supplementation is optimal. I concur with Dr. Heike A. Bischoff-Ferrari of the Harvard School of Public Health, who notes: "Recent evidence suggests that vitamin D intakes above current recommendations may be associated with better health outcomes. . . . An intake for all adults of [at least] 1,000 IU of vitamin D/day is needed."[88, 89]

VITAMIN K

Although vitamin K plays a role in bone health, deficiency does not seem to increase osteoporosis.[90] Because vitamin K stimulates blood clotting, which is already excessive in CFS/FMS patients (see Chapter 5), I do not recommend that those with CFS routinely take vitamin K.

Minerals

BORON (2 TO 3 MILLIGRAMS A DAY)

Boron is helpful in improving bone strength—especially when combined with adequate magnesium. It may also help cognitive function.

CHROMIUM (200 TO 500 MICROGRAMS A DAY)

Chromium (and glutathione) is critical for proper insulin function and preventing diabetes, and can also decrease many of the symptoms of hypoglycemia. It can even be useful in treating some cases of depression, particularly when carbohydrate craving is a prominent symptom. A study of 113 people found that chromium supplements reduced depression-related cravings for sweets and starches, and provided an overall general improvement in depressive symptoms.[91] Some physicians feel that it also helps cause weight loss.

COPPER (500 MICROGRAMS A DAY)

Copper is a double-edged sword. Although critical for antioxidant production (such as super oxide dismutase [SOD], one of the body's natural free-radical scavengers that reduces pain and inflammation), it also is a potent free radical trigger and is quite toxic in excess.[92] To strike an optimal balance, I recommend 0.5 micrograms a day of copper.

IODINE (150 TO 250 MICROGRAMS A DAY)

Optimal levels of iodine are critical for both healthy thyroid and breast tissue function. Iodine deficiency with secondary goiters used to be endemic in the United States until the mineral was added to wheat flour, and to a lesser degree salt. This eliminated much of the problem—until flour makers started adding bromine instead of iodine. This not only resulted in iodine intakes dropping by as much as half in the last decade, but the switch can worsen the effects of iodine deficiency, as bromine may block iodine's function.

One of the main problems caused by iodine deficiency is hypothyroidism, which can cause a host of problems. These include not only fatigue, weight gain, and pain but also infertility and miscarriages.

Iodine deficiency is also a common trigger for breast tenderness and fibrocystic breast disease, and I routinely supplement women who have these problems with iodine. It has even been suggested that seaweed, which is high in iodine, may lower breast cancer risk.[93] In fact, one of the upcoming studies planned by our foundation will be to check iodine, bromine, and fluorine levels (all related chemical "halides," which compete with one another) in tissue samples of women with breast cancer, fibrocystic breast disease, and healthy breasts. We suspect that low iodine, or excessive levels of bromides and fluorides, which may inhibit iodine, are factors that unnecessarily increase breast cancer risk.

MAGNESIUM (200 MILLIGRAMS A DAY)

Magnesium is involved in hundreds of different body functions, and is critically important in CFS/FMS. Unfortunately, the average American diet supplies less than 300 milligrams of magnesium per day, while the average unprocessed (e.g., Asian) diet supplies more than 600 milligrams per day. Magnesium is critical for producing energy in muscles. This means that low magnesium causes muscles to spasm and shorten, and this muscle shortening is a major cause of FMS pain. We frequently see marked pain relief, as well as increases in energy, with IV nutrient infusions that include magnesium. Magnesium is also critical for heart muscle function, and has been shown to improve both exercise endurance and cardiac function [94]—a key player in CFS.

Because of this, if your magnesium level is low, your muscles will stay in spasm and your fibromyalgia will not resolve. This is one of the reasons that taking magnesium is so critical. In addition, magnesium is important for the muscles' and body's strength and energy.[95] Most of your magnesium is inside your cells, but the blood test only measures the magnesium in your blood—making blood tests an unreliable measure. I suspect that magnesium has trouble getting into the cells in people with CFS/FMS. When CFS/FMS is properly treated, the magnesium may be better able to get inside the cells. The cells then soak it up like a thirsty sponge and your blood level may even drop—despite taking large amounts of oral and even intravenous magnesium. So keep in mind that magnesium blood tests do not drop below normal until severe magnesium depletion occurs,[96] and everyone with CFS/FMS, fatigue, or muscle achiness should take magnesium. An exception is if you have kidney failure with a blood creatinine level over 1.6 milligrams per deciliter (mg/dL)—very rare in CFS/FMS. Your doctor can help you determine whether supplemental magnesium places you at risk.

I generally recommend taking 200 to 450 milligrams of magnesium glycinate in conjunction with 1,800 milligrams of malic acid (discussed in Chapter 2) a day for eight months, and then cutting back to 200 milligrams a day of magnesium. If diarrhea and cramps are not a problem, you can take up to twice this amount. If you get diarrhea from the magnesium, cut the dosage back and then slowly increase it as is comfortable. Magnesium absorption is very difficult, which is why I like to use the glycinate forms.

Let's discuss some of the key functions of magnesium.

- Magnesium is critical for life. For example, one study showed that subjects who were in the highest 25 percent of serum magnesium values had a 40 percent decreased risk of dying during the study, with a 40 percent decrease in cardiovascular mortality and a 50 percent decrease in cancer deaths, compared to subjects whose magnesium levels were in the lowest 25 percent of the population.[97]
- Magnesium helps build bones, regulate body temperature, produce proteins, and release energy stored in muscles. Because of the latter, magnesium deficiency causes muscle spasm/shortening, contributing markedly to fibromyalgia, migraine headaches, and other pains.
- Magnesium deficiency likely contributes to brain fog. A study by Massachusetts Institute of Technology researchers found that magnesium helps regulate a key brain receptor that plays an important role in learning and memory. The finding indicates that magnesium deficiency may result in reduced ability to learn and memorize, while cognitive function may be improved by an abundance of magnesium.[98]

- Magnesium deficiency also contributes to obesity by causing insulin resistance. The average weight gain in CFS is 32.5 pounds, and this weight gain often triggers sleep apnea. Preventing insulin resistance, then, is one more benefit of magnesium supplementation.[99] Also, people with high magnesium intakes followed over fifteen years had a 31 percent lower chance of developing metabolic syndrome—a major cause of heart disease,[100] as well as a decreased risk of developing diabetes.[101]

Magnesium also:

- Helps protect against osteoporosis.[102, 103]
- Is associated with decreased inflammation levels (C-reactive protein, [CRP]), offering further heart protection.[104]
- Is associated with a 23 percent lower risk of colon cancer.[105]
- Improves asthma.[106]
- Decreases the frequency of migraine headaches.[107, 108] In fact, the quickest and most effective way to eliminate a migraine headache is by giving 2 grams of magnesium IV over five to ten minutes.
- Helps children with hyperactivity and attention deficit disorder when combined with vitamin B_6.[109]

For patients with CFS/FMS, magnesium (along with B vitamins and D-ribose) represents the most critical nutritional need.

MOLYBDENUM (250 MICROGRAMS A DAY)

This mineral can be helpful for those with allergies, especially for those with sensitivities to the sulfites found in wine. It may also help detoxify acetaldehydes, which are made by yeast.

SELENIUM (200 MICROGRAMS A DAY)

Selenium is critical for optimal immune function. This is important to both eliminate the many infections seen in CFS/FMS, and to prevent cancer.[110–112] Selenium is an antioxidant, and deficiency is associated with a shorter life, thyroid deficiencies, and immune dysfunction.[113] In fact, low selenium is one of the problems that causes an underactive thyroid with normal blood tests, as it is critical for converting inactive thyroid to the active form, which is not measured on the tests.

ZINC (15 TO 25 MILLIGRAMS A DAY)

Zinc, which has been shown to be deficient in FMS, is critical for optimal immune and antioxidant function. Recurrent infections cause high zinc losses, which then further weaken immune function.

Zinc may also help with cognitive function, especially when taken with stimulants that can help in CFS. One study gave forty-four children with ADHD either 55 milligrams of zinc or a placebo each day for six weeks along with Ritalin (which I think is overused in ADD and underused in CFS). While the behavior of all of the children improved during the study, those who had taken zinc had a more marked improvement. The study's authors believe that zinc may play a role in regulating the production of dopamine in the brain, which is associated with feelings of pleasure and reward and which has been linked to ADHD by other scientists. Dopamine is often low in CFS/FMS, and there is reason to believe zinc supplementation will be of marked benefit in these disorders as well.[114]

Amino Acids

Amino acid supplementation, especially with whey protein, has many benefits. Using partially denatured whey protein has been shown to increase glutathione production and has been helpful in CFS. In a study conducted at James Madison University in Virginia and reported in the journal *Medicine & Science in Sports & Exercise*, whey protein also increased endurance and decreased the muscle wear and tear that comes with intense exercise.[115] Whey protein also coats harmful bacteria, preventing them from adhering to the gut wall, where they can be infectious.

Although all of the amino acids are important, I will focus on the ones that are most critical in CFS/FMS. As is the case with most nutrients, optimal levels are good (and likely better than the RDA), but more is not always better. The vitamin powder has more than 7,500 milligrams of amino acids.

ARGININE (100 TO 200 MILLIGRAMS A DAY)

This key amino acid is another double-edged sword. Although it may help raise growth hormone, which would be beneficial in most CFS/FMS patients, arginine can also raise nitric oxide, which is postulated by Professor Martin Pall to be too high in CFS (for more on his theories see the notes at www.vitality101.com). My main concern with arginine is that it promotes the growth of some viruses in the herpes family, and therefore may also stimulate HHV–6 and Epstein-Barr viral growth. Therefore, I recommend that only the low levels recommended here be used in supplements for CFS/FMS.

METHIONINE (100 TO 300 MILLIGRAMS A DAY)

Although the amino acid methionine is a key part of the production of SAMe (a nutrient that is helpful in CFS/FMS), high levels seem to paradoxically decrease SAMe production and may also be associated with an increased heart attack risk.[116] Therefore, I recommend that only the low levels recommended here be added to supplements.

N-ACETYL-CYSTEINE (NAC)
(250 TO 650 MILLIGRAMS A DAY)

NAC is critical for making a key antioxidant called glutathione and for keeping vitamins C and E in their active forms. It has been speculated that glutathione deficiency may be a major root cause of CFS. Although taking glutathione by mouth has no effect on blood levels (it simply gets digested), taking NAC, glutamine (1,000 milligrams a day, which also helps bowel healing), and glycine (500 to 1,000 milligrams a day) plus vitamin C can markedly increase glutathione levels. Supplementing these three amino acids is especially important in CFS, as NAC, glutamine, and glycine levels can decrease by 30 to 50 percent in this disorder. For NAC, I recommend 650 to 1,000 milligrams daily for three to four months and then 250 milligrams a day for maintenance. Low glutathione levels may contribute to your immune dysfunction, including low "natural killer cell" activity, as glutathione protects your immune system from harm.

NAC has other benefits as well. In one study, taking high-dose NAC increased time to muscle fatigue by 30 percent while preventing a drop in glutathione.[117] It may even help to protect the heart muscle during a heart attack.[118] Antioxidant supplementation that includes NAC at doses of 600 to 3,000 milligrams a day may even significantly decrease symptoms of obsessive-compulsive disorder,[119, 120] which can trigger CFS/FMS. NAC also plays a role in detoxification. For three months, I would take 500 to 650 milligrams of extra NAC in addition to the 250 milligrams in the powder.

SERINE (500 TO 1,000 MILLIGRAMS A DAY)

In one study presented at the Myopain Research Conference in Italy, 500 milligrams a day significantly decreased symptoms of FMS. It supports antioxidant, brain, and immune function.

TAURINE (500 TO 1,000 MILLIGRAMS A DAY)

Taurine has been shown to increase energy, and can even be found in a few energy drinks. Unfortunately, most of these "energy drinks" largely contain caffeine and sugar—which are loan sharks for energy and should be avoided.

TRYPTOPHAN (100 TO 500 MILLIGRAMS A DAY)

Tryptophan aids the production of serotonin, which is critical for sleep and decreases depression. The law limits how much tryptophan can be added to supplements, since a toxic batch made many years ago in Japan caused a reaction called eosinophilia myalgia syndrome. However, the 100 to 500 milligrams recommended here should be sufficient.

TYROSINE (500 TO 1,000 MILLIGRAMS A DAY)

Tyrosine is critical for the production of adrenaline and dopamine, two neurotransmitters that are often low in CFS.

Cofactors

CHOLINE (100+ MILLIGRAMS A DAY)

This nutrient is critical for brain function and production of the neurotransmitter acetylcholine, which is also often low in CFS.

MALIC ACID (900 TO 1,600 MILLIGRAMS A DAY)

Malic acid is critical for energy production. This becomes especially important when added to magnesium or a powerful energy-producing compound called ribose (see Chapter 2).

INOSITOL (500 TO 1,000 MILLIGRAMS A DAY)

Inositol is a key component of your nerve coverings called the myelin sheath, and losses of inositol in the urine of diabetics likely contributes to their nerve pain and may contribute to fibromyalgia pain as well. Inositol is also helpful in treating anxiety. For CFS, inositol is critical to the production of SAMe, an expensive nutrient that has been shown to be helpful in CFS/FMS, depression, and arthritis. In fact, it has been estimated that combining the nutrients discussed in this chapter (which are in the Energy Revitalization System) results in your body making the equivalent of more than 400 milligrams of SAMe a day—a much more effective and less costly way to get this nutrient.

TRIMETHYLGLYCINE (BETAINE; 750 MILLIGRAMS A DAY)

Betaine acts as a methyl donor, which can be very helpful in CFS and for overall health, and also helps lower elevated homocysteine, a compound associated with increased risk of heart attacks and strokes.

Getting Optimal Nutritional Support Easily

All of the above key nutrients, in optimal levels, can be found in the Energy Revitalization System vitamin powder made by Enzymatic Therapy (see Appendix E: Resources). It has been designed to make optimal nutritional support easy and affordable for everyone, supplying more than thirty-five tablets' worth of nutrients in one drink and one capsule. I recommend you stay on it long term and adjust the dose to the level that feels best to you, using ½ to 1 scoop a day. Of course, you can also put together your own supplement strategy using these recommendations yourself, or in conjunction with a health practitioner.

As mentioned earlier, there are three other nutrients that are helpful in some situations. These are iron, calcium, and fish oil. In Chapter 2 we also discussed key energy nutrients that are used specifically to fire up your body's energy furnaces, especially my favorite new nutrient—ribose.

IRON

Iron is important because an iron level that is too high or too low can cause fatigue, poor immune function, cold intolerance, decreased thyroid function, and poor memory. I routinely recommend that all my chronic fatigue patients have their iron level and total iron binding capacity (TIBC) checked. Although not helpful by themselves, the iron level divided by the TIBC gives you a percent saturation, which is a useful measure. In addition, I recommend that patients have their ferritin blood level checked. These three tests all measure iron status. Some insurance companies balk at paying for all three tests, but the data and my clinical experience strongly support having them all done. Even if a person's iron percent saturation is low but still normal, he or she will often feel fatigued, despite not being anemic. The ferritin level, however, will pick up subtle deficiencies. Unfortunately, even minimal inflammation, such as a bladder infection, will falsely elevate the ferritin measurement, making it appear falsely normal. This is why all three tests are necessary to determine iron deficiency. Your holistic doctor should be able to help you read the results of these tests properly.

Once again, a "normal" iron test does not mean that you have enough iron. For example, one study reported in the British medical journal *The Lancet* showed that infertile females whose ferritin levels were between twenty and forty—a ferritin level over 9 is technically normal—were often able to become pregnant when they took supplemental iron.[121] Other research shows that low-normal iron levels cause poor mental functioning and immune function. This suggests that levels considered sufficient to prevent anemia are often inadequate for other body functions.

Although cosmetic issues may seem small relative to the debilitating nature of CFS, they are still important, as few of us would be happy with the severe hair thinning often seen in CFS/FMS. A review of forty years of research shows that iron deficiency contributes to hair loss and, according to Cleveland Clinic dermatologists, treatment of iron deficiency is important for restoring hair growth. In their opinion, "treatment for hair loss is enhanced when iron deficiency, with or without anemia, is treated."[122]

The Cleveland Clinic isn't alone in this opinion. George Cotsarelis, director of the University of Pennsylvania Hair and Scalp Clinic, has studied iron supplementation in women with various forms of hair loss. Cotsarelis and colleagues have found that women with hair loss have significantly lower iron stores than women without hair loss. Cotsarelis and Trost agree with our recommendations, saying that what most doctors consider a normal ferritin level is, in fact, too low. Ferritin levels of 10 to 15 ng/mL are within the "normal" range. Yet Cotsarelis says a ferritin level of at least 50 ng/mL is needed to help replenish hair. Trost and Bergfeld (from the Cleveland Clinic) shoot for 70 ng/mL. Iron supplements are not a cure for baldness. But as part of a multipronged approach, Cotsarelis and Trost say, supplements can be a big help.[123]

Because the normal lab ranges are not optimal, anyone whose ferritin level is below 40, or whose iron saturation is less than 22 percent, should be considered a prime subject for a trial treatment of iron therapy. Because too much iron can be very toxic, you should take a multivitamin without iron unless these blood tests show that you are low in that mineral (using my normal ranges—not the labs). In that instance, your doctor can help you raise your iron levels safely and without risk of developing toxicity. Although iron is important, it is also pro-oxidative (that is, it promotes free-radical activity) and can cause inflammation, arthritis, and liver and heart disease if the level is too high. This helps remind us that more is not always better. Nonetheless, although excessive iron can increase the risk of heart attack and stroke, so can low iron levels.[124]

A surprisingly large number of people display early hemochromatosis, or excess iron, in their iron studies. Early in the disease, fatigue and pain are often the only symptoms. If caught soon enough, hemochromatosis is remarkably easy to treat. Later, however, it is disabling and can be life-threatening. This is another reason to have your iron levels checked carefully.

Iron must be taken on an empty stomach; otherwise you will lose 85 percent of the absorption. Do not take calcium or iron supplements within six hours of your thyroid dose, as they block thyroid absorption. It is normal for iron to cause constipation and a black stool. You do not need to be alarmed unless it is overly foul-smelling, in which case it may indicate a bleeding ulcer and you should alert your doctor. Fortunately, if you take the iron every other day, you get almost as much benefit as taking it daily—with lower side effects. One good brand is Chelated Iron by Ultraceuticals.

CALCIUM

Although companies selling calcium would have you believe that every woman should be on it, it is actually a minor player in treating osteoporosis, and many other nutrient, hormonal, and lifestyle factors are much more important. In fact, the countries with the highest dietary calcium intakes also have the highest levels of osteoporosis. Many factors other than calcium intake cause osteoporosis, including high protein intake and inadequate exercise.

Since most people do not need it, and since it blocks thyroid absorption, I left calcium out of the vitamin powder. However, if you have loss of bone density through osteoporosis or osteopenia, I would then take 1,000 to 1,500 milligrams a day of calcium. The other time I recommend calcium is for those with plantar fasciitis (pain along the soles of your feet that is worse in the morning). Although the treatment protocol in this book usually makes the sole pain resolve, people have also found calcium supplementation to help plantar fasciitis. Since many calcium tablets do not dissolve properly in the stomach, chewable forms are best.

Many nutrients other than calcium are even more helpful in building bone density. An excellent approach is to use the vitamin powder

Ingredients found in Bone Health by Ultraceuticals		
	Amount per 6 caps	
Vitamin D	3,000	IU
Vitamin K$_2$	500	mcg
Vitamin K$_1$	100	mcg
Calcium	1,000	mg
Magnesium	400	mg
Manganese	3	mg
Strontium	340	mg
Boron	3	mg
Silica	200	mcg

plus a product called Bone Health, from Ultraceuticals, or use the ingredient list on page 184 to guide you in adding bone health to your supplement regimen.

FISH OILS

The two key omega-3 essential fatty acids in fish oil are eicosapentaenoic acid (EPA) and docohexaenoic acid (DHA), the latter being a major component of brain tissue. Perhaps the old wives' tales were right in calling fish "brain food."

Fish oil levels are low in CFS/FMS[125] and a series of patients with chronic fatigue syndrome was treated solely with a high EPA-containing

---

Fish Oil and Pregnancy

Although I do not recommend that women become pregnant while on the SHIN protocol, I would like to take a little time to discuss the importance of fish oils during pregnancy. When you are ready to conceive, you'll be taking prenatal vitamins or the vitamin powder to help promote healthy growth in your baby. It's a good idea to discuss with your holistic doctor how valuable fish-oil supplementation can also be during this time.

In a study of more than 11,580 pregnant women, high omega-3 fatty-acid intake late in pregnancy was shown to boost a baby's growth rate. However, a fish-rich diet does not seem to lengthen the pregnancy or cause preterm deliveries. In addition, infants born to moms with high blood levels of DHA at delivery had advanced attention spans (considered an indicator of IQ in babies) well into their second year of life.[130]

The benefits of fish oil continue to follow children throughout their lives. High fish-oil intake during pregnancy and lactation decreases the risk of the baby developing breast cancer as an adult. And, mothers who eat foods rich in omega-3 fatty acids during pregnancy and while nursing, and who continue to feed their babies such a diet after weaning, may dramatically reduce their daughters' risk of developing this cancer later in life, according to research presented at the American Association for Cancer Research. Remarkably, pregnant women with a history of asthma can also decrease the risk of their child getting asthma by 80 percent by taking fish oil during pregnancy.[131]

Omega-3 fatty acids also significantly decrease the risk of postpartum depression,[132] depression, schizophrenia, attention-deficit-hyperactivity disorder, (ADHD),[133] and bipolar disorder, yielding benefits for mom as well as baby.[134]

---

essential fatty acid supplement. All showed improvement in their symptomatology within eight to twelve weeks.[126] Even in healthy people, fish-oil supplements decreased anger, anxiety, and depression, and increased vigor—while also improving various types of attention, cognitive, and physiological functions, and mood.[127] Fish oils were also shown to significantly decrease stroke risk.[128] In addition, fish oil fights dry eyes,[129] often a major problem in CFS/FMS. If you have dry eyes or dry mouth, this is a good indicator of fish-oil deficiency. Because of high levels of mercury found in many types of fish, it is likely better to simply take mercury-free fish-oil supplements. Two excellent brands are Eskimo-3 fish oil by Enzymatic Therapy and omega-3 fish oil by Ultraceuticals.

Intravenous Nutritional Therapies

One of the most powerfully effective treatments that I have found for treating chronic fatigue syndrome and fibromyalgia is the use of intravenous nutritional support. As you know, less energy is produced in certain regions of the body, especially muscle tissue, when you have CFS/FMS. In fact, blood flow is actually shut down to those regions,[135] which then become starved for nutrients and loaded with toxins, leaving you achy and in pain. High-dose intravenous injections of magnesium, B vitamins, glutathione, vitamin C, and other nutrients force the blood vessels open in these closed-down areas, flooding them with nutrients and washing away the toxins. You'll find that when your doctor administers these injections, you'll feel a warm flush in the areas that have been most significantly affected by your illness.

I recommend that, if possible, all patients with CFS/FMS receive these IV therapies at least once a week for six weeks and then as needed. Along with ribose and the other supplements I've recommended (which should be continued while on the IVs), they can dramatically "jump-start" some of the body's systems and can markedly shorten the time it takes to begin feeling better. Many physicians refer to these therapies as Myers cocktails. If you have a physician who is willing to give them, I strongly recommend that you have them. This is a standard part of the treatment protocol at the Fibromyalgia & Fatigue Centers and is called the Standard IV. Physicians can see Appendix G for details on mixing and giving these IVs.

Don't Forget a Healthy Diet

Although I strongly recommend taking nutritional supplements to ensure obtaining the necessary nutrients, I also want to stress that a healthy diet is important. Eat a lot of whole grains, fresh fruits (whole fruit, not fruit juice), and fresh vegetables. Many raw vegetables have enzymes that help boost energy levels. You do not have to cut out all foods that might be bad or eat a diet that is impossible to follow. All you need to do is consume a diet that is reasonably healthy and low in caffeine and added sugar. The more unprocessed your diet is, the healthier you will be. Your body will tell you what's good for you by making you feel good.

Important Points

- Remove excess caffeine from your diet.
- Limit alcohol consumption to one to three drinks daily.
- Remove sugar and other sweeteners from your diet. Stevia, a sweet-tasting herb, and even saccharin (I do not recommend aspartame) can be used as substitutes. They taste good and are healthy.
- Use whole-grain flour instead of white flour whenever possible.
- Increase water intake so that your lips and mouth are not dry. Use pure water such as Dasani (in the United States—not the European brand) or a high-quality water filter (e.g., Multi Pure; see pure water, Appendix E).
- Take half to 1 scoop of the Energy Revitalization System vitamin powder (and B complex) by Enzymatic Therapy daily. This has more than fifty key nutrients in one drink and one capsule, and replaces more than thirty-five capsules of supplements. It is available in most health food stores and at www.vitality101.com. Or create your own supplement strategy using the recommendations in this chapter as a guide.
- Vitamin B_{12} injections can be helpful.
- Treat a too-low iron level with an iron supplement. A too-high iron level also needs to be treated properly.
- If you have osteoporosis or osteopenia, take Bone Health to increase bone density.
- Do not take calcium or iron supplements within six hours of your thyroid dose, as they block thyroid absorption.

- If you have dry eyes, dry mouth, depression, or inflammation, take mercury-free fish oil (e.g., Eskimo or Ultraceutical).
- In addition to taking supplements, eat a healthy diet that includes lots of fresh fruits and vegetables and a minimum of processed foods. Eat what makes you feel the best.

Questionnaire
(Check off treatments in Appendix B: Treatment Protocol)

___✓ 1. Do you have fatigue or pain? Check off #1—the vitamin powder—and #54—Myers/Standard IV.

_____ 2. Do you have dry eyes or dry mouth?

_____ 3. Do you have depression or inflammatory problems?

If yes to #2 or #3, take fish oil; check off #6.

_____ 4. Is your blood ferritin under 40 (or 70 if you have hair thinning) *or* is your iron percent saturation under 22 percent? If yes, check off #5—iron.

_____ 5. Is your B_{12} level under 540? If yes, check off #3—B_{12} shots.

_____ 6. Do you have osteoporosis or osteopenia (loss of bone density)? If yes, check off #56—bone health.

_____ 7. Do you have plantar fasciitis (pain along the soles of your feet that is worse in the morning)? If yes, check off #16—calcium.

_____ 8. Do you have frequent infections or do you use Tylenol often? If yes to either, check off #4—NAC.

PART 3

Pain Relief and Other Health Issues

Natural and Prescription Pain Relief for Fibromyalgia

7

*A*s noted earlier, treating sleep loss, hormonal dysfunctions, underlying infections, and nutritional deficiencies can get rid of most, if not all, fibromyalgia pain. Unfortunately, though, sometimes we cannot get to the underlying cause of the pain. This may be because of a viral infection we cannot fully treat yet or because we simply don't know what the trigger was. In such cases—and even in routine cases—it is important to have tools early in treatment that can be used to decrease or eliminate your pain. If needed, these can also be used long term.

The source of fibromyalgia pain varies from person to person. In most cases, it is triggered by a lack of energy in the muscles that leads to muscle shortening, stiffness, and pain. In such cases, muscle relaxants can be very helpful. Other times, pain is caused or aggravated by elevations in spinal fluid levels of substance P, the chemical messenger that transmits the sensation of pain. Changes in cell structures called N-methyl D-aspartate (NMDA) receptors in the brain, which play an important part in sensing pain, can also be involved in FMS, and may give us another avenue to fight the pain. Sometimes nerve pain, at times because tight muscles pinch the nerves, is the cause. The prescription medications Elavil, Neurontin, and lidocaine are especially helpful for treating nerve pain.

Another important component of fibromyalgia pain is called central sensitization. This is when the pain signal actually is triggered or amplified by changes in the brain cells themselves. I liken it to babies in a nursery. When one starts crying, they may all start in. Similarly, when pain becomes chronic, brain cells in the area of the ones sensing the pain signal begin to fire as well, amplifying the pain. Even normal touch can then also become painful (this is called allodynia). Research has shown that when the same pain stimulus is given to someone with fibromyalgia and to a healthy person, a much larger area in the pain centers lights up on the brain scan in the person with FMS.

For most people, the pain is a mix of the above, and many treatments described in this chapter will help several kinds of pain. As you know, I like to use natural therapies first but will prescribe prescription medications when needed. We will therefore discuss the natural therapies first, followed by medications. We will then briefly discuss the many other types of pain that are common in CFS/FMS, such as migraines, arthritis, and disc pain.

Research shows that in half of those with fibromyalgia, treating with the SHIN protocol eliminates their pain after three to four months. During this time, the herbs used for sleep, such as those found in the Revitalizing Sleep Formula, act as muscle relaxants. Other herbs discussed later in this chapter are also helpful for pain. I also like to begin treatment with a prescription muscle relaxant medication called Skelaxin and a pain medication called Ultram. This way patients can get immediate pain relief while waiting for the SHIN protocol to begin working.

I do *not* recommend using Motrin family medications (NSAIDs) in FMS, as they are minimally effective and are estimated to kill more than 16,500 Americans unnecessarily each year by causing bleeding stomach ulcers. Fortunately, there are safe and more effective natural alternatives. Long-term use of acetaminophen, found in Tylenol and many other over-the-counter medications, should be avoided because it depletes your body's glutathione—an amino-acid compound that is a critical antioxidant for people with CFS/FMS.

Natural Pain Treatments

Many natural treatments available to help with pain. Some are taken internally, others applied externally. They can be used in conjunction with conventional medical treatments.

HOMEOPATHIC REMEDIES

Rhus toxicodendron (Rhus tox) is a homeopathic treatment that helps a small percentage of fibromyalgia patients with their pain. However, because it is homeopathic, it has almost no side effects and is inexpensive, so it may be a good place to begin. Follow the directions and dosage recommendations on the bottle for about a week to judge whether this remedy will work for you. The tablets are probably the easiest form to use. Be sure to let them dissolve under your tongue—don't chew them. You can take a tablet every fifteen minutes for the first two hours and then four to six times a day. For inflammatory/injury pain, arnica homeopathic creams can be very helpful. My favorite is called Traumeel.

HERBAL TREATMENTS

Pain often disrupts sleep, which is critical for pain relief. As we discussed in Chapter 3, the best herbal/natural remedies for sleep include extracts of wild lettuce (28 to 112 milligrams), Jamaican dogwood (12 to 48 milligrams), Passionflower (90 to 360 milligrams), valerian (200 to 800 milligrams), hops (30 to 120 milligrams), and Suntheanine (50 to 200 milligrams). All six of these are combined in the Revitalizing Sleep Formula. Although the package says you can take one to four capsules an hour before bedtime, you can also take up to three capsules three times a day for muscle pain and/or anxiety. Even though these herbs help sleep, they will also leave you calm but usually not sedated during the day.

Many other natural therapies can be helpful for pain, including inflammatory and muscle pain. My three favorite pain-relieving herbals are willow bark, boswellia, and cherry. All three of these can be found in combination in a number of products, including the End Pain formula by Enzymatic Therapy and the Pain Formula by ITI (see Appendix E: Resources). Begin with one to three tablets (even though the box says one to two) up to three times a day as needed. Although there may be some immediate relief, its most powerful effects begin at one week and build over six weeks. Continue treatment until maximum benefit is achieved, about four to six weeks, and then taper down to the lowest effective dose. These herbs may also be taken individually at the dosages recommended on pages 194–196.

WILLOW BARK is the original source of aspirin, but when used as the entire herb it has been found to be much safer and is often more effective. The active ingredient is salicin, and it acts as a COX (cyclooxygenase enzyme) inhibitor, decreasing inflammation. Yet unlike the aspirin and Motrin family medications, willow bark does not cause gastritis and ulcer bleeding. Although no studies have been performed specifically addressing fibromyalgia, the studies on willow bark are quite consistent in their effectiveness in reducing chronic pain, and their findings can be applied to FMS.

In one study, 210 patients with severe chronic low back pain were randomly assigned to receive an oral willow bark extract with either 120 milligrams (low dose) or 240 milligrams (high dose) of salicin, or a placebo, in a four-week blinded trial. In the last week of treatment, 39 percent in the group receiving the high-dose extract were pain free, 21 percent in the group receiving the low-dose extract were pain free, and only 6 percent in the placebo group were pain free. The response in the high-dose group was evident after only one week of treatment.[1] The researchers then studied 451 patients with low back pain, using salicin at 240 milligrams or at 120 milligrams, or standard orthopedic/NSAID (e.g., Motrin) care for four weeks. Forty percent of the patients in the 240-milligram group and 19 percent in the 120-milligram group were pain free after four weeks. In the standard treatment group using NSAIDs, only 18 percent were pain free. The study showed that willow bark was not just far more effective and safer than standard prescription therapies, but also decreased the cost of care by approximately 40 percent.[2]

Another review found that willow bark extract has comparable anti-inflammatory activity to higher doses of acetylsalicylic acid/aspirin (ASS), in addition to reducing pain and fever. No adverse effects on the stomach lining (e.g., indigestion, ulcers) were observed, in contrast to aspirin. A daily dose of willow bark extract standardized to 240 milligrams salicin per day was also significantly superior to placebo in patients with osteoarthritis (the normal wear-and-tear type of arthritis) of the hip and the knee. In two open studies against standard active treatments as controls, willow bark extract exhibited advantages compared to NSAIDs, and was about as effective as Vioxx.[3] Another placebo-controlled study found that willow bark (salicin 240 milligrams a day) was more effective than placebo in treating osteoarthritis after only two weeks of therapy.[4] Other studies also show willow bark to be safe and effective for general pain.[5–8]

All of this makes willow bark a wonderful natural pain medicine. It is safe and effective for arthritis, back pain, and likely many other types of pain. I would begin with six tablets of the End Pain daily (to get 240 milligrams of salicin) until maximum benefit is seen. At that point, you may be able to lower the dose to 120 milligrams or less a day and/or take it as needed.

BOSWELLIA SERRATA, also known as frankincense, has been used in traditional Ayurvedic medicine for centuries. Boswellia has been found to be quite helpful in treating inflammation and pain[9–14] and it also does this without causing ulcers, as aspirin family medications often do.[15] It has been shown in studies to be helpful for both rheumatoid arthritis[16] and osteoarthritis.[17]

One study evaluated thirty patients with osteoarthritis of the knee. Patients were given 1,000 milligrams of an extract of Boswellia or a placebo for eight weeks and then the groups were switched for the next eight weeks. All of the patients on the Boswellia showed significantly decreased pain and improved ability to walk. In fact, the improvement was quite remarkable—the pain index fell by 90 percent after eight weeks, with a similarly dramatic increase in function.[17] This is discussed at more length in the patient-oriented newsletter *Nutrition and Healing* by Jonathan Wright, M.D. (www.wrightnewsletter.com).

Boswellia has demonstrated significant anti-inflammatory properties, blocking two inflammatory chemicals—a quality that is unique to this herb and that makes it helpful for treating asthma and colitis, as well as pain.[18–22] Boswellia does not appear to have any major side effects that resulted in people withdrawing from the studies but did rarely cause minor gastrointestinal disturbances or rash. A common dose is 150 to 350 milligrams three times a day.

CHERRY FRUIT (Prunus cerasus) contains compounds that inhibit COX-1 (inflammation)[23] and has both antioxidant and anti-inflammatory properties. Although there are not as many human studies on the use of cherries as on the use of Boswellia, many people find that simply eating ten to twenty cherries a day helps relieve their arthritis considerably. Early research, as well as how many people continue to take this supplement (which to me is a significant indicator of effectiveness), suggests that cherry fruit holds a lot of promise.[24, 25] Research even suggests that in addition to pain relief, cherry fruit may also inhibit colon and perhaps other cancers.[25] About 2,000 milligrams of cherry fruit extract (present in six tablets of the End Pain herbal formula) contains the active components present in ten cherries or one quart of cherry juice.

I recommend beginning with both the End Pain and the Revitalizing Sleep Formula for six weeks. The dose can then be adjusted as needed. There are other herbs, in addition to the three found in the End Pain formula, that can be helpful for treating the CFS/FMS pain.

GINGER can have substantial health benefits for people with CFIDS/ FMS. Sometimes, fresh ginger, high in the compound gingerol, and dried ginger, high in shogaol, have different effects. I will note the uses where this distinction is important. The benefits of ginger include the following:

- *Relief of muscle and/or joint pain.* Like aspirin and ibuprofen, many components of ginger are potent inhibitors of inflammatory substances such as prostaglandins. Ginger is also thought to inhibit substance P, a pain mediator that is known to be elevated in FMS. For substance P inhibition, dried ginger seems to be most effective. In a study of ten patients with muscle pain and forty-six patients with arthritis (both rheumatoid and osteoarthritis), 100 percent of muscle pain patients and 75 percent of arthritis patients noted relief. The recommended dose was 1,000 milligrams of powdered ginger a day. Many patients took 3,000 to 4,000 milligrams a day and noted quicker and better relief using the higher dose.[1] Try using the fresh ginger and then a slice of dried ginger to see which works better for you.
- *Decreased nausea, vomiting, and diarrhea.* Ginger decreases bowel spasm while improving gastric motility (moving food from the stomach to the bowels). These are often major problems in CFS/FMS, resulting in bloating after eating. Ginger can also inhibit diarrhea. In addition, in several studies, fresh (for example, roasted) but not dried ginger was found to inhibit stomach ulcers caused by aspirin and ibuprofen. It is a strong antioxidant, and can inhibit certain bowel infections (salmonella and vibrio). Taking 500 to 1,000 milligrams of ginger is effective to calm general stomach upset.
- *Increased thermogenesis (warming of the body).* Fresh ginger works much better for this.

- *Relief of migraine headaches.*
- *Disequilibrium* (for example, motion sickness). Although likely not as effective for vestibular (inner ear) dizziness, in which you feel like you are spinning in a circle, ginger inhibits the nausea associated with dizziness. For motion sickness, it works best when you take 1,000 milligrams four hours before travel.
- *Increased blood pressure.* This can be helpful for people with CFS/FMS, who often have low blood pressure. Only dried ginger works for this purpose.
- *Decreased risk of heart disease.* Ginger is a platelet inhibitor (like aspirin and vitamin E) and may also lower cholesterol.

Ginger tea preparations are among the most popular ways to take ginger. To make the tea, boil 10 grams of chopped fresh ginger (about a quarter-inch slice) and add stevia to sweeten it, as desired. Some people find the ginger brews better if they allow the chopped ginger to dry out slightly before using it (just keep a bag of ginger slices in your refrigerator). Once you finish drinking the tea, eat the ginger that remains. You can also purchase packets of ginger tea crystals. I wouldn't worry very much about the small amount of sugar in these products relative to the amount of ginger—as long as ginger is the first ingredient listed on the package. These products supply about 5,000 milligrams of ginger per cup of tea.

Minced ginger is also available in a liquid base for cooking (similar to jarred minced garlic). Or, if you like the sharp taste of ginger, candied ginger cubes might be a good choice. If you use fresh ginger in cooking or to make tea, do not peel it until just before use or some of the volatile (active) oils will evaporate.

You can also take 1,000 milligrams of dried ginger extract one to four times a day or 500 to 1,000 milligrams of dry powder three to four times a day—with the dose decreased to the lowest effective dose in four to six weeks. These initial, higher doses can be more effective for pain; side effects of ginger are minimal, but include nausea and heartburn.

DIETARY SUPPLEMENTS

- Ribose and magnesium kick-start energy production. In our CFS/FMS study, significant pain relief was experienced in those taking ribose. Magnesium is also critical for muscle relaxation, which in turn aids pain relief.

- The supplement 5-Hydroxy-L-Tryptophan (5-HTP), a form of the amino acid tryptophan, raises serotonin levels, and can be very helpful for pain. In two studies in which fibromyalgia patients were given 100 milligrams of 5-HTP three times a day, their symptoms markedly improved, so it is well worth trying. It can also help you lose weight. Give it six to ten weeks to work.

- Glucosamine is a cartilage compound that has been shown in several controlled studies to be helpful for osteoarthritis. Although the exact way it works is not certain, it appears to stimulate cartilage production by bone cells. It tends to be more helpful for arthritis pain than for fibromyalgia pain, but it is worth trying. Take 750 milligrams two times a day for six weeks—it takes that long to find out if it is going to help. When the maximum benefit is seen, reduce the dose to the lowest dose that maintains the benefit.

  To give just one of many examples of glucosamine's effectiveness, in a head-on study of two hundred osteoarthritis patients using 1,500 milligrams a day of either glucosamine sulfate or 1,200 milligrams a day of ibuprofen (Motrin), the Motrin worked better for the first two weeks. After that, the glucosamine was as effective as the Motrin. The glucosamine group also had significantly fewer and milder side effects than the Motrin group.

  Another important point is that Motrin and other nonsteroidal anti-inflammatory drugs do not slow down the progression of arthritis, and may actually make the arthritis worse. Glucosamine may actually help heal the arthritic joint, and benefit often persists after the glucosamine is stopped. I would use glucosamine sulfate (*not* chloride), as the sulfate may also be helpful in both joint repair and improving the body's mitochondrial function.

- Methylsulfonylmethane (MSM) is a form of sulfur that has been reported to be helpful for some people with fibromyalgia. It can take as much as 12 to 15 grams a day (12,000 to 15,000 milligrams, or twenty-four to thirty capsules) to see the benefit. I usually use 6 grams a day in the beginning, as it is best to always use the lowest dose possible of any supplement. If MSM helps within three to six weeks, then you can reduce the dose to the lowest dose that maintains the benefit. Taking it with vitamin C probably helps the absorption of the MSM.

- Essential fatty acids (EFAs), which are the building blocks of fats and oils, have an anti-inflammatory effect and can be beneficial for pain.

Symptoms of EFA deficiency are many and varied, and include fatigue, poor memory, recurrent respiratory infections, gas, bloating, arthralgias (aches and pains), constipation, cracking nails, depression, dry hair and skin, and inadequate saliva, tears, and vaginal lubrication. If you have dry eyes, dry mouth, dry hair, and/or dry skin, these symptoms may suggest an essential-fatty-acid deficiency, and taking these in the form of mercury-free fish oils can be very helpful for pain and inflammation. Because of their importance, I am going to discuss them in more detail.

Essential fatty acids play an important and yet poorly recognized role in human health. They are involved in many functions, including hormone production, immune function, the regulation of inflammation and blood flow, and the amount and wateriness of saliva, tears, and other bodily fluids. EFAs also are part of the makeup of the membranes surrounding every cell in the body.

Most Americans get only about 10 percent of the amount of EFAs they need for optimal well-being. This is despite the fact that the average person's fat intake has increased by about fifty pounds a year in the last century. Unfortunately, food-processing techniques have essentially removed the EFAs from our food supply because oils are produced at high temperatures, and previously healthy vegetable oils are hydrogenated, or saturated, to harden and stabilize them. These processing steps both eliminate the EFAs and make it difficult for your body to use the EFAs it does get.

Fats and oils are not the same thing. Fats usually refer to saturated fats, which are solid at room temperature. Saturated means that the hooks (bonds) that connect each of the atoms in the fat molecules are all in use, and there is no room for any new atoms to attach. This makes the fat molecules straight and rigid, and thus hard. Oils usually refer to unsaturated fats, which are liquid at room temperature. These unsaturated fats are either monounsaturated or polyunsaturated. Monounsaturated fats have one open hook, and polyunsaturated fats have several open hooks where molecules can attach. This makes them more flexible (fluid). This is where things begin to get technical: If the first open hook (double bond) is six carbon atoms from the end of the fat molecule, it is called an omega-6 fatty acid. Most vegetable oils are omega-6 oils. If the first open hook is three carbon atoms from the end, the molecule is an omega-3 fatty acid. Fish oils and flaxseed oil are omega-3 oils.

How your body is able to use the fat depends on whether it is a saturated fat or an omega-3 or omega-6 fatty acid. In many processed foods (for example, margarine) the unsaturated fats are changed from their healthy natural state, in which they are known as cis-fatty acids, to an unnatural unhealthy state, in which they are called trans-fatty acids. These trans-fatty acids can cause heart disease, obesity, immune suppression, and decreased testosterone levels, while worsening fatty acid deficiencies. Despite advertising hype to the contrary, margarine is probably less healthy than butter, and I recommend not using it.

Differentiating between these fats is important because they are the building blocks of cell membranes, the balloonlike walls that enclose all cells in the body. These membranes perform the critical functions of allowing in and keeping in water, minerals, and other nutrients. In addition, the regulatory hormones and neurotransmitters—molecules that tell the cells what they need to do—function by fitting into receptors located in the cell membranes. The membranes are made up of fatty acids and a phosphorus molecule, usually choline or serine. The type of fat available to your body when it makes cell membranes is critical. Your body likes to use omega-3 and -6 fatty acids because these are more fluid and more easily allow the passage of hormones, neurotransmitters, and other fluids in and out of the cells. However, when omega-3 and omega-6 fatty acids are not available, your body has to use saturated fats. This results in rigid, poorly functioning cellular walls that can make it hard for the hormones and neurotransmitters to function properly.

EFAs are also critical for making an important class of hormones called prostaglandins. These hormones regulate inflammation, pain, bowel function, fluid balance, mood, allergies, and the production of some other hormones. Because of its effect on prostaglandin levels, borage or evening primrose oil can help PMS as well. For more information on these and EFAs in general, see the *From Fatigued to Fantastic!* notes at www.vitality101.con.

To treat possible essential-fatty-acid deficiency, I recommend taking Eskimo-3 (Enzymatic Therapy) or omega-3 (Ultraceuticals) fish oils, which are mercury and toxin free, at a dose of three to nine capsules a day. Take these for three months. If dry skin, dry hair, dry mouth, and/or dry eyes improve, then you probably had a fish oil deficiency. After three months, you can decrease the above regimen to three capsules of fish oil a day and/or three servings a week of tuna, salmon, or herring. As an added benefit, fish oil helps people's moods. For example depression that does not respond to Saint John's wort or antidepressant medications will sometimes improve with omega-3 fatty acids.

BODYWORK

There are many forms of bodywork that can eliminate pain by stretching your tightened muscles. My favorites include Trager, Rolfing, myofascial release, chiropractic treatments, and acupuncture. Some physical therapists are simply too rough or unfamiliar with fibromyalgia and can aggravate symptoms. If any bodywork therapist hurts you, let them know so they can ease back and work more gently. Remember, "No pain, no gain" is a good recipe for hurting yourself. However, a skilled practitioner can effectively help you treat your illness. As you research which techniques and practitioners, are right for you, keep these guidelines in mind:

- Rolfing should be done only by a certified Rolfer with a lot of experience, as some people with minimal training claim that they do Rolfing and can work too aggressively.
- When talking with a physical therapist, ask if he or she knows how to do Dr. Janet Travell's spray-and-stretch technique. This approach uses a cold spray to briefly block pain, allowing the muscle to be easily and comfortably stretched. This technique takes time to learn, and knowledge of the technique may indicate a more thorough, dedicated practitioner. Structural issues and trigger points that may contribute to pain will be discussed later in this chapter.
- Prolotherapy is a technique that may relieve joint pain in people with loose ligaments who can hyperextend their joints and have "loose," elastic skin. The technique consists of injecting weak ligaments with a substance that causes inflammation. The end result of this therapy is to strengthen the ligament, thereby reducing pain. For a detailed article on prolotherapy, see the *From Fatigued to Fantastic!* notes at www .vitality101.com.
- Magnets have been helpful for many patients with pain. Although some physicians feel they are simply placebos (and some poorly made

ones are), research has shown that they can increase blood flow to painful areas and decrease pain. I generally recommend starting with spot magnets for localized areas that hurt a lot, as well as magnet shoe insoles and the universal chair pad. If the spot magnets help in two months, then consider purchasing a mattress pad. The mattress pads are more expensive and, for some patients, too strong to start with. Many people, though, have been pleased that they started with a mattress pad because it offered substantial relief. A number of different companies sell magnets and related products (see Appendix E: Resources).

Prescription Medications

Although natural remedies can be helpful, the pain experienced by fibromyalgia patients is often severe enough to warrant the addition of prescription therapies. All of the natural therapies I've discussed can be combined with the prescriptions below, and can decrease the amount of medication needed while increasing safety and decreasing side effects. I also discuss how to treat other pains commonly seen in fibromyalgia, such as nerve pain, migraines, and arthritis. As always, I recommend working with a holistically trained physician who is familiar with both natural and prescription therapies.

PRESCRIPTION PAIN CREAMS AND LOTIONS

Many people with fibromyalgia also have a few painful body areas that are especially distressing but they shy away from taking pills, as they are sensitive to prescription drugs. That's why I often recommend topical pain lotions. After two weeks of use, you can actually get the same tissue concentrations in the local muscles and tendons topically as you can when taking medications by mouth—without the side effects. Many compounding pharmacies make these topical pain gels/lotions/creams (regular pharmacies are usually not familiar with them), and they are happy to guide your physician. I like to use ITC Pharmacy (see Appendix E: Resources). Simply ask your doctor to call them to prescribe the pain lotion or if you have nerve pain, the nerve pain lotion. These typically include five to six pain medications. By rubbing a thin layer of the lotion or gel into the skin over painful areas, you can often eliminate your worst pain spots. Sometimes using these products for seven to fourteen days in one spot will relieve the pain, or even make that area of pain go away permanently—and then you can march through other pain spots, eliminating them a few at a time. You can use these products on up to three or four silver-dollar-size areas at a time, three times a day. The cost is approximately sixty-six dollars for a 30-gram tube, which lasts quite a while. For a more detailed discussion of the many topical pain options available (and other pain issues), see my book *Pain Free 1–2–3.*

PRESCRIPTION ORAL MEDICATIONS

- *Tramadol (Ultram).* I have found tramadol to be the single best pain medication for fibromyalgia. It affects both serotonin and endorphin (narcotic) receptors, and is considered minimally addicting, although I've never seen addiction with it in my practice. The recommended regimen is one to two 50-milligram tablets up to four times a day as needed for pain. The most common side effects are nausea and vomiting (when people use more than six tablets a day), and sedation. These effects generally wear off with continued use, and can often be avoided altogether by starting with a low dose and slowly working up to the level that most effectively treats your pain.

MUSCLE RELAXANTS

- *Metaxalone (Skelaxin).* This muscle relaxant is nonsedating and is helpful in around half of the fibromyalgia population. You will usually know within one week whether Skelaxin will work for you. Take one 800-milligram tablet four times a day as needed for pain. It can be taken with Ultram.
- *Tizanidine (Zanaflex).* This muscle relaxant can be sedating, so many people take it at night to relieve the pain, spasms, muscle cramps, and tightness that may inhibit sleep. The usual dose is one 4-milligram tablet up to three times a day for pain. Zanaflex can sometimes cause nightmares; if this occurs, discontinue use, as the problem usually does not go away until the medication is stopped. Do not take it (or lower the dose to 2 to 4 milligrams) while on the antibiotic Cipro.

ANTIDEPRESSANTS

Antidepressants such as venlafaxine (Effexor), duloxetine (Cymbalta), paroxetine (Paxil), fluoxetine (Prozac), and sertraline (Zoloft), tried in the order listed, can sometimes be effective in treating fibromyalgia pain—even when no depression is present. In fact, most of the CFS/FMS patients I treat with antidepressants are not depressed. However, these medications are effective because they raise serotonin, which lowers the chemical that transmits pain (called substance P). It takes six weeks to see their full effect.

It's best to start with low doses and then work up to higher doses to see the optimum effect. This is especially true if you are taking Effexor for nerve pain, which often takes 225 milligrams per day to work. Your doctor can help you establish the best dose. Although drug interactions are possible, I have not found this to be a major problem. If you have a chronic fast heart rate and anxiety, however, these can be exacerbated when serotonin levels go too high because of serotonin-raising treatments—especially when several of them are taken together. This is called serotonergic syndrome and can be life-threatening. As I discussed earlier, for patients with a fast pulse, I recommend that all serotonin-raising medications be reviewed and, if needed, the doses lowered for about a week to see if the heart rate comes down. If the heart rate does indeed drop, your doctor will need to adjust your medications.

Some of the more common treatments that can raise serotonin include:

- Almost all of the antidepressants (including Elavil)
- Trazodone (Desyrel)
- Tramadol (Ultram)
- Saint John's Wort
- Tryptophan or 5-HTP

TRICYCLIC ANTIDEPRESSANTS
(AMITRIPTYLINE, DOXEPIN, ETC.)

AMITRIPTYLINE (ELAVIL) is especially good for nerve pain, pelvic pain, vulvadynia (pain in the vulvar area), interstitial cystitis, and proctalgia fugax (episodic rectal pain due to muscle spasm). The main side effects are weight gain, sedation, restless leg syndrome, heart palpitations, and dry mouth. Elavil can also worsen neurally mediated hypertension (NMH), a type of low blood pressure syndrome experienced by some people with CFS/FMS. Because these medications, except doxepin (Sinequan), tend to be high in side effects, I use them mostly for severe nerve pain and pelvic pain syndromes.

INTRAVENOUS (IV) NUTRIENTS AND LIDOCAINE

Intravenous treatment with the anesthetic lidocaine, especially when given with intravenous nutritional therapies (called the Standard IV at the Fibromyalgia Fatigue Centers or more commonly known as Myers cocktails), can be a blessing for both easing muscle and spastic colon pain and helping raise energy levels in people with CFS/FMS. (For more information about Myers cocktails, see Appendix G.)

Intravenous lidocaine may first be given in a test dose of 40 to 50 milligrams infused over a thirty-minute period. The Myers cocktail can be given at the same time, in a different IV bag but through the same needle. If the lidocaine is well tolerated, you can take 100 milligrams the first day, as long as your blood pressure remains stable and there are no severe side effects. The treatment can be sedating—a sleepy feeling is common, and I often let patients take a nap on the table afterward—and you should not drive after a lidocaine infusion.

If the first treatment is well tolerated, we give a maximum of 100 to 120 milligrams an hour to a dose of 300 to 400 milligrams at a sitting, if needed. The effect seems to increase over the first four times that it is given. I usually infuse a dose of at least 200 milligrams during a single two-hour session before deciding that it is not effective for a particular patient.

Intravenous lidocaine can be taken as often as needed. Many people find that they need a treatment every one to three weeks. If lidocaine is administered at much higher doses than those mentioned here, abnormal heart rhythms or seizures can result, so at higher doses patients are sometimes hooked up to a heart monitor during the treatment. Some people feel that giving lidocaine without a monitor is controversial, but in my experience, at low levels it has been quite safe, and IV-administered lidocaine has been found to be safe and effective for pain in many studies and reports.[27–30]

Lidocaine can also be used in topical creams, but I do not find it to be effective this way. However, using a patch containing lidocaine that you apply over painful areas can be helpful. This patch is called Lidoderm and is available at any pharmacy by prescription. You can exceed the labeled dose slightly, using up to four patches at a time and leaving them on for up to sixteen hours a day. Give it two weeks to see the full effect, though it usually works more quickly.

NEURONTIN, GABITRIL, AND LYRICA

These medications work by increasing the effect of gamma-aminobutyric-acid (GABA), a "calming" neurotransmitter (brain chemical). They are often effective for fibromyalgia pain, allodynia, pelvic pain syndromes, and nerve pain, and are helpful for sleep and restless leg syndrome (see Chapter 3). They are not addictive but, like any medication, should be tapered off slowly if they've been taken for more than two to four months. I prefer to prescribe Lyrica only if Neurontin and Gabitril are not effective, as Lyrica is more expensive and can cause marked weight gain in some people. Lyrica can be very effective, however, and may be the first medication to be specifically approved by the FDA for treating fibromyalgia, and it is currently under review for this indication.

These natural and prescription therapies for fibromyalgia pain are generally highly effective. Nonetheless, some people have more persistent and severe pain, and it is important to note that there are dozens of other effective treatments as well, but they are simply beyond the scope of this book. For more information on these, I refer you to my *From Fatigued to Fantastic!* notes at www.vitality101.com (use the password FFTF) or my book *Pain Free 1–2–3*. In addition, these sources contain detailed information (and the numerous scientific study references supporting them) on how to eliminate many different kinds of pain. These include:

- Nerve pain
- Arthritis
- Migraine and tension headaches
- Osteoporosis
- Back pain
- Pelvic pain
- Indigestion
- Spastic colon
- Carpal tunnel syndrome

In most patients, these can be relieved effectively (and without surgery) using a mix of natural and prescription therapies.

Structural problems can also contribute to pain (e.g., uneven hip heights), and treating these can be very helpful. We will finish this chapter with a brief discussion of these issues, followed by an exploration of trigger points and myofascial pain by Dr. Hal Blatman, a highly respected pain specialist.

Structural Issues

Although herbal therapies and medications may often eliminate fibromyalgia pain, it is also sometimes necessary to treat structural problems. For example, if the left hip is higher than the right hip, the left shoulder is often lower than the right shoulder. This is the body's attempt to maintain balance, but it puts a significant strain on other muscles. Using a small insert (for example, a heel lift or orthotic) in the shoe of the short leg to make the hips the same height can help those strained muscles and eliminate one of the causes of pain. Or, if you find that one hip is lower than the other when you sit, using a cushioning support under the low side of your behind will make the hips more even, again reducing strain on overtaxed muscles. Many possible structural issues may be contributing to muscle spasm and pain; often, a chiropractor or a physical therapy physician (a physiatrist) can be of benefit. As noted earlier in the chapter, there are many different types of structural therapies.

A form of neuromuscular reeducation called Trager, developed by Dr. Milton Trager, has been beneficial for my more severe fibromyalgia patients. If your fibromyalgia persists despite the treatments discussed in this book, you should consider calling the Trager Institute (see Appendix E: Resources) to locate the closest practitioner. The best kinds of Trager practitioners are instructors and tutors, who have reached a high level of expertise in the technique.

Rolfing is another technique that can be effective for FMS pain. Also known as structural reintegration, Rolfing is deep-tissue manipulation and massage. It is designed to relieve muscular and emotional tension and rebalance muscles. If done right, it can be comfortable; if done incorrectly, it hurts. A lot of people who say they are Rolfers are not fully trained in the technique. If someone does something that hurts, tell him or her to stop. The one exception to this is a different technique called ischemic compression, in which the practitioner pushes on a spot with thirty pounds of pressure for forty-five seconds. It hurts like hell, and then feels better. You can also do this on your own more comfortably using a device called a Thera Cane (see Appendix E: Resources). This simple and often overlooked technique can be helpful for treating tender spots. If you push on these spots for thirty to forty-five seconds, applying about twenty to thirty pounds of pressure (for example, with your thumb), they will often be tender and then the pain will subside. This can often be done in the context of a massage. Although not recommended for dozens of tender areas at one time, it can be helpful if a few nagging spots remain after treatment. To locate a Rolfing practitioner in your area, contact the Rolf Institute (see Appendix E: Resources).

Many patients have also found a technique called myofascial release to be effective. If you decide to see a physical therapist, make sure that you pick someone who is both knowledgeable and gentle. It's a good sign if they know the spray-and-stretch technique of Dr. Travell discussed earlier. I have seen too many patients made worse by physical therapists who were too rough. With fibromyalgia, gentleness is often much more effective than roughness.

Acupuncture is another type of treatment that can be helpful. Because it approaches health and illness from a different perspective than traditional medicine does, it can often be effective for illnesses that resist traditional measures. Many practitioners combine acupuncture with herbal and homeopathic remedies to make their treatments even more effective.

Chiropractic also can be helpful in releasing the muscles. Unfortunately, however, if you don't treat the perpetuating factors that caused the muscles to shorten in the first place, they'll go right back to being shortened a few days after the treatment. That's why so many excellent chiropractors add nutritional, hormonal, antifungal, and other natural treatments to their practices. A special form of chiropractic, called Atlas chiropractic, focuses on the atlas vertebrae in your neck. This may be especially helpful if you have overactive knee reflexes or if your symptoms get worse when you turn your head upward to look at the ceiling for twenty seconds (if you have these symptoms, also read about cervical stenosis and the Chiari I Malformation in Chapter 9).

Additionally, yoga and many other forms of body and energy work have been very helpful for our patients. Try several and see which feels best to you. Many patients find that bodywork also releases suppressed feelings

Natural and Prescription Pain Relief for Fibromyalgia   209

and memories from their muscles. Experience, feel, and embrace these. Your awareness, experience, and release of these feelings are important parts of the healing process.

Trigger Points and Myofascial Pain in Fibromyalgia

Because trigger points and their role in pain management are poorly understood, I have asked the preeminent pain specialist Dr. Hal Blatman to discuss these. Dr. Blatman is president of the American Holistic Medical Association, director of the Blatman Pain Clinic in Cincinnati, and author of *Winners' Guide to Pain Relief* (available online at www.winoverpain.com). His book contains many examples showing where to look for the cause of each specific area of pain you are having, and local treatments that may be helpful in reducing the pain pattern.

Structural Aspects of Pain Treatment

Medical students learn theories about what causes pain and then go on to practice medicine and treat and teach their patients. Unfortunately, most people do not know that what doctors are taught about the mechanisms of pain are just theories. While these theories may work and be helpful, they do not deserve their automatic credibility and often lead people to unnecessary surgeries and medications.

The first theory of pain concerns inflammation and includes words like "arthritis," "tendonitis," and "bursitis." Indeed, when we go to the doctor complaining of pain in a joint, we often expect to be told we have a "touch of arthritis." Additionally, we sometimes like to speak to the doctor like we know something about our condition. This often leads us to say we have inflammation instead of pain, because as consumers we are taught to assume that pain must come from inflammation. The truth is that unless the body part is red and swollen, it may be more accurate to simply complain of pain.

The focus in medical training on inflammation and arthritis leads doctors to believe that if they can show an abnormality on an X-ray that is close to the location of the pain, then they can attribute the pain to the abnormality noted on the X-ray. Except for fractures, this is generally a mistake and requires a leap of faith that physicians have no right to make. The more I see and learn, the more I am convinced that pain mostly comes from muscles and not from arthritic changes in joints, which may have more to do with restricting motion than causing pain. As a resident in orthopedic surgery, I saw patients with bone-on-bone hip X-rays who had very limited hip motion yet no hip pain.

Another theory of pain that doctors are taught involves depression, and this is true—just not in the way most doctors think. Doctors are presented, for example, with a case study of a middle-aged woman who has "hurt" for a few years. What's the diagnosis for this vague chronic pain? Depression. However, in this instance it is most likely that the cause and effect—depression to pain—is backward. Pain physiologically causes depression, as the mood and depression center in the brain is bombarded with pain darts from the muscles. When the level of pain is high enough, it will cause depression no matter what else is going on in life. The part of the muscle that sends this pain dart is the myofascial trigger point, and this is a common cause of pain in fibromyalgia patients.

Doctors are also taught about neuropathic pain, the pain that comes from nerves. It was originally thought that nerves had to be cut or otherwise injured to cause this kind of pain. Doctors are only starting to make the connection among neuropathic pain, myofascial pain, and fibromyalgia. The referral pain pattern from myofascial trigger points is sometimes diagnosed as neuropathic pain. Most drug therapy for this condition is based on using seizure medications, and many times these are helpful.

Another pain theory that doctors are taught is that pain radiating from the neck down the arm, or from the lower back down the leg, must come from a disc in the neck or lower back that is pushing on a nerve. However, so-called sciatica, for example, is more often caused by trigger points in the buttock muscles than by a slipped disc or pinched nerve. A stiff neck is caused more often by trigger points in the neck and upper shoulder/back muscles than a pinched nerve in the neck. But doctors know how to look for the slipped or compressed disc, and unfortunately for many people, they also know how to fix it. For every person helped by spine surgery, there are more who are just as miserable afterward.

The most unfortunate theory doctors are taught is the supratentorial theory of pain. It basically states that if all tests are normal and you still think you hurt, you must be making it up. Doctors should never assume that something is not real just because it cannot be proven with the results of a test. There are so many potential causes of pain that there is no way current diagnostic testing can reveal everything. The shameful part of this theory is that many patients are told that their pain is in their head. Their families don't take them seriously, and they even start to doubt themselves.

During my years of practicing medicine, I have come to understand that these theories are incomplete and don't help us diagnose or treat pain as well as we would hope. Many times these theories allow insurance companies to justify denying claims, and cause patients and their families untold grief and doubt about the reality of a loved one's symptoms. When most people with fibromyalgia go to the doctor, the actual cause of their suffering doesn't match anything their doctor has been taught. This means that even well-meaning doctors are usually unable to help their FMS patients beyond prescribing a few medications for depression and sleep.

The diagnosis of fibromyalgia can be tricky. Patients and physicians are taught to use "tender points" as a significant examination finding. It is assumed that the number of tender points can be used to determine the diagnosis of FMS and response to treatment. Unfortunately, tender points are highly overrated and not very important; they are simply specific places on the body that medical doctors have agreed cause pain when pressed. They have meaning in research, and little meaning in medical practice. What are much more important are the causes, diagnosis, pain referral patterns, and treatment of myofascial pain. Unfortunately, physicians are not taught much about myofascial pain in medical school or in training programs.

In my experience, at least 60 to 70 percent of fibromyalgia pain is caused by trigger points in muscle. These trigger points are small knots that form in the muscles as a tissue response to injury. The injury can be a strain, bruise, or cut. The knots create taut or ropy bands of muscle. They restrict motion, cause spasms, and generate a tremendous amount of pain. Sometimes this pain feels like a sharp hot poker, and other times like burning, numbness, tingling, and aching. There can even be more than one sensation at the same time. What is more significant than the trigger point itself is that every trigger point causes pain in, or refers pain to, some other place in the body. Trigger points in the upper shoulders and back of the neck, for example, cause headache from the back of the head to the forehead and sinuses. Lower back pain and sciatica pain down the leg are caused by trigger points in the buttocks.

No one with FMS has only one trigger point. In general, most of the overall body pain is caused by referred pain from the entire "orchestra" of trigger points, all playing at the same time. The reality is that how you feel depends on how loudly the orchestra of trigger points is playing, and which solo artist or ensemble just stood up to play. This is determined by how you have used your body in the past three days (which muscles you overused), what the weather is going to do tomorrow, how you slept last night, and what you have eaten in the past few months.

Fortunately, there is a lot that you can do to help reduce myofascial pain, which comes from these trigger points. There are some fundamental dietary considerations that I have found to be universally true in my patients. Foods that always increase pain and inflammation include soda, sugar, wheat, white potatoes, and fruit juice. Aspartame and partially hydrogenated oil are ingredients to be totally avoided. If you are treating your FMS and do not see favorable results, these foods and chemicals can be to blame. In some cases, one soft drink (or even a glass of OJ) per day can insure that your body will not be able to heal. If you proceed to make these changes in your lifestyle, cutting out sugar and wheat should be done gradually over a couple of months. Otherwise, you may go through an unpleasant withdrawal period.

Dealing with the trigger points themselves is fairly straightforward. The more "active" the trigger point, the more pain it causes locally and the more pain it refers. There are several techniques that will make trigger points less active. These techniques include:

Acupressure (pushing on the trigger point)
Myofascial release (bodywork that stretches the muscles)
Stretching
Application of medication through the skin over the trigger point

Trigger point acupuncture

Chiropractic adjustment

Injection of trigger points with lidocaine

In my experience, the quickest and most effective treatment to inactivate trigger points is a trigger point injection with lidocaine (Novocain). There is no added benefit in most people to injecting cortisone. Novocain is generally helpful, but dry needling and acupuncture also work.

The most important technique for people at home and at work is to push on the trigger points. This is called acupressure, and it makes trigger points smaller. Be careful when you push on these tender knots in your muscles, and only cause a level of discomfort that you can relax with. This is called a "good" hurt. After pushing on the trigger points, they will be less active, and the muscles will then be a little softer. At this time, the muscles are more ready to be stretched. Slowly and gently stretching the muscles will help keep them from tightening back up. Working on yourself in this way for a few minutes several times each day will give you more control over the pain that runs your life.

Additionally, everyone with fibromyalgia should try a ten- to fifteen-minute detoxification bath using a cup each of sea salt and baking soda. Rinse off afterward. This will be helpful when your skin hurts, when you are miserable, and when changing your diet leaves you feeling more achy.

In the thousands of pain patients I have treated over the years, there are less than a dozen whom I've not been able to help get adequate pain relief. Unfortunately, most physicians are simply not taught how to treat pain effectively. The good news is that there is a new specialty called physiatry, which specializes in pain management, and many other practitioners have also taken special training to learn how to effectively treat you. I recommend going to a member of the American Academy of Pain Management (www.aapainmanage.org) to find a pain specialist. In addition, physicians at the Fibromyalgia & Fatigue Centers nationally (see Chapter 12 and www.fibroandfatigue.com) are specially trained in treating fibromyalgia pain.

Important Points

- Most CFS/FMS pain can be eliminated.
- Getting eight hours of solid sleep a night, and treating low thyroid function, nutritional deficiencies, and underlying infections (especially yeast) often eliminate the root causes of the pain.

- The Revitalizing Sleep Formula herbal is an excellent muscle relaxant, and the End Pain natural herbal formula is good for relieving many kinds of pain. I would use the two together, or develop a similar herbal plan, allowing six weeks to see the full effect.
- Try natural and prescription treatments individually and/or in combination, as needed. Dozens of effective ones are available. For more detailed information, see my book *Pain Free 1–2–3* and/or the *From Fatigued to Fantastic!* notes at www.vitality101.com.
- Ultram, Skelaxin, Neurontin, and Lyrica are excellent pain medications for CFS/FMS. Avoid Tylenol and Advil family medications.
- If you have severe or persistent localized pains, get the book *Winners' Guide to Pain Relief* (available online at www.winoverpain.com) to learn about structural treatments you can do on your own for pain relief.
- I recommend going to a member of the American Academy of Pain Management (www.aapainmanage.org) to find a pain specialist. In addition, the guidelines in Chapter 12 will help you find a physician near you or at the Fibromyalgia & Fatigue Centers nationally who is specially trained in treating fibromyalgia pain.

Questionnaire

1. Do you have widespread FMS pain?

   If yes, check off #12, 64, 65, 70, and 75.

2. Do you have a few localized areas of pain that are especially problematic?

   If yes, check off #71 and 72.

3. Do you have severe vaginal or bladder pain?

   Read the sections on vulvodynia and interstitial cystitis in my *Pain Free 1–2–3*, and check off #17, 22, and 83.

4. For other pains such as back pain, carpal tunnel syndrome, migraines, arthritis, nerve pain, and indigestion, see my book *Pain Free 1–2–3* and/or the *Pain Free 1–2–3* notes at www.vitality101.com and check off the recommended treatments and #83.

8 *More Natural Remedies*

*A*fter the highly technical information in earlier chapters, I think you'll be happy to join me in exploring more simplified, down-to-earth natural remedies. These treatments are often dramatically helpful for CFS/FMS.

It pleases me that there has been an increase in the use and acceptance of herbal remedies. This renaissance has been especially true in Europe and Asia, where the explosion of interest in herbal remedies has been associated with a major increase in scientific research. In Europe, the German government's Federal Health Agency has created the Commission E, an independent group that evaluates the safety and effectiveness of various herbal therapies. It has published a series of more than four hundred articles that help physicians make informed decisions on how to use these tools (available from the American Botanical Council; see Appendix E: Resources). As a result, Germany uses more than three times as many herbal remedies as the United States does. Hopefully, this country will eventually catch up with both Europe and Asia. While the German government actually promotes education and awareness for its physicians, the U.S. Food and Drug Administration (FDA) has prohibited manufacturers from making any therapeutic claims for herbal remedies or even directly supplying the scientific data supporting the use of herbal remedies or information on their proper use with the products unless the company pays the more than $400 million dollars it takes to go through the FDA process. Unfortunately, this is not financially feasible for a product that is not patentable.

Because the quality control of herbals is quite variable, a movement is under way to standardize herbal preparations by making sure that they have a specific amount of the active agent. So if the label says standardized, you have a better chance that the herbal will be effective. If it has the complex wording I use in discussing that herbal product—for example, 24 percent glycosides—better yet. Except for looking to see if these complex words are on the label of the herbal remedy, feel free to ignore the few complex names in this chapter.

Let's review the use of herbal remedies to treat some problems often seen in CFS/FMS.

For Anxiety

Given the severity of the illness and the difficulty finding a physician familiar with CFS/FMS, anxiety is often a common problem in these syndromes. In addition, many of the metabolic problems (such as hypoglycemia from an underactive adrenal or chronic pain) that accompany CFS/FMS can also accentuate anxiety.

Having spent the last thirty years providing effective treatment for those with disabling diseases such as chronic fatigue syndrome, fibromyalgia, and chronic pain, I know how devastating severe anxiety can be. Unfortunately, all that most doctors have to offer are medications such as Valium and antidepressants. These are not just often ineffective, but they are also rife with side effects. Fortunately, herbal remedies can be helpful, and I have found these to be dramatically effective in treating anxiety in my practice. Patients are amazed at how highly effective these remedies are at restoring a naturally calm and peaceful state of mind. What is even more remarkable is that patients find that these herbs actually increase their energy and mental clarity. Let's look at a few of the more helpful ones.

L-THEANINE

L-THEANINE is an herbal remedy that helps insomnia and calms anxiety, while keeping one energized and clear-minded. It does so by increasing the calming neurotransmitter gamma-aminobutyric acid (GABA) while stimulating the production of alpha brain waves, which are associated with a meditative, awake yet relaxed state of mind.[1] L-theanine also naturally stimulates the release of the "happiness molecules" serotonin and dopamine. As it balances out the excess stimulation caused by caffeine,[2] it's only a matter of time until you go to your local Starbucks and the barista asks, "Would you like one pump of Suntheanine or two?" For more information on L-theanine, see Chapter 3. Take between 50 and 200 milligrams of the Suntheanine form (by Taiyo International) to produce relaxation within thirty to forty minutes, without inducing drowsiness.

VITAMIN B COMPLEX

VITAMIN B$_1$ (THIAMINE) is critical for proper brain function, mental clarity, and energy production, as well as for preventing the production of excess lactic acid (lactate). Research has shown that excess sensitivity to high levels of lactic acid is intimately involved in causing anxiety attacks in those who are prone to them. Dr. Janet Travell, who during her lifetime remained the world's leading expert on pain management, discovered that vitamin B$_1$, in very high doses, decreases anxiety and improves mental clarity by overcoming metabolic blocks and helping your body work more effectively—instead of by numbing you. It takes two to six weeks to see the benefits. Take 500 milligrams of vitamin B$_1$ three times a day for anxiety.

VITAMIN B$_3$ (NIACIN) is known as a natural tranquilizer. In a study on rats, niacin had similar effects to Valium on the turnover of serotonin, noradrenaline, dopamine, and GABA in the areas of the brain that are thought to be affected by anxiety—without being addictive. Some experts go so far as to call niacin "nature's Valium." Niacin also helps decrease excess lactic acid levels and episodes of low blood sugar/hypoglycemia (from adrenal fatigue). Take 10 to 100 milligrams of the niacinamide form daily.

VITAMIN B$_6$ (PYRIDOXINE) deficiency can contribute to anxiety, as this vitamin is critical for the production of two brain chemicals (neurotransmitters) that prevent anxiety (GABA and serotonin). Take 25 to 100 milligrams daily.

VITAMIN B$_{12}$ Many individuals require superhigh levels to get adequate levels into the brain, where B$_{12}$ is needed. Take 500 to 1,000 micrograms a day.

VITAMIN B$_5$ (PANTOTHENIC ACID) is another B vitamin that is critical for the treatment of adrenal fatigue. As noted earlier, adrenal fatigue is a common trigger for hypoglycemia-induced anxiety. If you get irritable when you're hungry, crave sugar, crash with stress, and/or have low blood pressure with dizziness on standing, you probably have adrenal fatigue. Take 50 to 1,000 milligrams daily.

Optimal and often high-dose levels of B vitamins create an important foundation for the treatment of anxiety.

MAGNESIUM

Most Americans are deficient in magnesium, a key mineral critical for more than three hundred chemical reactions in the body. In fact, magnesium has been called the antistress mineral. Magnesium relaxes muscles, helps sleep, and relieves tension. Clinically, we have seen that dropping magnesium levels can trigger hyperventilation/panic attacks (and even seizures, if very severe) and that these are often relieved with magnesium therapy. Take 200 milligrams a day.

PASSIONFLOWER EXTRACT

This is one of the best-known herbs for the treatment of anxiety. Passionflower was first cultivated by Native Americans. Spanish conquerors first learned of passionflower from the Aztecs of Mexico, who used it as a sedative to treat insomnia and nervousness. The plant was taken back to Europe, where it became widely cultivated and introduced into European medicine. In fact, in South America when people are anxious, their friends often tell them to "go get a passionflower drink." Take 100 to 200 milligrams one to four times a day, as needed.

MAGNOLIA

Magnolia bark has a long history of use in traditional Chinese formulas that relieve anxiety without leaving you feeling like you've been drugged. Magnolia extract is rich in two phytochemicals—honokiol, which exerts an antianxiety effect, and magnolol, which acts as an antidepressant—and can also alleviate stress without sedating you. Dozens of animal studies have shown that it is a nonaddictive, nonsedating stress buster, even at low doses.

The good news is that you can now be calm and energized, and have a clear mind—naturally. The components above can be taken individually or more easily found in combination in several products such as Calming Balance from Health Freedom Nutrition, or Tranquility from Ultraceuticals (see Appendix E: Resources). For severe anxiety, begin with two to three capsules of either three times a day. Although some effect is seen within a half hour (so it can also be used on an as-needed basis) the effects continue to powerfully increase over two weeks with continued use. Once your anxiety is under control, the dose can then be lowered, or it can be taken when needed. People find it helpful to have effective natural anxiety relief without side effects including brain fog.

The Kava Kava Controversy

Kava kava (or simply kava), a member of the peppercorn family, has been one of the South Pacific's most revered herbs and intoxicants. In several of that region's cultures, it was central to many social celebrations and was often used as a remedy for a number of physical ailments. Uses included soothing the nerves, counteracting fatigue, inducing relaxation, aiding in weight loss, and treating cystitis, urinary tract congestion, and rheumatism. Hawaiian kahunas (medicine men) used it extensively for ailments such as "general debility (especially in children), weary muscles (a great restorer of strength), chills and head colds, difficulty in passing urine, and sharp blinding headaches." Overall, kava was "found to reduce fatigue, allay anxiety, and to produce a generally pleasant, cheerful, and sociable attitude . . . [sometimes] bordering on intoxication."[3] Kava was traditionally prepared as a drink from the chewed or ground-up herb. When used ceremonially, kava was usually taken on an empty stomach in the evening.

In the United States, it is usually taken in capsule form. A single dose containing 150 to 210 milligrams of kava pyrones is the usual recommended dose to induce sleep. Most capsules contain 30 percent kava pyrones, so a 250-milligram capsule has 75 milligrams of kava. Thus, to get

150 to 210 milligrams of the pyrones, you would take 500 to 700 milligrams of the extract at night for sleep. At this dose, many people find that it relieves insomnia and induces a deep, restful sleep with clear, epic-length dreams. Upon waking, they report feeling rested.[3]

When used for anxiety, the usual dose is one 100-milligram capsule three times a day. The effect begins in about one week and increases over the next eight weeks. Interestingly, while several placebo-controlled studies have shown kava to be as effective for anxiety as prescription medications like amitriptyline (Elavil) and diazepam (Valium), unlike the sedating prescription medications, it was not found to cause any significant side effects. Surprisingly, it actually improved mental functioning and clarity. Research also shows kava to be an excellent muscle relaxant. It seems to work by a mechanism similar to that of lidocaine (Novocain), which has been shown to be beneficial for CFS/FMS.[3-4]

Although most people do not get any side effects when using kava alone for short periods, there are several cautions. Kava may increase the effect of other sedative medications. If you do combine kava with other sedatives, you should do so only if it does not severely impair functioning. The German Commission E monograph on kava suggests it not be used in pregnancy or nonsituational depression (that is, depression for no apparent reason).[4]

A second concern with kava is that taking prolonged high doses may cause a dry, scaly rash that begins on the face and moves downward. Visual sensitivity to bright light may also occur. Taking the B vitamins may decrease this, as can staying in the dose range discussed above. If you take kava kava and a rash occurs, stop taking the kava or lower the dose immediately.

Although there have been a few rare reports of liver inflammation with chronic use, these are so unusual relative to most medications (e.g., acetaminophen) that I still consider it acceptable to use. Nonetheless, this rare side effect has made the use of kava controversial. Like a number of natural treatments, you should take kava kava only under the care of a holistic physician.

For Depression

Happiness has its own biochemistry, which can be powerfully balanced and enhanced naturally. Using the SHIN protocol will help achieve that balance, through a good night's sleep (Chapter 3), hormonal supplementation (Chapter 4), and overall nutritional support (Chapter 6). Research has also shown that walking briskly each day is as effective as Prozac for depression.

It is also critical that your body has the building blocks to make the three key "happiness" neurotransmitters that your body needs: serotonin, dopamine, and norepinephrine. Many natural products are helpful for depression, and as is often the case, it is critical to begin with proper nutrition. Let's review these, beginning with the basics.

- B_{12} and folate/folic acid seem to be especially important. These two nutrients together contribute strongly to the production of both serotonin and a powerful depression-fighting nutrient called SAMe. Approximately one-third of patients with depression have been found to be deficient in folic acid, and this by itself can cause depression, as can B_{12} deficiency. In fact, studies of high-dose folic acid have shown this nutrient to be effective as an antidepressant. Take 500 to 2,000 micrograms of vitamin B_{12} and 400 to 1,200 micrograms of folic acid a day to be sure that optimal levels are getting into the brain where they are needed.
- The B vitamins riboflavin and niacinamide are critical for energy production. Depression is a common symptom of riboflavin and niacin deficiency. Take 25 to 100 milligrams of each daily.
- Vitamin B_6 levels are often quite low in depressed patients, and this is especially problematic in women taking birth control pills or estrogen—both of which can deplete vitamin B_6. Vitamin B_6 is critical for the production of serotonin, dopamine, and norepinephrine. Take 25 to 100 milligrams daily.
- Magnesium deficiency is the single most important nutritional deficiency in the United States. It contributes to pain, fatigue, and increased risk of heart attacks, in addition to depression, as magnesium is critical in more than three hundred different reactions in the body. Take 200 to 400 milligrams a day.
- Serotonin is made from 5-hydroxytryptophan (5-HTP), and dopamine and norepinephrine are made from tyrosine. Studies have shown 5-HTP to be as effective as prescription antidepressants, but much better tolerated. Another placebo-controlled study has shown tyrosine to also be as effective as prescription antidepressants without side effects. In addition, if 5-HTP is given without tyrosine, it often stops working after a few months.

 Do not take 5-HTP without your holistic doctor's okay if you are also on prescription antidepressants, as the combination may raise serotonin too high. Because it can be stimulating, tyrosine is best taken early in the day. Take 200 to 400 milligrams of 5-HTP and 500 to 1,000 milligrams of tyrosine a day.

- The effectiveness of Saint John's wort as an antidepressant has been documented in twenty-five double-blind studies with a total of more than fifteen hundred patients. Those studies showed the herb to be as effective as prescription antidepressants, without the side effects. In addition, it helped improve sleep, lower anxiety, and raise self-esteem in study participants. Take 300 to 500 milligrams three times a day.
- Magnolia bark helps depression as well as anxiety.

Although some effect is seen within two to three weeks of starting these natural antidepressants, the effects continue to powerfully increase over six weeks with continued use. Once your depression is under control, the dose can then be lowered, and you can ask your physician about tapering off your antidepressants.

These nutrients and herbs can be tried individually or can be found in combination in Happiness 1–2–3 from Health Freedom Nutrition and in In Harmony by Ultraceuticals (see Appendix E: Resources). Both products contain 5-HTP and Saint John's wort, so consult with your holistic physician if you are also taking prescription antidepressants, to maintain safe serotonin levels.

For Memory and Circulation

Ginkgo biloba extract has been shown to have multiple benefits. These include:

- *Improving memory.* This effect has been shown in healthy young volunteers and in older adults in several placebo-controlled studies.[5-7] Many CFS/FMS patients also find that ginkgo helps their memory. In twelve healthy males, electroencephalogram (EEG) testing showed that taking 120 to 240 milligrams of ginkgo biloba extract improved alpha brain wave activity in a way that supported better cognitive function.
- *Improving circulation.* In general, ginkgo improves circulation in the brain and legs. More than forty controlled studies have shown this. In the process, ginkgo may also decrease tinnitus (ringing in the ears) and headaches, as well as Raynaud's syndrome, in which spasms in the arteries of the fingers in response to cold cause pain and extreme

coldness. This is sometimes seen in people with CFS/FMS. Ginkgo may also lower cholesterol and help angina.

- *Improving the decreased libido and erections and the delayed orgasm sometimes seen with antidepressant use.* Dosages of 60 to 80 milligrams of ginkgo three times a day for six weeks are required for this.
- *Decreasing the breast tenderness and mood shifts of premenstrual syndrome (PMS).*[7A]
- *Helping relieve loss of balance and vertigo.*[8, 9]
- *Helping asthma and bronchitis.* In China, ginkgo is made into a tea for this purpose.
- *Helping depression.* Doses of 80 milligrams, taken three times a day, may be effective for this.

The ginkgo you buy should be a 50:1 extract standardized to contain 24 percent glycosides (it will say this on the label). For most purposes, 40 milligrams three times a day is the standard dose. Treating depression, however, requires 80 milligrams three times a day. It takes six weeks to see the effect of treatment. Serious side effects are uncommon, as are drug interactions. In fact, the side effects seen with ginkgo in studies were often less than those seen with placebo.

For Occasional Energy Boosts

Tyrosine is an amino acid (one of the building blocks of protein) that is used to make the neurotransmitter norepinephrine. This brain chemical is thought to be low in people with CFIDS/FMS. Tyrosine may be considered for occasional use, and acts as a stimulant without significant side effects.[10] Take 500 to 4,000 milligrams daily for energy.

For Antiviral Protection

For people with CFIDS/FMS, the main use of lemon balm, also known as melissa, is to improve sleep (see Chapter 3). However, the herb can also be used topically as an antiviral against cold sores if used early in the outbreak.[11]. Use Loma-hephan cream applied two to four times a day for five to ten days.

For the Flu

Elderberry extract can help ease flu symptoms and shorten the duration of the illness. In one study, 90 percent of patients who took elderberry extract were completely well in two to three days versus six days for the placebo group. Take four tablespoons a day for three days. Children should take no more than two tablespoons a day for three days.

For High Cholesterol

Cholesterol-lowering medications can be very problematic in CFS/FMS patients, depleting coenzyme Q_{10} and triggering or aggravating muscle pain. As an alternative for my patients, I recommend the following herbal combination treatment:

- Inositol hexaniacinate, 650 milligrams three times a day
- Chromium, 800 to 1,000 micrograms a day
- Berberine, 900 to 1,200 milligrams a day
- Policosanol, 20 to 40 milligrams a day
- Deodorized garlic, 500 to 1,000 milligrams a day, or 1 to 2 cloves of fresh garlic a day

These can be taken individually or found in combination in Chol-less from Ultraceuticals. They can also be taken along with cholesterol-lowering medications. Give these herbals six weeks to work. In addition, add oats, which can also help lower cholesterol, to your diet by eating oatmeal or a cereal such as Life or Cheerios. Your holistic doctor can advise you on how to effectively lower cholesterol without drugs.

For Loss of Libido

This is a common problem, found in 73 percent of CFS/FMS patients. For women, I recommend the following treatment combination:

- Maca root extract, 400 to 800 milligrams a day
- Rhodiola rosea extract, 150 to 300 milligrams a day
- Ashwagandha root extract, 250 to 500 milligrams a day
- Siberian ginseng extract, 150 to 300 milligrams a day
- Ginkgo biloba extract 50 to 240 milligrams a day
- Diindolymethane (DIM), 100 to 200 milligrams a day
- Macuna pruriens extract, (15 percent L-dopa), 100 to 200 milligrams a day

These can be tried individually or many of these can be found in combination in Desire by Ultraceuticals or Hot Plants for Her by Enzymatic Therapy. For men, I recommend:

- Maca root extract, 400 to 800 milligrams a day
- Rhodiola rosea extract, 150 to 300 milligrams a day
- Epimedium extract, 100 to 200 milligrams a day
- Longjack extract, 50 to 100 milligrams a day
- Panax ginseng, 100 to 200 milligrams a day
- Ginkgo biloba extract, 50 to 240 milligrams a day
- Diindolymethane (DIM), 100 to 200 milligrams a day
- Macuna pruriens extract (15 percent L-dopa), 50 to 200 milligrams a day
- Tribulus terrestris extract, 100 to 200 milligrams a day

These can be tried individually or many of these can be found in combination in Potency Plus by Ultraceuticals or Hot Plants for Him by Enzymatic Therapy.

For Osteoporosis

Because of hormonal deficiencies and inability to exercise, we often see loss of bone density (osteoporosis and osteopenia) in CFS/FMS. Fortunately, natural remedies can be more effective than prescription medications for these problems. I recommend:

- Vitamin D, 2,000 to 3,000 IU a day
- Vitamin K, 500 to 600 micrograms a day
- Calcium, 1,000 milligrams a day
- Magnesium, 200 to 400+ milligrams a day
- Boron, 2 to 3 milligrams a day
- Silica, 200 micrograms a day
- Strontium, 170 to 640 milligrams a day

Strontium deserves special mention. This mineral is highly effective at improving bone density. I am not speaking about strontium–90, the very dangerous radioactive compound released during nuclear testing. The strontium available in health food stores is nonradioactive and safe— even in high doses. Studies using strontium in the treatment of 353 osteoporosis patients showed a dramatic 15 percent increase in spine bone mineral density (BMD) over two years in patients using 680 milligrams of strontium (2,000 milligrams of strontium ranelate) a day.[12] A placebo-controlled study with 1,649 osteoporotic women showed that new fractures decreased by 49 percent in the first year of treatment, and bone mineral density in the lumbar spine increased by an average of 14.4 percent after three years. There was an 8.3 percent increase in hip BMD as well.[13] Other forms of strontium have shown similar benefits, and 170 to 680 milligrams of elemental strontium daily appears to be a good dose. (I suspect the 680-milligram dose used in the studies is higher than is needed.) Early data suggest that strontium may also be helpful in the treatment of osteoarthritis. Although it took three to thirty-six months of therapy, taking strontium was associated with a marked reduction in bone pain in osteoporosis patients.[14]

All of the above can be found individually or can be found in combination in Bone Health from Ultraceuticals. In addition, be sure to optimize estrogen, testosterone, and DHEA-S levels as discussed in Chapter 4 and to increase the amount you walk as able.

A Word of Caution

While herbs are generally safe when used correctly, there are several that can cause liver inflammation, and chaparral has even caused liver failure. Some other herbs that may cause liver disease include germander, comfrey, mistletoe, margosa oil, maté tea, gordolobo, yerba tea, Jin Bu Huan, and pennyroyal. And there are many more. Always follow label instructions and talk to your holistic doctor about what herbal supplements you are taking. If you have unexplained mild elevation of your liver blood tests (SGOT and SGPT [ALT and AST]), stay off herbs for three months and then repeat the test to be sure levels have returned to normal.

If you are interested in learning more about herbs in general, two excellent resources are the American Botanical Council and the *Quarterly Review of Natural Medicine* (see Appendix E: Resources). I also invite you to sign up for my free e-mail newsletter at www.vitality101.com, which keeps you up to date on the newest research and developments in maintaining overall health. It also reviews a different illness each issue—explaining how to use the best of natural and prescription therapies.

In addition, don't forget how helpful yoga and other forms of bodywork, energy work, and other structural therapies can be for anxiety, pain, depression, and overall well-being. We have placed an article by qigong master Ken Cohen in the *From Fatigued to Fantastic!* site notes at www.vitality101.com, in which he explains how to use qigong to treat CFS/FMS.

Important Points

- Hundreds of natural remedies are available to help treat medical problems and maintain optimal health. These are often more effective, and almost always safer and cheaper, than prescription medications.
- An outstanding natural remedy for both anxiety and insomnia is L-theanine from green tea. Use only the Suntheanine form, which is the only one most reliable companies will add to their products.
- Excellent natural remedies are available for osteoporosis, anxiety, depression, high cholesterol, loss of libido, pain, and many other problems.
- Strontium can be more effective than many medications for osteoporosis.

Questionnaire

1. Do you have high cholesterol? If yes, check off #75A.

2. Do you have anxiety? If yes, check off #7.

3. Do you have depression? If yes, check off #58.

4. Do you have loss of bone density (osteoporosis or osteopenia)? If yes, check off #69.

5. Do you have loss of libido? If yes, check off #60.

9   *Other Areas to Explore*

Most CFS/FMS patients obtain full resolution of, or at least substantial improvement in, their symptoms with the approaches I have discussed so far. However, some patients still suffer significant persistent disabilities. Several physicians have found success with other treatments, and many of these are worth exploring. And, most importantly, there are three critical areas that although not "high tech" are important to repeat and stress. These are:

1. Keep your attention on what feels good and makes you happy.
2. Exercise (once you are on treatment).
3. Be gentle with yourself.

Let's begin by exploring other treatments, in order of priority, that can be very helpful in a subset of patients.

Overcoming Food and Environmental Sensitivities

Although many of my patients' food and other sensitivities resolve when we treat their underlying yeast overgrowth, parasitic infections, and underactive adrenal glands, problems sometimes persist and need to be treated. These kinds of sensitivities can be hard to isolate because of the many different reactions that they can cause. In addition, some reactions are subtle, while others can be confused with other medical conditions. To further complicate matters, many people are sensitive to food additives that they do not even know are present. Two important examples of these are monosodium glutamate (MSG) and aspartame (the artificial sweetener).

Unfortunately, most food allergy blood tests are simply not reliable. They are expensive and often leave people with the incorrect belief that they are allergic to everything. I find that most food allergy tests are better at making people crazy than at distinguishing true allergies. This was confirmed by a study done at Bastyr University.[1] They found that when an individual's blood was sent to a number of laboratories doing food allergy testing, each lab gave markedly different results from the same blood sample. The same individual patient was found to be allergic to anywhere from 22 to 76 percent of foods tested, depending on which lab did the test. Even when several vials of blood from one person—but labeled with different names—were sent to a single lab, they still gave different results. Because of this, I consider most food allergy blood testing to be unreliable; however, there are a few laboratories that may be helpful. For example, ELISA/ACT Biotechnologies Laboratories (previously known as Serammune Physicians Laboratories) may be more reliable, as duplicate tests on the same person have been consistent in the past.[2]

The best approaches that I have found for determining what allergies/sensitivities, if any, are present are:

- *Nambudripad Allergy Elimination Technique (NAET).* When done by a gifted practitioner, NAET is a remarkably powerful and easy way to not just test for sensitivities, but to also quickly eliminate them.
- *An elimination diet.* In an elimination diet, the most common problem foods are eliminated from the diet for two weeks. The foods that seem to cause the most problems are milk, wheat, eggs, soy, citrus, monosodium glutamate (MSG), aspartame, sugar, alcohol, chocolate, and coffee. People with food allergies usually go through withdrawal when they cut out the foods to which they are allergic, and they may feel worse for the first seven to ten days. But once they get over the hump, they often feel dramatically better. The eliminated food groups are then reintroduced, adding one every few days, to isolate the spe-

cific problem foods. These problem foods are left out of the diet for a few months and then are slowly reintroduced, since the sensitivity will often have decreased. Once reintroduced, the problem foods are initially eaten every three to seven days to see how they are tolerated.

- *Sublingual neutralization.* Many physicians who practice what is called environmental medicine use sublingual neutralization, among other approaches, and are very skilled at treating food allergies. In sublingual neutralization, dilutions of the allergic substance placed under the tongue will reproduce and later eliminate the allergic symptoms. Although I don't use these approaches, and although they are controversial, I have seen them work wonders for many people.

I prefer to use the first two of these approaches, especially NAET, which I find to be the simplest and most effective way to look for and eliminate food and environmental sensitivities, and food allergy elimination diets to be the least expensive. Let's review both of these a bit further.

NAET was developed by Devi S. Nambudripad, M.D., Ph.D., R.N., chiropractor, and acupuncturist. She developed a system that combines acupressure and applied kinesiology (AK muscle testing) to look for and eliminate underlying sensitivities. When your body is allergic or sensitive to something, and a practitioner tests, using many different vials (each containing the homeopathic signatures of a specific substance), the energy in your acupuncture/meridian system weakens when you hold the offending substance. When that happens, your muscles may also weaken, and this weakness can be tested for using AK, thereby determining to what things your body is sensitive. Stimulating certain acupuncture points while you hold the vial can then desensitize your body to that substance, eliminating that allergy (see www.NAET.com for more information).

I highly recommend NAET in my practice, and am myself a true convert to its effectiveness. As a (slightly) younger man, I had horrible ragweed allergies (hay fever). A friend and NAET practitioner in Annapolis kept saying that she could help. But, being a typical arrogant doctor, I of course told her that there was "no way that voodoo would help"—a response that reflected the cynicism a lot of people feel toward alternative therapies. One day, however, when I was especially miserable, she said, "Stop being a nitwit and let me treat you." A single twenty-minute treatment later, I felt as though someone had turned off a faucet in my nose. My severe lifelong hay fever was gone. That was nine years ago, and my hay fever has never returned. I was so impressed that I flew to Los Angeles to meet Dr. Devi and later married the woman in Annapolis who treated me.

Since then, I have learned more about how powerful NAET can be, even seeing autism improve with the treatment. Our foundation funded a recently completed study using NAET for autism. After one year of fifty treatments, twenty-three of the thirty autistic children were improved and back in regular schools as opposed to zero of thirty in the untreated control group. The results were so impressive that a second study may move forward in the future through the Complementary and Alternative Medicine (CAM) section of the NIH.

If you find yourself sensitive to many foods or other substances, I recommend going to www.naet.com to get more information and to find a practitioner near you (there are more than eight thousand worldwide). Each treatment can eliminate one allergy, and I recommend you allow the practitioner to treat for the ten most common allergen groups before going after specific allergens. It usually takes ten to fifteen visits to begin seeing the benefits, as most people usually have multiple sensitivities, and twenty-five to fifty treatments to complete the treatment course. If you have only a single allergen (e.g., hay fever or cat dander), then, like me, you may only need one to three treatments.

Multiple Food Elimination Diet

An elimination diet can be difficult but is inexpensive and can help isolate the foods to which you have sensitivities. The diet I prefer only eliminates the more common offending foods. For detailed information on how to do this kind of diet, see the *From Fatigued to Fantastic!* notes at www .vitality101.com.

Some people, however, prefer to do a more limited elimination diet in which they eat and drink nothing but rice, lamb, and distilled water for ten to fifteen days. This is a very restrictive diet, and I recommend that it be done only under the supervision of a health-care practitioner (such as a naturopath). Should you decide to try this extreme elimination diet, you'll want to be sure that you are still maintaining good nutrition. Jeffrey Bland, a well-known nutritional biochemist, has developed a powder that supplies necessary nutrients from low-allergy sources, such as rice. During the initial seven to ten days of the elimination diet, it allows you to avoid all

allergic foods. If your symptoms resolve during this time span, you are jus-
tified in suspecting that you have food allergies. You can then begin rein-
troducing the different foods as described on pages 230–231 to determine
exactly which ones are causing problems for you. Although Dr. Bland's
food product costs about three hundred dollars, it can help determine food
sensitivities. However, you should not use this approach if you have very
severe CFS—for example, if you are bedridden—because you need to
strengthen your body as much as possible before you go through the withdrawal phase of treating food allergies. For more information on Dr.
Bland's powder, contact Metagenics (see Appendix E: Resources).

Neurotoxins—Biotoxin-Induced Illnesses

Neurotoxin-induced illness is a concept developed by Ritchie Shoemaker, a physician and researcher who practices in Pocomoke, Maryland.
Dr. Shoemaker theorizes that the production of toxins can be caused
by many different processes, including Lyme infections; exposure to water-
damaged buildings (sick building syndrome), ciguatera (fish toxin), and
marine algae; injuries; and even certain genetic illnesses. These toxic chemicals (called ionophores because they can move from cell to cell) can stay in
your body even after the initial infection or trigger is gone. Normally, the
body is able to excrete most toxins through the liver and kidneys to eliminate them from the body. What makes these toxins unique is that they are
small enough to be easily reabsorbed in the gut, and are excreted only by
the liver. The liver excretes the toxins into the bowel so that they can be
eliminated from the body with your stool. Unfortunately, these toxins are
then reabsorbed from the bowel and therefore cannot be eliminated (they
continue to recirculate to the liver and then back to the blood).

These toxins can cause or be associated with multiple hormonal and
immune changes. Dr. Shoemaker finds that most CFS/FMS patients have
hypothalamic dysfunction associated with low melanocyte-stimulating
hormone (MSH) and VEGF levels, as well as multiple other hormonal
problems (including those I discussed earlier in Chapter 4). In addition,
numerous changes are seen in immune-system molecules such as Complement 4A (C_4A) elevation, which he uses to monitor therapy. Although he
uses literally dozens of tests to diagnose patients and monitor the effectiveness of treatment, and the science behind what he does is complex (and rea-

sonable), I discuss a simplified overview of his treatment protocol, which many patients find helpful. For those who would like more detail, I refer you to his recent study,[3] described at www.vitality101.com, and Dr. Shoemaker's Web site at www.chronicneurotoxins.com.

What Tests Should You Start With?

Although no blood tests are currently available to directly measure these toxins, there are numerous tests that can look for their effects and help you and your physician monitor therapy. There is an extensive set of baseline tests that Dr. Shoemaker recommends. If one would like to begin with a markedly simplified approach (my recommendation, not his) that focuses more on how to get well than on understanding the detailed biochemistry, one should begin with the following tests (although much of the information below, except for the VCS vision test, is more for your physician than for you, so feel free to skip over the complex parts):

1. *VCS vision test.* Dr. Shoemaker feels that your nervous system is sensitive to these toxins. The retina in the back of the eye is part of the nervous system, and he uses a test that examines the body's ability to discern different shades of black and gray. This VCS vision test can be done on his Web site for about ten dollars. Although it may be positive in some healthy people, and negative in 8 percent of CFS/FMS patients (it is positive in 92 percent), it is a helpful test to monitor his treatment.

2. *Do a special culture of your nose.* Using a sterile cotton swab, the doctor gets a sample from deep inside your nose (at least 2 inches). This has to be cultured using an API-STEP culture technique done in some hospital microbiology labs. If the culture shows colonization with a coagulation-negative staph bacteria resistant to at least two antibiotics, see the treatment on page 237.

3. *Western blot for Lyme,* C4A (Complement 4A—should be under 3,000) and, to screen further for Lyme, a C3A (if the C3A and C4A are both positive, suspect Lyme infection).

4. *If you want to have tests to document the problem* and with which to monitor treatment, consider an MSH (low), VEGF (low), and MMP9

(high; use 85 to 332 for the normal range). However, I still think that how you feel is the best monitor of your progress.

Dr. Shoemaker monitors dozens of other tests in his patients as well, but the biggest part of his treatment can be done with what we've recommended here.

What Is the Treatment?

Below is a simplified form of the treatment protocol Dr. Shoemaker recommends to his patients:

STEP 1

Because the liver is able to pull the toxins out of the body and excrete them into your bowel, the trick is to keep the toxins in your bowel so that they go out in the stool. Fortunately, there is a medication called Questran (cholestyramine), which is a powder that acts like a sponge and soaks up the toxins. Dr. Shoemaker recommends that people take one scoop or one packet four times a day. Those who are going to improve with this treatment alone will usually start feeling better within a month, or at least have their vision test go from positive to negative. Insomnia, pain, and spastic colon symptoms can also sometimes improve quickly with this treatment.

As a caution, be aware that if you have underlying Lyme disease, the Questran will cause a severe flare-up. Because of this, if the Lyme test *or* both the C4A and C3A tests are positive (which can be seen with Lyme), he recommends treating with doxycycline 100 milligrams twice a day for three weeks followed by the medication Actos, 45 milligrams a day for seven days just before beginning the Questran. Continue the Actos for three more days along with the Questran.

If the Questran does not eliminate the symptoms and normalize the vision test after one month, continue the Questran for one more month. However, if you are better after one month (two months for Lyme patients), decrease the Questran to twice a day until symptoms resolve, the vision test is normal, and the C4A blood test is normal. Then you can stop treatment. If symptoms then recur, it suggests that something (e.g., persistent infection or being in a "sick building") is still making neurotoxins. This should then be treated as well.

The main problem with Questran is that is soaks up everything. This means that you will likely not absorb a lot of the medications or supplements you are taking if they are taken at the same time as the Questran. Because of this, take the Questran on this schedule:

- Take your vitamins and medications (except iron and sleep meds) first thing in the morning. Wait 30 minutes before taking the Questran and then another twenty to thirty minutes until eating breakfast. When lowering the dose to two times a day, skip the a.m. Questran dose.
- Take your next two doses of Questran (each day) as close to a half hour before lunch and dinner as you can. Eating makes your body pour the neurotoxin-containing bile into your gut. Eating a half hour after the Questran puts the medicine right where it needs to be to soak up and bind the neurotoxins.
- Take your last (fourth) dose at bedtime. Take any sleep aids one hour before bedtime so they can be absorbed before you take the Questran.

Mix each dose of Questran in 4 ounces of water. Drink 12 ounces of water after taking the Questran. Constipation is normally a problem while on Questran, so drink a lot of water and eat a few prunes each day. Also, take high-dose magnesium or vitamin C or other laxatives as needed, since you want to move the bound neurotoxins out of your body. Dr. Shoemaker uses 70 percent sorbitol, 1 to 3 teaspoons three times a day as needed for constipation.

It is not uncommon for people to have their symptoms worsen—sometimes dramatically—when a chronic infection is first killed. This is called a die-off (Herxheimer) reaction, and was first noted in the early days of treating syphilis. Since then, it has been seen in many infections, including fungal infections. Interestingly, some people also experience this when they begin Questran to remove toxins. Dr. Shoemaker finds that if people's symptoms worsen while on the Questran, they are more likely to have Lyme disease. He uses a medication called Actos (taken at a dose of 45 milligrams a day for seven days before restarting the Questran and continuing for three days after resuming Questran), which can decrease the die-off reaction. Because people with CFS/fibromyalgia tend to be sensitive to medications anyway, you may choose to begin with one teaspoon of Questran once or twice daily for one to two days and then increase the dose to decrease the risk of getting a severe die-off reaction.

Although the Questran has about 1 teaspoon of sugar per scoop, it is still okay to use in this situation. Using unsweetened cranberry juice (add stevia) instead of apple juice, or simply mixing it with water if even minimal sugar is a problem will decrease the amount of sugar you are getting as well. You can also get Questran lite with NutraSweet. This first step with Questran will be adequate treatment for only 9 percent of patients, but is critical for the following steps to work. If the patient's symptoms persist despite the Questran, Dr. Shoemaker then recommends doing each of the treatments in the order below until he or she feels well.

STEP 2

If the nasal swab culture is positive for a coag-negative staph bacteria resistant to at least two of the antibiotics tested against it, Dr. Shoemaker recommends that his patients be treated with the following three antibiotics simultaneously for one month:

1. Rifampin, 600 milligrams each morning with food
2. Bactroban nasal cream or spray, applied deep in both nostrils three times a day
3. Either doxycycline (100 milligrams two times a day), Ceftin (250 milligrams two times a day), or Cipro (500 milligrams two times a day), depending on what the test shows that the infection is sensitive to.

Stay on Questran twice a day during this stage as well, and recheck the nasal culture a week after discontinuing the antibiotics. Around 50 percent of patients will be feeling better by this stage.

STEP 3

If you are not adequately improved, Dr. Shoemaker recommends that you look for wheat (gluten) allergies. Do this by checking blood tests for anti-gliaden IgA and IgG antibodies and transglutaminase IgA antibodies. If the transglutaminase IgA antibodies are positive, you have celiac sprue (a genetic wheat allergy) and need to see a gastroenterologist. If this test is negative, but either the anti-gliaden IgA or IgG antibodies are positive, you must avoid gluten (wheat products) for six months. This is a difficult diet; a dietitian can show you how to construct gluten-free menus. In addition, Dr. Shoemaker believes that this condition is usually associated with a mold-contaminated indoor exposure. He recommends a test called the EPA Relative Mold Index (ERMI), available from the Mycometrix Company in New Jersey for about three hundred dollars a kit. Use it to check your home and work space and other places where you spend a lot of time. If the test scores positive (over 10), it suggests that you may be suffering from sick-building syndrome. If so, there are four key steps to treatment:

1. Remove yourself from the contaminated environment.
2. Remove the source of the moisture causing the mold overgrowth (e.g., fix any leaks).
3. Decontaminate with the help of mold-removal experts.
4. Install HEPA filtration.

Once these are completed, it is reasonable to repeat the Questran as in Step 1. If the C4A level and symptoms stay low after this, you are in good shape. If they go back up, it suggests persistent toxic exposure.

STEP 4

If symptoms persist, check a matrix metallo-proteinase-9 (MMP-9) and VEGF blood tests. If the MMP-9 is between 332 and 1,500, Dr. Shoemaker treats with Actos (a diabetes medicine that can also be used in nondiabetics) at a dose of 45 milligrams a day plus a low amylose diet (low in simple carbohydrates) for one month. If the MMP-9 is higher than 1,500, he treats for two to three months. If the MMP-9 is normal, or symptoms persist after this treatment and normalization of the MMP-9, he then goes to Step 5.

STEP 5

If the VEGF is under 31, Dr. Shoemaker continues the Actos and adds fish oil (1 to 2 tablespoons a day; I recommend Eskimo-3 or the Omega-3 brands of fish oil, which are mercury free) and creatine (take 1.5 grams a day for every ten pounds that you weigh) for one more month.

STEP 6

In less than 10 percent of patients, there is a persistent C4A elevation and symptoms persist. In this group Dr. Shoemaker uses injections of a hormone that stimulates new blood-cell formation called Procrit, giving 8,000 units twice a week for five doses. If you still do not feel better, specialized testing to look for neurologic disorders may be necessary. If you initially improve on Procrit and then relapse, he suggests resuming Procrit at a dose of 4,000 to 6,000 units each three to five days as needed.

Although Procrit raises the low red blood cell mass seen in CFS, this is not why it works here. Levels of Procrit need to stay elevated to suppress elevated C4A, and giving it weekly is not frequent enough. In fact, a study giving the injections weekly improved the red blood cell mass without improving symptoms of CFS.[4] However, Dr. Shoemaker's twice-weekly approach normalized C4A levels and markedly decreased brain fog in CFS.[5]

For more information on Dr. Shoemaker's work and to do the VCS vision test, visit his Web site at www.chronicneurotoxins.com.

Seasonal Affective Disorder

If your fatigue is a problem mainly from October to May, is less pronounced on sunny days, and is associated with increased sleep, weight gain, and carbohydrate craving during the winter, you may suffer from sunlight deprivation. This malady is known as seasonal affective disorder (SAD), or the winter blues.

SAD is treatable with a light box, which is available by mail order (see Bio Brite in Appendix E: Resources). Use a 10,000-lux box positioned at a forty-five-degree angle in relation to your face and about eighteen inches away. Spend thirty to forty-five minutes in front of the box every morning from September through May. Add a half hour at night, if necessary. Experiment to find the times of day and session lengths that feel best to you. You do not have to sit still in front of the box, but can do table work such as reading or writing.

If you have trouble waking up in the morning, attach a bright (about 250-lux) bedside lamp to a timer and program it to turn on two hours before your alarm is set to go off. Portable light visors are also available by mail order. Most patients find that it takes one to six weeks of light treatment to see any results.

Serotonin deficiency has been put forward as a possible cause of SAD. Serotonin is a neurotransmitter that is particularly connected with the process of sleep. Medications that raise the serotonin level, such as fluoxetine (Prozac), have been shown to be effective against SAD.[6] In addition, as discussed in Chapter 6, vitamin D from sunshine can have major immune system and other benefits.

Medications

Many medications can cause fatigue as a side effect. If you are on a medication and your fatigue has been worse since you started taking it, talk to your physician about alternative measures or about just stopping it. This is especially important if you are on cholesterol-lowering medications (as discussed in Chapter 8) or high blood pressure medications. If on the latter, let's discuss which ones are likely to make you feel better instead of worse.

Interestingly, a blood pressure–raising enzyme called angiotensin-converting enzyme (ACE) has been found to be elevated in some CFS/FMS patients.[7] Despite this, their blood pressure may still be low, due, for example, to underactive adrenal glands. According to some physicians, CFS/FMS symptoms and depression have improved in a few patients who were given the ACE inhibitor captopril (Capoten) for hypertension. Other doctors have found that some CFS/FMS patients improved with nimodipine (Nimotop) or amlodipine (Norvasc), calcium channel blockers that relax the blood vessels to allow more blood and oxygen to get to the brain and heart. If your blood pressure is high, you might consider a trial of Nimotop or, if that is too expensive, Norvasc, followed by a trial of hydralazine (Apresoline) and then a trial of quinapril (Accupril) or captopril (Capoten), for two weeks each, to see which feels the best to you. If your ACE levels are high, it may also suggest the presence of antibiotic-sensitive infections within your cells (as occurs in another immune illness called sarcoidosis), and a trial of antibiotic therapy as discussed in Chapter 5 may be warranted. More importantly, if you have CFS/FMS and high blood pressure, you are at high risk of having sleep apnea (see page 70).

Detoxification

Many toxic substances, such as mercury from dental fillings, monosodium glutamate (MSG), pesticides, and others too numerous to list, can contribute to CFS/FMS and keep you from healing properly. Many practitioners use detoxification techniques to rid your body of these toxins. Detoxification may be as simple as sitting in a sauna for thirty to sixty minutes a day. Be sure to drink plenty of water while in the sauna and rinse off immediately afterward so that the skin does not reabsorb the toxins. The dry heat also helps tight muscles to relax. If you decide to invest in a home sauna, especially if you are chemically sensitive, the far infrared sauna made by High Tech Health is an excellent choice (see Appendix E: Resources). For more information on detoxification, I recommend Dr. Majid Ali's book *The Canary and Chronic Fatigue*.

The Goldstein Protocol

Dr. Jay Goldstein, a well-known researcher working on brain chemistry and CFS/FMS, has come up with a list of recommended treatments that may be helpful. Because the agents he uses act directly on the disordered blood flow in the brain, Dr. Goldstein finds that patients generally know what effect each medication will have within one hour—and even within minutes for some agents.[8] He has several books that may be too technical for the casual reader; however, the determined reader will find information that can sometimes help not only brain fog, but also pain and fatigue. A newsletter summarizing how to use his treatments is also available at www.vitality101.com. Your physician may help you find relief using the Goldstein protocol.

Guaifenesin

Paul St. Amand, an endocrinologist at UCLA, has proposed that a defect in eliminating/metabolizing phosphates is the underlying cause of fibromyalgia. Dr. St. Amand finds that using an over-the-counter medication called guaifenesin helps eliminate these phosphates, resulting in pain relief. I have found that a small percentage of patients improve with this treatment approach, but most do not. My main concern with the treatment is that you cannot use anything with natural salicylates (aspirin compounds) while on it—eliminating virtually *all* herbals and even makeup. It takes many months to work, and people often experience flare-ups during treatment.

If not for having to eliminate all herbals, I would add this to my protocol. Nonetheless, it can help and is a very inexpensive approach that people can do on their own. Dr. St. Amand's book *What Your Doctor May NOT Tell You About Fibromyalgia* explains how to follow his protocol, and more detailed information is also available in the *From Fatigued to Fantastic!* notes at www.vitality101.com.

Multiple Chemical Sensitivity Syndrome

I believe this syndrome is an extreme subset of chronic fatigue syndrome. In multiple chemical sensitivity syndrome (MCS), the body has given up and is reactive to almost everything in the environment. Many, if not most, CFS/FMS patients have multiple allergies and sensitivities to environmental chemicals and medications. However, while this is common, it is *not* MCS.

Patients with MCS cannot live in a normal house because they can become deathly ill if a new carpet is put in, if the walls are painted or wallpapered, or if pesticide is sprayed. They can become ill just from washing the dishes or reading a book. They can react negatively to any or all of the thousands of chemicals with which we normally come in contact in our daily lives.[9] People who have this extreme problem do have treatment options available to them, however. To learn more, you may want to read *Tired or Toxic?* by Sherry Rogers, M.D. (see Appendix E: Resources). In addition to using the SHIN protocol, you may want to consult NAET practitioners and environmental medicine physicians.

Chiari Malformations and Cervical Stenosis

Rarely, CFS/FMS can be caused by compression of the spinal column or the base of the brain. Neurosurgeon Mike Rosner found that two unusual malformations of the skull or spinal canal could compress the brain and/or spinal cord, causing symptoms that mimicked those of CFS/FMS. When the compression was surgically released, CFS/FMS patients with these malformations sometimes saw a decrease in their pain and fatigue.

The Chiari 1 Malformation (CMI) is a condition in which the back of the skull is underdeveloped, compressing the cerebellar tonsils located at the back of the brain. These tonsils are then squeezed out of the opening at the base of the skull by at least 3 to 5 millimeters (0.12 to 0.2 inch). This is called tonsillar herniation. As with CFS/FMS, CMI can be genetic. There are also situations in which the brain stem is compressed without tonsillar herniation. The second malformation is called cervical stenosis (CS) and is a compression of the spinal cord in the neck because the spinal tube is unusually narrow. Both can cause symptoms that mimic those of CFS/FMS.

While it is not known how common these problems are, it is a current topic of debate. Based on magnetic resonance imaging (MRI) scans as read by radiologists, CMI and CS are not much more common in people with CFS/FMS than in healthy people. On the other hand, the physical examinations of people with CFS/FMS often show abnormalities that are also seen in CMI or CS. Because of these two seemingly opposite findings, some people suggest that CMI and CS are rare in people with CFS/FMS, while others believe that they are common.

Let me put this in perspective. In disc disease, X-rays and MRIs by themselves are not reliable in making the diagnosis. The same problem occurs with CMI and CS. Given fifty spine MRIs of patients with and without disc disease, radiologists cannot reliably tell which group of patients has severe pain and which group is healthy and pain free. Indeed, if you were to lie and tell the radiologist that the healthy group of patients had severe back pain, the MRI report would usually be read as showing several areas of disc disease. This is not to put down radiologists. The radiologists I've had the honor of knowing and working with have been superb. It simply shows the limits of our technology.

Like disc disease, the diagnosis of CMI and CS needs to be made by a combination of MRI, symptoms, and physical exam findings that all match up. Unfortunately, many of the symptoms of CFS/FMS are similar to CMI/CS symptoms, making it harder to tell whether CMI/CS is rare in CFS/FMS patients or whether they *all* have CMI/CS. As research and clinical experience show that more than 85 percent of CFS/FMS patients improve with nonsurgical therapies, it is likely the former. However, because the MRI test shows normal-size bony structures in most CFS/FMS patients yet neurologic examination suggests CMI or CS, it could be that swelling of the brain or spinal cord tissue causes compression, despite a normal-size skull or spinal canal. A whiplash injury or other head and neck injuries, the head being bent backward during surgical intubation for an extended period, infections, and/or hormonal or nutritional deficiencies could each account for all the above findings. It may be analogous to carpal tunnel syndrome—a result of nerve compression that improves by decreasing tissue swelling with thyroid or B_6 supplementation—without surgery.

Although the exam for CMI and CS is complex, there are some screening tests that can simplify things and help you determine whether you need an MRI. Here are some examples:

- You have overactive knee reflexes (present in most CFIDS/FMS patients) and the reflex gets even more active if checked with your head extended backward while sitting up, so your head is looking up at the ceiling.
- You have a lot of trouble with the hand-flip exam: with the palms of your hands down in front of you (parallel to the ground, with one hand on top of the other and touching), repeatedly quickly turn the top hand over back and forth. This means the upper palm, alternating with the back of the upper hand, will be touching the back of the bottom hand. Flip the top hand back and forth around five to ten times.
- Your ablility to feel something cold diminishes markedly as a cold object moves from your face to your neck to midchest—for example, while your skin is touched with a cool spoon or other metal object. The spoon should not slide down, but three areas should be touched for one to two seconds each.

If two of these three tests are positive and you have not gotten better on the SHIN protocol and the other treatments we've discussed, I would consider a referral to Dr. Rosner for evaluation. He is in North Carolina at 828-684-1076. It makes sense to me to treat this condition without surgery before spending thousands of dollars on MRIs and even more on surgery, with its attendant risks.

There are also some other helpful tests that you can do yourself:

- Almost all CMI/CS patients have intense pain at the base of the skull that radiates to the head and neck. This is also common in people who have CFS/FMS without CMI/CS. In CMI/CS, though, it is more likely to be much worse when the head is tilted all the way back for thirty seconds while sitting, so that your head is facing the ceiling. In this position it is also likely to be worse when coughing. In addition, if you have nystagmus (the eyes, while wide open, involuntarily flit back and forth or in a circular motion) when the head is tilted back, this also suggests CMI/CS. Have someone watch your eyes while you do this.

- If you can do a fairly quick tandem walk for fifty feet, according to Dr. Rosner, you probably do not have CMI. The tandem walk test is similar to the test for drunk drivers. Put one heel just in front of the toes of the other foot with each step you take. Try to walk a twenty-five to fifty-foot straight line doing this.

- While sitting, lift one foot three to six inches off the ground. Have someone push down on the top of your thigh with one hand, trying to push the foot back down, while you resist strongly for a few seconds (don't have your partner push down hard enough to hurt). You can also do the pushing yourself. If the foot can be pushed down easily, it's suspicious for CS. However, similar results can be seen with generalized weakness in FMS.

- About 50 percent of people with CMI and CS have no gag reflex. Use a spoon, pen (not the point), or similar object to test your gag reflex. Put the object all the way into the back of your throat and move it against the right and left wall to test for gagging.

- Dr. Rosner reports that about 50 percent of his patients have a positive Romberg test. With your feet together, stand up straight, close your eyes, and hold your arms straight out in front of your body with the palms up for about fifteen to twenty-five seconds. Have someone watch you. If there is a lot of swaying from side to side, the Romberg test is positive.

If treatment for CFS/FMS fails to help you and you have a positive MRI for CMI/CS, I would seek a doctor who has a lot of experience treating CMI/CS in people with CFS/FMS. Otherwise, you run the risk of having the CMI/CS diagnosis missed or having surgery that is not effective because it does not remove enough bone to fully relieve the compression of the brain tissue. I have only needed to refer fewer than seven of my more than three thousand patients for evaluation for surgery for these issues; it is rarely needed.

Ampligen and IV Gamma Globulin

Researchers are also studying treatment with high doses of *intravenous* gamma globulin and Ampligen, both of which are immune-function enhancers. These treatments cost many thousands of dollars per year, and I do not think that most patients need them. Ampligen, for example, increases the time CFS patients can walk on a treadmill by only 18 percent (less than two minutes) over placebo. At forty thousand dollars per six months and with unknown long-term risks, this treatment is way down on my list of recommendations (and not even in my top 270 recommended treatments). When the FDA approves it, though, you will hear a lot about it, as there will be a lot of money to be made.

I do find that weekly intramuscular (versus *intravenous*) injections of 2 cc of gamma globulin (Gammar) for six weeks (or longer if needed) can often dramatically help patients with recurrent infections (see page 135). Alternatively, one can use 4 cc every other week or even weekly, and this may be even more effective. These low-dose shots, luckily, are not as expensive, and even 1 gram a week for six months has been shown to help.[10] I highly recommend them if you have suspected infections that have not otherwise responded to treatment, and save the IV form for cases of genetic gamma globulin deficiencies.

The Future Is Hopeful

Although the SHIN protocol can help more than 85 percent of those with CFS/FMS, we are constantly looking for other issues that need to be addressed and treatments that can help. Eventually, we will achieve our goal of finding effective treatment for everyone.

Important Points

- Check for food sensitivities, then temporarily remove suspect foods from your diet or eliminate them with desensitization techniques such as NAET.

- Consider a VCS vision test at www.chronicneurotoxins.com to look for neurotoxins and treat, if necessary.
- If symptoms worsen and you get severe pain when you tilt your head all the way back, consider CMI/CS.
- Ask your doctor for alternatives to medications that have fatigue as a side effect.
- Treat high blood pressure with Nimotop, Apresoline, or Accupril (and check for sleep apnea). Use natural alternatives instead of cholesterol-lowering medications, when possible.
- If you feel worse between September and April, consider the possibility of seasonal affective disorder.
- Patients have benefited from gamma globulin shots, kutapressin/Nexavir shots, intravenous nutritional support, and a variety of treatments developed by Dr. Jay Goldstein.
- Consider detoxification with a far infrared sauna from High Tech Health (see Appendix E: Resources)
- When you can, begin an exercise program. Walking or warm-water swimming exercises are excellent for beginners.
- Get plenty of fresh air and sunshine (without burning).
- Do not try to make up for lost time as you start to feel better.

Am I Crazy?
Understanding the
10   Mind-Body Connection

We have a bad habit in medicine. If a doctor cannot figure out what is wrong with the patient, the doctor brands that patient a "turkey." Imagine calling an electrician because your lights do not work. The electrician checks all the wiring, can't find the problem, and says, "You're crazy. There's nothing wrong with your lights." You flip the switches and they still do not work, but the electrician just says, "I've looked. There's no problem here," and walks out the door. This is analogous to what many CFS patients experience. I apologize for the medical profession's calling you crazy just because we cannot determine the cause of your problem. It is inappropriate and cruel.

Fortunately, the Centers for Disease Control (CDC), one of the major governmental agencies responsible for CFS (and other) research, is spending millions of dollars on advertising to dispel the misconception that CFS is all in your mind. It is working hard to teach both doctors and the public that CFS is both a very physical and devastating illness. Hopefully, getting treatment will be easier in the future.

Research has proven that people with CFS and those without CFS have similar rates of psychiatric disorders.[1] What you have is clearly a real and physical illness. And, like most other physical processes—such as diabetes, heart disease, cancer, and ulcers—it has an associated psychological component. In my practice, I frequently see CFS patients who seem to be caught on the horns of an emotional dilemma. These patients find themselves in situations in which they are unable to make a choice between two or more alternatives—for example, between working and having children or between staying with or leaving their spouse. These conflicts come in an infinite variety, and defending yourself against acknowledging a conflict can sap your energy. In my experience, when people start to feel better physically, they find it easier to deal with their emotional issues. However, you do not have to resolve every conflict. If you have something that you cannot settle at the moment, you might find it helpful to simply acknowledge the conflict instead of suppressing it. Tell yourself, "Yes, I have these two areas that are in conflict, and I cannot reconcile them now." Many people find that after a while, when they simply acknowledge the problem, a solution comes from a new perspective.

Other people have been convinced that who they are and what they feel and want are not okay, and they tie themselves into emotional knots trying to find a way to get permission to be themselves. *For those of you suffering under the illusion that you are not okay, let me put out a simple proposition. If you are not directly harming another person or severely harming yourself, whoever you are and whatever you want to do or be is simply and inherently okay.* It might also help you to understand that you may sometimes mistake uncomfortable feelings such as disappointment or sadness for fatigue. Try to be aware of when you do this. There is no such thing as an inappropriate feeling. You have the right to feel whatever you feel. Does this mean that you are crazy? No. It simply means that, like all human beings, you have emotional issues to deal with as part of your growth process.

Unfortunately, some patients become so frustrated by being told that their CFS is "all in their head" that they are in a catch–22. They feel that if they acknowledge that they also have emotional issues just like everyone else, they are validating the doctors who say that their illness is all emotional. Rest assured, however, that the research study done at my clinic in Maryland, along with research performed at the CDC and elsewhere, further proves that CFS/FMS are real and physical. This is so because people who received the active treatment improved dramatically and those receiving placebo did not. Chronic fatigue syndrome and fibromyalgia are real, physical diseases. If it was "all in your head" the placebo group would have improved as much as the active group. This means that anyone who says it's all in your head is no longer simply a nitwit. Now they are unscientific nitwits. Give yourself permission to be human. You are no more and no less crazy than anyone else.

Part of getting well is "lightening up." There is a traditional Zen metaphor relating to this truth that describes "worry" as an old man carrying a load of feathers. He is nearly crushed under their weight not because they are heavy, but because he thinks that he is carrying rocks. Like this old man, we can often become weighed down by "rocks" of our own imagining. Many of the worries we carry around sort themselves out as soon as we let go of them. Although things may not always work out the way we would like them to (CFS patients often describe themselves as "control freaks"), they usually work out for the best. Because of this, it helps to have or reclaim a sense of humor.

I am a firm believer in psychological counseling—if and when you feel that it would be helpful. This is especially pertinent in CFS/FMS. As many as 70 percent of you have suffered physical or emotional abuse—as opposed to 15 percent of "healthy" people.[2] Counseling is helpful for anybody who is growing and changing. People who are growing frequently come across areas that are difficult and with which it is usual and natural to need help. As is true for any disease, when you treat the physical component, you must also treat the underlying psychological issues. If you do not, the disease will simply manifest itself in another way.

Although about 12 percent of CFS patients also have depression, only a small minority have depression as the cause of their fatigue. The "depression" caused by CFS/FMS is often simply frustration and stress. This gives you a simple way to distinguish whether you also have depression. CFS/FMS patients usually have a lot of interests and are frustrated by their lack of energy. However, if you have depression that causes fatigue, you probably have few interests. I discuss ways to lift depression, naturally and with prescription drugs, throughout the book, but specifically in Chapter 8.

Whether or not you are depressed, you may consider some type of therapist for emotional support and guidance. Be careful whom you choose, however. Make sure "psychotherapist" is one word—not two! Talk to your friends and relatives to find somebody who is good. Your physician may also be an excellent resource. There are many good therapeutic approaches, but my own personal bias is for a therapist who takes a transpersonal psychology or Jungian approach. I have found one physician, Brugh Joy, to be extraordinarily skilled at helping people understand their deep psyches (see Appendix E: Resources). Dr. Joy runs workshops in the mountains of

Arizona, and I cannot recommend these workshops strongly enough. To me, they seem more effective than regular counseling. Remember that these workshops do not treat the physical symptoms of CFS/FMS, but rather focus on personal growth. I also recommend the telephone counseling by the Reverend Bren Jacobson (see Appendix E: Resources), who has provided a sidebar on the power of asking for what you want, at the end of this chapter. By using your chronic fatigue and fibromyalgia as a springboard for personal growth, you can find your CFS turning into a blessing. I found this to be the case for me. My CFS/FMS gave me a firsthand understanding of the problem and a powerful incentive to learn how to overcome it. It has also led me into wonderful areas of growth.

The Mind-Body Connection

All illnesses have a psychological component. Although the highly stressed executive may have a bacterial infection such as *Helicobacter pylori* or excess acid causing his or her ulcer, it helps to remove the three telephones from his or her ear while treating the infection and excess acid.

I find that most people with CFS/FMS are mega-type-A overachievers. As a group, our sensitivity and intuitive abilities are high. We often had low self-esteem as children, and tended to seek approval, sometimes from someone who was simply not going to give it. This, combined with our sensitivity to the feelings of others, caused us to avoid conflict and to try to meet other people's needs—at the expense of our own. Many of us closed off our feelings and our empathetic nature for a while because we were too young to handle their intensity. Because of our need for approval and our low self-esteem, we often drove ourselves to being the best at what we did, or tried to be all things to all people. Not being able to say no because we wanted to avoid conflict or loss of approval led us to feel as though we could not defend our emotional boundaries, and left us feeling drained. We responded to fatigue by redoubling our efforts, instead of resting as our bodies tried to tell us to do. As we depleted our energy reserves—sometimes while feeling great on an adrenaline "high"—we encountered the physical trigger to our disease ("blew our fuse"), whether it was an infection, an injury, childbirth, or something else. This trigger, combined with physical problems such as yeast overgrowth or hormonal deficiencies and, often, a genetic tendency to the disease, set the process in motion.

What can we do about it? First, we can recognize that all this helped us grow and achieve. One of the fun parts of working with people with CFS/FMS is that they are especially intelligent and inquisitive. People with diabetes, high blood pressure, or even cancer don't usually come in having done a computer search on their illness. CFS/FMS patients often have. It is great to work with patients who can teach me, as well as allow me to teach them.

CFS/FMS forces us to take care of our needs first. After all, you don't have much choice when taking a shower uses up all of your energy for the day. Taking care of yourself first is an important lesson for you to learn and to continue, even when you get well. Start by easing up on yourself. It's okay to recognize that you tend to be a perfectionist and maybe even a bit controlling. But we also beat up on ourselves by feeling that we're never quite good enough. I find it helpful to begin with the following prescription:

- No blame
- No fault
- No guilt
- No judgment
- No comparing yourself with other people
- No expectations

This applies to yourself and others. It is okay to feel anything you feel. Whatever you feel is totally valid. Own your feelings as *your* feelings, however, and recognize that they may not have much to do with the person they are directed at. Feel the feelings, then let go of them. Don't blame the person you're feeling them toward. Don't feel guilty or blame yourself (or others) for anything—this includes not feeling guilty when you catch yourself blaming someone else.

In the beginning, you may catch yourself blaming, finding fault, judging, or laying a guilt trip on yourself and/or other people hundreds of times a day. This is normal. When you catch yourself doing it—even if it's three days later—just drop it in midthought. Don't beat yourself up for it. Just recognize that it's an old pattern that you have decided to change. Over the next few weeks, it will happen less and less. Eventually, it will be uncommon. Even then, when you catch yourself blaming, feeling guilty, making comparisons between yourself and others (or comparing two other people), simply gently let go of it—without blame. Doing so allows your whole view of reality to change.

What happened? When you were judging others, you were in truth judging yourself and projecting it outward. These judgments were often views and expectations that had been placed on you by others, such as your parents, school, religious institutions, or society. Most likely, this happened early in your life and you internalized it. By letting go of blame, fault, comparisons, guilt, and judgment toward others, you stop judging yourself. Hence the truism "Judge not, lest ye be judged" (being a good Jewish lad, I get to know these lines). When you release these old expectations/programs, that's when the fun can begin.

Once you have done this, use your feelings (not your brain) to figure out what you want. Although our minds are wonderful tools, they are too subject to outside programming to know what we want. Your feelings know, though. If something feels good from a centered place when you picture or do it, it's probably what your inner self (whether you call it your psyche, soul, or whatever) really wants to do and be. If it feels bad, then you don't want to do it, no matter how much your brain is saying you should. Stop "shoulding" on yourself! Instead, as you start feeling better with treatment, use your energy to do the things that feel good. Because of your CFS/FMS (and associated low energy), you've likely managed to survive not doing most of the things that feel bad for years. Let those things stay undone. Pace yourself as you add in the new things that feel good, and check with your feelings frequently. Don't make up for lost time by trying to do too much.

One day, a friend of mine, Jeffrey Maitland, Ph.D., sent me an article entitled "Stone Agers in the Fast Lane." In it, he gives a very well-thought-out discussion on how certain psychological patterns can lead to CFS/FMS. I was really ticked off because he beat me to the punch. On the other hand, I knew he was brilliant because he had independently come to the same conclusions I had. I think you'll enjoy the article. It is in the *From Fatigued to Fantastic!* notes at www.vitality101.com. In addition, for more information on psychologically getting from where you are to where you want to go, I invite you to read my book *Three Steps to Happiness! Healing Through Joy*, which can also be found at www.vitality101.com.

The Fatigued to Fantastic Prescription

- No blame
- No fault
- No guilt
- No judgment
- No comparing yourself with other people
- No expectations

Continually shift your thoughts and actions to things that feel good. Let go of thoughts and stop doing things that feel bad. Then allow space and time in your mind and life for what you want to manifest. As your body begins to heal from CFS/FMS, you'll find that your inner self feels better too.

Natural Treatments for Anxiety and Depression

While working on the psychological issues above, it is also helpful to have highly safe and effective natural therapies that you can use for both anxiety and depression. Fortunately, there are many natural products that my patients have found to alleviate both anxiety and depression, and these are discussed in Chapter 8: More Natural Remedies.

ENERGY THERAPIES FOR ANXIETY

An interesting phenomenon is occurring. Although Western medicine has focused largely on biochemistry (drugs) and ignored energy medicine (e.g., acupuncture), this is changing. The body's energy system is being explored more aggressively (though without the thousands of years of associated philosophies that have developed along with acupuncture)—with surprising results. One of these was the development of NAET to eliminate sensitivities, as discussed in Chapter 9. Another is the use of a remarkably simple technique called the Emotional Freedom Technique (EFT), which can often eliminate phobias and the stress of old traumas in minutes. Although hard to believe until you have experienced it yourself, people are amazed as the phobias or old traumas simply melt away. Because of its effectiveness and simplicity, EFT use is growing rapidly among psychologists, physicians, and other health-care practitioners. For more information on EFT, read the excellent book *Getting Thru to Your Emotions with EFT* by Phillip Mountrose and Jane Mountrose and/or go to Gary Craig's Web site at www.emofree.com.

SAFE AND HIGHLY EFFECTIVE
NATURAL TREATMENTS FOR DEPRESSION

By looking at American society today, one would think that there is a massive epidemic of Prozac deficiency. Millions of Americans are complaining of being unhappy and depressed, yet most doctors simply throw a pill at the problem. I prefer to go after the underlying causes, while using natural therapies to support the biochemistry of happiness. When you do this, most depression can be effectively treated—without the side effects caused by prescription antidepressants.

I'M TIRED OF BEING DEPRESSED
AND WANT TO BE HAPPY! HOW SHOULD I BEGIN?

Let's look at both the physical and psychospiritual components—which is a good approach for any illness.

From a psychological perspective, depression usually represents repressed anger, which has been turned inward. This is why choosing to allow yourself to be angry or even to sometimes go into a rage can be healthy when you're depressed—even if the people around you don't like it. You can tell when the anger is healthy because it will feel good. Remember though, that you are choosing to be angry, and what you are angry about is nobody else's fault (so don't beat up others with your anger). When you don't allow guilt to get in the way, notice how your depression decreases and you feel better after a good fit of anger.

THREE GUIDELINES FOR RELEASING ANGER AND OVERCOMING
DEPRESSION, SO YOU CAN ACHIEVE HAPPINESS

Having worked with thousands of ill patients over the last thirty years, I have found that there are three steps that will psychospiritually help you get past depression and leave you feeling happy:

1. Feel all of your feelings without the need to understand or justify them. When they no longer feel good, let go of them.

2. Make life a "no-fault" system. As discussed above, this means No Blame, No Fault, No Guilt, No Judgment, No Comparing, and No Expectations on yourself or anyone else. This means you'll be changing habits of thinking. For example, if you find yourself judging somebody, simply drop the judgment in midthought when you notice it. And no judging yourself for judging others.

3. Learn to keep your attention on what feels good. We sometimes are given the misconception that keeping attention on problems is more realistic. That is nonsense. Life is like a massive buffet with thousands of options. You can choose to keep your attention on those things that feel good. You'll notice that if a problem truly requires your attention at any given time, it will feel good to focus on it. Otherwise, you're living your life as if you have two hundred TV channels to choose from, but you're only watching the ones you don't like.

WHAT CAN I DO TO FEEL BETTER WHILE I'M DOING THESE THINGS?

Happiness has its own biochemistry, which can be powerfully balanced and enhanced naturally. As with so many aspects of health, overall nutritional support is essential, as is exercise. In fact, research has shown that walking briskly each day is as effective as Prozac for depression. Use herbal support if needed to get eight hours of sleep a night, as well. Also, as noted earlier, thyroid hormone helps depression—even in those with normal thyroid blood tests—but only the T_3 form and not the T_4 form found in Synthroid.[3] There are also many herbals and nutrients that are effective for both anxiety and depression. If these don't help, it is reasonable to try prescription antidepressants like Prozac, Paxil, and Wellbutrin. Fortunately, by using the approach we've discussed, most people find that they can once again feel happy—naturally.

I'd like to give you one of the most important pieces of guidance I can give you. Be gentle with yourself, and only do and keep your attention on what *feels* good! Many of you can also find comfort and guidance from spiritual books written by those in your religious tradition who teach you to love and honor yourself. In addition, for those with a New Age perspective, I recommend the best-selling book *Ask and It Is Given* by Jerry Hicks and Esther Hicks.

Being Gentle with Yourself

When you first begin recovering, reserve the energy that is slowly returning for activities that make you feel good. Most of the things that you have left undone can remain that way. Many probably do not ever need to be done.

Although you likely view your illness as an enemy, let it become your ally. Many people with CFS have been caught in role entrapment. Such people were taught that they have to be the perfect spouse or the perfect parent or the perfect employee. The superwoman complex is a good example. CFS can be your body's way of getting out of the roles in which you are trapped. Most of us have so bought into society's expectations of us that we have taken them on as our own. What we fail to recognize is that because of its tremendous rate of acceleration, our current society is an aberration. There has been no other stable society during the last three thousand-plus years, nor are there many others presently on the planet, in which "normal" change occurred so rapidly. Despite all of our modern conveniences and labor-saving devices, which were supposed to give us more free time, most people find that they are running ever faster. Whereas one parent used to be home to take care of the children while the other parent worked outside the home, now often both parents must work outside the home to maintain the family's standard of living.

Because our whole society is trapped in roles, this chaos may seem normal. It is not. It is abnormal. Although some people thrive on it, more people every day are becoming burned out and "blowing fuses." I suspect that the physical processes that make up CFS and fibromyalgia are manifestations of this—and that we are just beginning to see the tip of the iceberg.

As you get well, you will need to reclaim your own natural speed and pace of life. This may (or may not) mean a somewhat lower standard of living, but you may have been living with that for several years now anyway. On the plus side, it may also mean that your children will have a parent who is happy and present, and that your life will be more fulfilling. Many people live their lives like hamsters, running faster and faster on the exercise wheels in their cage while going nowhere. Give yourself permission to step off the wheel. These are important points. Remember, life is supposed to be fun.

I'd like to finish this chapter with a guest article by Rev. Bren Jacobson. Despite being both intuitive and knowledgeable, he is modest and has a wonderful sense of humor. This can be helpful in assisting you to get through feelings and subjects that seem to be dragging you down. Even though I read extensively from a wide range of medical journals and sources (which is how the information in this book was amassed), whenever I would bring new studies up with Bren he would already know about them—and have even more details on the study and other studies on the topic.

In addition to doing pastoral/psychological counseling, Reverend Bren's broad knowledge base about both the human body and psyche allows him also to serve as a consultant, researching many difficult and so-called "untreatable" medical topics for people. He is also able to guide them in how to combine the best of complementary and standard therapies—often bringing help, clear guidance, and hope to people whose physicians could not. For either pastoral or psychological counseling by phone, or for consultations, he can be reached at 410-224-4877. He is an excellent resource (see Appendix E: Resources).

Ask for What You Want

Bren Jacobson

"Man is born free, but everywhere he is in chains."—Jean Jacques Rousseau

As a counselor for the past thirty-five years, I have worked with many, many people who have overcome chronic fatigue syndrome and fibromyalgia. Through this experience, I have come to the conclusion that enlisting the aid of someone who can see the situation in a more detached and objective way is one of the quickest ways you can find your way out of the maze of CFS/FMS. Just treating the body without bringing the mind, emotions, and spirit into balance is, at best, a partial solution and often only a temporary one. Enlisting the aid of a guide or counselor, meanwhile, can help you figure out what you want and how to most effectively express those desires so as to enlist the help of others. This is not because one is broken and needs to be fixed, but because it is a shortcut to returning to a healthy and vital life and it enriches one's life and relationships.

One of the most consistent problems that people have is that they do not directly ask for what they want. This problem is particularly relevant, not to mention ubiquitous, in those who suffer from CFS/FMS, and if not properly dealt with will definitely impede their recovery from this condition.

As Dr. Teitelbaum has noted, it is common for those who suffer from these conditions to have been type A overachievers prior to becoming ill. CFS/FMS sufferers may thus have extreme difficulty accepting the transition from being the caregiver, competent and in charge and juggling many balls at once, to being in a state of dependency and unable to perform the simplest of daily chores. You may feel guilt at not being able to shoulder your fair share of the burden in the office and/or home setting. You may find yourself caught in a bind: you need more help than you did before you got sick, and you may have more difficulty asking for it.

The reasons people find it difficult to let others know what they desire begin early in our development. As children, we find it natural to ask for what we want. However, as we grow older, we find that when we do express what we want, others frequently do not fulfil our wishes. Even worse, they may tell us that our desires are unrealistic, opportunistic, or an imposition on them. In order to avoid the feelings that often result from such rejection, we may unconsciously develop a strategy of not directly asking for what we need or want.

There are two major problems with this strategy. The first is that most of the time we simply do not get what we want or need, for the obvious reason that no matter how observant and accommodating the people in our lives may be, they are rarely mind readers. The second major complication of this strategy is that it undermines and harms the relationships that are important to our well-being.

Those with chronic fatigue and fibromyalgia further suffer from this predicament because they often look healthy and may be met with skepticism, doubt, and some unwillingness to acknowledge the extent of their problems by associates, friends, family, and health-care providers. If this were not bad enough, the CFS sufferers may encounter ignorance and misbelief by a medical establishment that does not know what is wrong with them or mistakenly believes that their problems do not exist or that there is no treatment for their illness. You may have been told that you should see a therapist or take antidepressants, that you should go on a vacation (which you have neither the will nor the energy to do), or that you will have to tough it out and learn to live with it. All of these struggles lead unendingly into more stress, feelings of failure, discouragement, and frustration.

Many people with CFS/FMS, then, come to an impasse and crisis. Their predicament now is that their inability to function adequately leads to more psychological and physical stress, which causes more frustration and which then creates further stress—until the entire situation spirals out of control. If this unholy mess were not bad enough, the stress causes muscle tightness that precipitates pain, which leads to sleeplessness, which generates more stress, which creates more pain, and so on.

But just as there are many ways of breaking up and diminishing destructive physical patterns in the body, there are ways of breaking up and diminishing the psychological patterns that threaten to keep us enmeshed in pain. First, we can learn not to be ashamed of wanting help, and second, we can learn how to ask for that help in ways that will be beneficial to ourselves and also to our relationships with others. It's not easy to overcome the cultural indoctrination that we all must be superhuman men and women. However, the ultimate reward for acknowledging and validating our wants and needs can be high. When we are able to ask for the most basic of wants and needs, we may find that we discover inner wants, needs, desires, and yearnings we never knew existed.

How do you more directly and effectively ask for what you need and want? You may wish to begin by cultivating self-acceptance. Your wants and needs are valid. Articulate those needs and wants to yourself. Then approach the person you are asking for help with candor and respect. This is obvious, but it is amazing how often we forget it. You may also want to think about the possibility that there may be a number of ways for you to get what you need and want. Be open to brainstorming with others.

Of course, just because we know what we need and want and are able to express those needs in a clear and effective way does not necessarily mean that we will always get those needs met. Those who we ask have their own needs, time constraints, and difficulties, and it is unlikely that they will always be able or willing to come to our aid every time we ask for help. No one person has the time, knowledge, understanding, patience, sensitivity, intelligence, and will to minister to all of our needs. Therefore, it is helpful to develop a network of resources, information, and people that we can rely upon. Ideally, this network would include friends, family, a significant other, some kind of spiritual community, and health-care providers. It is best not to exclude any possible source of help. I have on many occasions received comfort and even inspiration from to- tal strangers whom I encountered on a given day.

As you learn to ask for what you need, you may want to explore the related issue of setting limits and learning to say no. Most of you know that this is one of the things that can be gravely difficult. You may have a long history of trying to be all things to all people. This can frequently cause setbacks in your recovery. I would simply like to recommend a book that addresses this predicament in an effective, humorous, and enjoyable manner: *The Book for People Who Do Too Much,* by Bradley Trevor Greive. And while you are at it, you might practice what I have been talking about by asking someone close to you, very sweetly, if they would be a dear and pick it up for you the next time they are in a bookstore.

The importance of achieving a mind-body-spirit balance cannot be underestimated for those struggling with CFS/FMS. Working with a counselor may help you better define your needs and goals and communicate them effectively with those in your support network.

I end with a quotation that I learned many years ago. It is not meant to serve as advice but rather as a thought to be contemplated and an idea to be played with.

The secret is to be
And not to wonder
How to be.

Stop trying
To be
And realize
That you
Are!

Important Points

- CFS and fibromyalgia are physical processes with physical causes. However, like most illnesses, they also have psychological components that must be treated.
- CFS patients both with and without depression and anxiety have been helped by the new generation of antidepressants, such as Zoloft, Prozac, Paxil, and Effexor. Natural remedies, however, can be more effective with many fewer side effects.
- Consider therapy for emotional support and guidance. The Reverend Bren Jacobson does superb counseling by phone (410-224-4877).
- Get into a "centered" space, then constantly shift your attention and actions to things that (in that centered space) feel good.

11 *Losing Weight with CFS and FMS*

*I*n addition to the myriad other problems you have to bear, two recent studies of ours found that fibromyalgia and CFS patients have an average weight gain of thirty-two pounds. Because of the metabolic problems that occur in these syndromes, it is almost impossible to lose weight and keep it off until you receive proper treatment. It is much easier to lose the weight and keep it off, however, when one understands that there are many things that contribute to this problem. For people with CFS/FMS, simply altering your diet is not enough to lose weight. A large percentage of you have found that it is impossible to lose weight and keep it off no matter what you do.

There are several ways that CFS/FMS is contributing to your inability to lose weight. Both physical stresses (e.g., infections, nutritional deficiencies) and emotional/situational stresses can result in a metabolic chain reaction that results in weight gain. With effective treatment of their CFS/FMS, most people find that their weight gain stops and that usual weight-loss measures will finally work.

So What Caused the Weight Gain?

Let's begin with poor sleep. The expression "getting your beauty sleep" actually has a basis in fact. Deep sleep is a major trigger for growth hormone production. Growth hormone stimulates production of muscle (which burns fat) and improves insulin sensitivity (which decreases the tendency to make fat), while also decreasing fibromyalgia symptoms. Thus, getting the eight to nine hours of sleep a night that the human body is meant to have can powerfully contribute to your staying young-looking and trim. Poor sleep also causes lower levels of the hormone leptin, which regulates hunger.

In addition, as we've noted elsewhere, the hypothalamic "circuit breaker" that gets suppressed with stress also controls our hormone system. This results in inadequate levels of thyroid and adrenal hormones. The thyroid is like your body's gas pedal—regulating how many calories you burn—and low thyroid can dramatically trigger weight gain. The adrenal glands are the body's stress handlers. In the beginning of your illness, chronic stress and depression result in elevated cortisol levels, which can directly cause weight gain. Continuing excessive stress may result in exhaustion of the adrenal glands over time. As it is the job of the adrenal glands to maintain blood sugar levels in the time of stress, adrenal exhaustion can result in episodes of hypoglycemia (low blood sugar). If you get periods where you feel that somebody had better feed you NOW or you're going to kill them, you are likely hypoglycemic and would benefit from adrenal support. Unfortunately, an underactive adrenal gland causes people to become hypoglycemic and to crave sugar and eat more than they normally would. This leads to further weight gain.

Infections can also contribute to weight gain. Clinical experience has shown that fungal overgrowth stirs sugar cravings and leads to weight gain. Although we do not know the mechanism for this, we have repeatedly seen excess weight drop off once this overgrowth is treated and eliminated.

Another major problem is carnitine deficiency, a problem that is present in most CFS/FMS patients. Unfortunately, this deficiency forces your body to turn calories into fat, and makes it almost impossible to lose fat. Simply taking supplemental carnitine does not help adequately, however, as it does not transfer into cells optimally in this form. I do recommend that people take 1,000 milligrams of *acetyl-L*-carnitine daily for four months, as cells can absorb this form easily, leading to energy production and weight loss.

Last but not least, many people with CFS/FMS have insulin resistance—meaning they need high blood levels of insulin to maintain a normal level of blood sugar. Unfortunately, high insulin levels increase your body's production of fat. If weight gain is a problem, check a fasting blood insulin level. To do so, do not eat after midnight, then have your lab check your insulin level first thing in the morning. If the insulin reading is higher than ten, your doctor may decide to prescribe the diabetes medication Metformin, which improves insulin sensitivity even in nondiabetics. This drug can not only help weight loss, but also improve other symptoms of CFS/FMS. In females, if insulin levels are high, and DHEA-S and testosterone levels are also elevated, you may have PCOS (polycystic ovarian syndrome—another cause of CFS/FMS). I treat PCOS with Metformin and Cortef. Be sure to take the vitamin powder recommended earlier or B complex supplements if on Metformin; otherwise it will cause a vitamin B_{12} deficiency.

So How Can You Go About Treating These Problems So That You Can Lose Weight and Feel Better?

1. Cut down the sugar and simple carbohydrates in your diet and increase your water intake. If your mouth feels parched and you are not taking a medication that causes dry mouth, then you are thirsty and need to drink more water (even if you already drink like a fish).
2. Sleep; get eight to nine hours of solid sleep a night.
3. Treat low thyroid or adrenal function, if applicable.
4. Treat yeast/candida overgrowth, if present.
5. Get optimum nutritional support. When you are deficient in vitamins or minerals, your body will crave more food than you need, and your metabolism will be sluggish. As mentioned, take 500 to 1,000 milligrams of acetyl-L-carnitine daily along with the energy revitalization system.
6. Treat insulin resistance, if present.

It is not unusual for people to shed thirty to fifty pounds by simply treating these metabolic factors.

12   *Finding a Physician*

*H*aving developed an effective treatment protocol for fibromyalgia and chronic fatigue syn-
drome over the last thirty years, and having proven it to be effective in two
studies—one a well-done randomized, double-blind, placebo-controlled
trial—my colleagues and I have now turned our attention to our goal of
making effective treatment available to the well over 50 million people
worldwide who suffer from these illnesses. Training and encouraging physicians so that people will have proper access to care has been a full-time
job—to the point that I am now a member of the "Two Million Mile
Club" on a major airline. Fortunately, writing this chapter is now much
easier than it was six years ago, and people all over the country can finally
get the care they need.

People ask me how they can talk their doctor into giving them the treatments they need. In most cases, the answer is that you can't. Most doctors,
appropriately enough, will not do the things that they are not properly
trained in. This does not make them bad physicians. If you came to me and
said, "Dr. Teitelbaum, I would like you to do a heart bypass operation on
me," I would say, "I'm sorry, I am not trained in this, and I can't." If you then
gave me a copy of a book called *From Bypass to Fantastic* and a scalpel, well,
you still would not want me performing surgery on you. This would not
make me a bad physician, and your doctor not treating you for CFS/FMS

does not make him or her a bad physician, either. The best thing to do is to go to a physician who specializes in treating these complex syndromes.

Holistic Physicians

In the past, these doctors were simply not available or, at best, were hard to find. This has changed. Now, as CFS/FMS is going mainstream, and more physicians are being trained in complementary medicine, it is getting easier to get the treatments you need. For example, there is now an American Board of Holistic Medicine that has certified more than one thousand practitioners, and part of their certification is in the treatments discussed in this book. In addition, more states are recognizing that naturopaths trained in four-year programs are competent as physicians, and should have the legal right to also give IV therapies and prescribe natural hormones and other medications.

Most physicians who know how to help CFS/FMS patients are considered holistic. These doctors usually have advanced training in using natural therapies and also spend a lot of time exploring the scientific literature. They also allow the longer visits needed to treat CFS/FMS. Unfortunately, because of the way insurance company payments are made, many doctors cannot afford to sustain a practice based on just a few long visits per day. They need to fit as many patients in to their office as possible, in the least amount of time. Because of this, most physicians who can effectively deal with these illnesses do not participate with insurance. Fortunately, the biggest expense is for testing and medications, which are often covered.

When Looking for a Physician, Consider the Following Questions

1. Does he or she specialize in treating CFS/FMS and recognize it as a real and physical illness?
2. Will he or she prescribe the medications needed for you to get eight hours of sleep a night?
3. Does he or she use bioidentical hormones based on your symptoms, even if the tests are normal?

4. Will he or she treat for candida with Diflucan for six weeks?
5. Does he or she give nutritional IVs (e.g., Myers cocktails)?

If the answer to these five questions is yes, you have a physician who is likely to be able to help you.

Finding a Holistic Physician

Holistic doctors are much more likely to know how to help CFS/FMS patients. To find these, I recommend the three organizations below.

American Board of Holistic Medicine
Certifies physicians as having advanced training in the use of natural therapies. Their Web site lists more than one thousand physicians.
www.holisticboard.org

American Holistic Medical Association (AHMA)
4101 Lake Boone Trail, Suite 201
Raleigh, NC 27607
919-787-5146
www.holisticmedicine.org

American College for Advancement of Medicine
P.O. Box 3427
Laguna Hills, CA 92654
http://www.apma.net

More Good News

In addition to these resources, a national chain of Fibromyalgia & Fatigue Centers was established in 2004. Several years ago, Bob Baurys, a prominent businessman, came down with chronic fatigue syndrome. He went through the same difficult experience working with physicians that most of you have gone through. He was finally lucky enough to find a physician who was trained in using the protocols in this book and he recovered. This businessman was shocked that people with CFS and fibromyalgia did not have proper access to care—especially having gone through the process himself. Fortunately, what this businessman does is to set up health-care systems with his compassionate associate, Sue Hrim, RN.

When I traveled to these centers in 2006 to evaluate their program, I was deeply impressed with the level of care they were able to provide. They had created what I have been working to see happen for decades, and it felt as if this was the culmination of thirty years of my work. I am now national medical director of the Fibromyalgia & Fatigue Centers (FFC), sixteen centers across the country (www.fibroandfatigue.com). The centers accept patients from around the world and, after an initial in-person visit, they can manage care via phone if you do not live near a center. Since opening their first center in Dallas in January 2004, the Fibromyalgia & Fatigue Centers have treated more than five thousand patients and have an 80 percent success rate within four visits to the centers.

So that you have an idea of what you should expect from your doctor in CFS/FMS care, I will give you an overview of the treatment at the centers. Because CFS/FMS are complex diseases that involve multisystem disturbances and abnormalities, your physician should spend time with you, at least an hour at the new-patient visit, then dedicate at least thirty to sixty minutes for follow-up appointments. Your doctor should do a comprehensive evaluation and extensive lab work in order to develop a treatment plan unique to your specific needs.

The approach at the FFC includes a six-step integrated program that works to address the underlying dysfunctions that cause your illness. They use a patient-centered, holistic plan of care that treats the whole body. No matter which physician you choose, you'll want to be sure that he or she is similarly interested in your complete recovery, not just a remission of symptoms. As you know, successful treatment of these diseases requires a plan tailored to the individual. Your treatment, then, may occur in one order, while another person's might occur in a completely different order. And of course, multiple steps are often initiated simultaneously. Be sure that your physician uses a similar flexible approach.

At the FFC, we use steps that follow the protocol in this book. Generally, these can be broken down as follows:

1. Stabilize the patient by addressing pain and sleep disturbances.
2. Enhance the mitochondria by improving nutrition.

3. Balance the hormones by evaluating hypothalamic, thyroid, adrenal, ovarian/testicular, and pituitary function.
4. Evaluate infectious components and treat underlying infections.
5. Address unique etiologies such as neurotoxins and coagulation defects.
6. Provide an individualized maintenance program with the minimal amount of medications and supplements needed to keep you well.

Use these steps as guidelines when talking with prospective health-care providers about their treatment methods and strategies. For more information on how to find a doctor, as well as on the Fibromyalgia & Fatigue Centers, see Appendix E: Resources and www.fibroandfatigue.com.

Getting Insurance Coverage for Labs and Medications

As I've noted, most physicians specializing in CFS/FMS do not work with health insurance companies. Nonetheless, I find that if people have prescription coverage, most of the medications will be covered. For those of you without prescription insurance coverage who have low incomes (common in CFS/FMS), many, if not most, of the medications you'll need may be supplied for free by the drug companies. For more information on this important option, go to www.PPARx.org (see Appendix E: Resources).

Lab tests are also usually, but if you have to battle with your insurance company, the information in Appendix C can be helpful. It tells you what tests your insurance should cover, based on your symptoms. If you do not have insurance, or your insurance does not cover the cost of the testing, it is a good idea to call different laboratories to see what they charge, as the price can vary markedly. With many labs you'll be able to negotiate a 50 percent discount if you are willing to pay for the tests at the time of service, but this must be negotiated before they draw your blood.

Fighting your physician or insurance company is not a good use of your precious energy. In the long run, you will do better finding physicians who will work with you. Remember, CFIDS, fibromyalgia, and other chronic fatigue states are now treatable illnesses. You will do best using your energy to find a physician who wants to work with you to help you move beyond your disease.

Other Helpful Tools

Treating CFS/FMS can be complicated and time-consuming. In addition to using the worksheet in this book to develop your personalized treatment plan, you can also use the educational programs at www.vitality101.com. Because of the expense involved in creating and maintaining these Web-based computer programs, we do have to charge a modest amount for using these programs. However, we want everyone to be able to access effective treatment, so those on medical assistance (Medicaid) may access the programs for free. Simply e-mail us in the question-and-answer section of the Web site for details.

To help determine whether you want to use these programs, you can expect to find:

1. *The long-form program.* This will obtain a detailed history from you, including lab test results, and will create:
   - A complete medical record of your case for your physician (except, of course, for the physical examination—which is usually unremarkable for people with CFS/FMS).
   - A list of probable factors contributing to the illness in your specific case.
   - A program of natural remedies (again, tailored to your specific case) that can help you begin a major part of treatment on your own.
   - A prioritized list of the prescription treatments most likely to help you.
2. *The short-form program.* If you do not need a complete medical record for your physician, I recommend that you do the "short-form program," which is less expensive and much easier to fill out. Although it will not create a complete medical record of your case, it will analyze your symptoms and lab tests to create:
   - A list of probable factors contributing to the illness in your specific case.
   - Natural remedies (again, tailored to your specific case) that can help you begin a major part of treatment on your own.
   - A prioritized list of the prescription treatments most likely to help you.

In many ways, the latter program is similar to what you will have created using this book, but it will also analyze your lab tests to further help you determine exactly what you need to do to get well. If your physician is open-minded, you may be able to encourage him or her to give you the treatments you need based on either the computer program or the protocol you filled out while reading this book. Give your doctor a copy of Appendix G: For Physicians and a copy of the research study from my Web site as well, as these documents may encourage your health-care practitioner to work with you.

We have finally reached the point where the care you need is available from well-trained physicians. Won't it be nice to have a doctor who knows more than you do?

Important Points

- It is best to see a physician who is an expert in treating CFS and fibromyalgia, as these are complex syndromes.
- The Fibromyalgia & Fatigue Centers is a national chain of treatment facilities whose physicians are expertly trained in treating these syndromes. They are familiar with everything in this book and much more. For information, see www.fibroandfatigue.com.
- There is a computerized educational program available at www.vitality101.com that can analyze your symptoms and blood tests to help you determine what treatments are most likely to help you get well.
- In addition, you can sign up for a free e-mail newsletter at www.vitality101.com that will keep you up to date on the newest developments in treating CFS, fibromyalgia, and pain. There is a second newsletter that will also update you on using the best of natural and standard medicine to maintain optimal health.

Conclusion

"The person who says it cannot be done should not interrupt the person doing it."

—Chinese proverb

Old mind-sets are often difficult to change. It took many years for chronic fatigue syndrome and fibromyalgia to be recognized as real and physical processes. As time goes on and more physicians become aware of these illnesses, patients will no longer have to accept being labeled crazy because of a few physicians' ignorance.

We are entering the next stage.

Chronic fatigue syndrome and fibromyalgia are now treatable. This simple fact needs to be demonstrated and reported over and over again to become accepted by physicians. Over time, it is hoped that even more physicians will learn how to treat CFS/FMS and how to encourage and support their fatigue patients. Others, sadly, will continue to keep their heads stuck in the sand. It is all right to ignore these doctors who ignore you. You will be better off spending your energy tending to and taking responsibility for your physical and emotional needs so that you can attain and then maintain optimum health. This is especially true because you can now get the help you need.

Your illness may have been treated as being "all in your head" for a long time, but do not fall into the trap of ignoring your emotional and psychological needs. Many CFS patients have been overachievers in an effort to compensate for childhood low self-esteem. Love yourself for having had that low self-esteem, love yourself for having been an overachiever, then let go of both these experiences. Take the "shoulds" placed on you by your family, and society and drop them. Love yourself for having had them, and then love yourself for letting go of them. Although CFS is devastating, even this dark cloud has a silver lining. It has taught you what you do not have to do, and has given you space to explore who you truly are. You have earned the right to be yourself.

As you start feeling better, slowly add activities to your life that make you feel good. If you do something that makes you feel poorly, stop doing it. Joseph Campbell, a world-renowned teacher of the mythology of and paths for personal growth in many diverse cultures, was asked how people can stay true to themselves. Put succinctly, his advice was: "Follow your bliss." Perhaps a "should" led you to become an accountant, doctor, or lawyer, but your bliss truly lies in being an artist, mother, poet, or dancer. Perhaps the opposite is true. If you do what makes you feel happy and excited, you will get yourself on the right track. Whatever you do, however, do not try to make up for lost time by trying to do too much. The few lingering symptoms of your illness will effectively let you know when you are pushing too hard. Recognize that your illness may have been a valuable teacher.

As your chronic fatigue resolves and you begin to feel well again, let your friends, the media, and your former physicians (most CFS/FMS patients have seen quite a few) know. Because in the past there was no single expensive drug for the treatment of CFS/FMS, millions of pharmaceutical dollars had not yet been spent on publicity. For better or worse, this is changing as drug companies realize that we are a big market. Even the CDC (Centers for Disease Control) is spending millions of dollars on an advertising campaign to teach doctors and the public that CFS/FMS are real and devastating diseases. These changes will help to insure that those who have suffered with the illness will be better able to get the understanding and help they need.

I know it's been a long, hard road for you but, as the song says, "The times they are a-changin'!"

It's time to get your life back NOW!

Study Abstracts of Effective Treatment Modalities for Chronic Fatigue Syndrome and Fibromyalgia

The full text of studies #1 and 3 can be seen at www.vitality101.com.

Study #1: Published as lead article, Journal of Chronic Fatigue Syndrome, *Vol. 8, No. 2, 2001, pp. 3–24*

Effective Treatment of Chronic Fatigue Syndrome and Fibromyalgia—a Randomized, Double-Blind, Placebo-Controlled, Intent-to-Treat Study

Jacob E. Teitelbaum, M.D.; Barbara Bird, M.T., CLS;
Robert M. Greenfield, M.D.; Alan Weiss, M.D.;
Larry Muenz, Ph.D.; Laurie Gould, B.S.

No outside funding.

ABSTRACT. Background: Hypothalamic dysfunction has been suggested in fibromyalgia (FMS) and chronic fatigue syndrome (CFS). This dysfunction may result in disordered sleep, subclinical hormonal deficiencies, and immunologic changes. Our previously published open trial showed that patients usually improve by using a protocol that treats all the above processes simultaneously. The current study examines this protocol using a randomized, double-blind design with an intent-to-treat analysis.

Methods: Seventy-two FMS patients (thirty-eight active; thirty-four placebo; sixty-nine also met CFS criteria) received all active or all placebo therapies as a unified intervention. Patients were treated, as indicated by symptoms and/or lab testing, for: (1) subclinical thyroidal, gonadal, and/ or adrenal insufficiency; (2) disordered sleep; (3) suspected NMH; (4) opportunistic infections; and (5) suspected nutritional deficiencies.

Results: At the final visit, sixteen active patients were "much better," fourteen "better," two "same," zero "worse," and one "much worse" versus three, nine, eleven, six, and four, respectively, in the placebo group (p<.0001, Cochran-Mantel-Haenszel trend test). Significant improvement in the FMS Impact Questionnaire (FIQ) scores (decreasing from 54.8 to 33.2 versus 51.4 to 47.7) and Analog scores (improving from 176.1 to 310.3 versus 177.1 to 211.9 [both with p<.0001 by random effects regression]), and tender point index (TPI) (31.7 to 15.5 versus 35.0 to 32.3, p<.0001 by baseline adjusted linear model) were seen. Long-term follow-up (mean 1.9 years) of the active group showed continuing and increasing improvement over time, despite patients being able to wean off most treatments.

Conclusions: Significantly greater benefits were seen in the active group than in the placebo group for all primary outcomes. Using an integrated treatment approach, effective treatment is now available for CFS/FMS.

Study #2: Published in Journal of Alternative and Complementary Medicine, *November 1, 2006; 12(9): 857–62.*

The Use of D-ribose in Chronic Fatigue Syndrome and Fibromyalgia: A Pilot Study

J. E. Teitelbaum, C. Johnson, and J. S. Cyr

Objectives: Fibromyalgia (FMS) and chronic fatigue syndrome (CFS) are debilitating syndromes that are often associated with impaired cellular energy metabolism. As D-ribose has been shown to increase cellular energy synthesis in heart and skeletal muscle, this open-label uncontrolled pilot study was done to evaluate whether D-ribose could improve symptoms in fibromyalgia and/or chronic fatigue syndrome patients.

Design: Forty-one patients with a diagnosis of FMS and/or CFS were given D-ribose, a naturally occurring pentose carbohydrate, at a dose of 5 g t.i.d. for a total of 280 g. All patients completed questionnaires containing discrete visual analog scales (VAS) and a global assessment pre- and post-D-ribose administration.

Results: D-ribose, which was well tolerated, resulted in a significant improvement in all five VAS categories: energy; sleep; mental clarity; pain intensity; and well-being, as well as an improvement in patients' global assessment. Approximately 66 percent of patients experienced significant improvement while on D-ribose, with an average increase in energy on the VAS of 45 percent and an average improvement in overall well-being of 30 percent (p < 0.0001).

Conclusions: D-ribose significantly reduced clinical symptoms in patients suffering from fibromyalgia and chronic fatigue syndrome.

Study #3: Published in Journal of Musculoskeletal Pain,
Vol. 3, No. 4, 1995, pp. 91–110

Effective Treatment of Severe Chronic Fatigue: A Report of a Series of Sixty-four Patients

Jacob Teitelbaum, Barbara Bird

ABSTRACT. Objectives: To determine the underlying causes of severe chronic fatigue states and the effect of concurrently treating the underlying etiologies.

Methods: Sixty-four patients with a median of three years of severe fatigue, which markedly limited their activity, were studied. These patients were characterized by a mix of symptoms including recurrent sore throats, swollen glands, increased thirst, sleeplessness, achiness, and poor memory and concentration without apparent cause. They presented in our office during 1991–1993 and were selected by consecutive sampling. The patients were assessed and treated for the processes noted below.

As fatigue is purely subjective, the patients determined whether they showed worsening, no significant change, significant but incomplete improvement, or much improvement [that is, fatigue no longer a problem].

Results: Forty-six patients had at least three or more contributing problems. Fibromyalgia was present in forty-four patients. Overt or subclinical hypothyroidism or hypoadrenalism was suspected in thirty and forty patients, respectively. Superinfections associated with immune dysfunction (e.g., bowel parasites or yeast overgrowth) were suspected in thirty cases. Improvement with micronutrient supplementation was noted.

Depression, anxiety/hyperventilation, and situational stresses were considered to be the primary processes in four, four, and three patients, respectively.

Treatment resulted in complete resolution of fatigue in 57 percent and significant but incomplete improvement in 39 percent of the patients. Improvement was seen at a median time of seven weeks.

Conclusions: Severe chronic fatigue states are multifactorial processes that, in many patients, respond well to treatment.

Originally published in the *Journal of Musculoskeletal Pain* 3 (1995): 91–110. Used courtesy Haworth Press.

The SHIN Treatment Worksheet

Treatment Protocol "Short Form"—CFS/FMS

Many of the products mentioned below can also be ordered from 800–333–5287 or www.vitality101.com.

Below is a listing of the more common treatments used in treating CFS/FMS. If you would like, a more comprehensive form with more than 280 options can be seen and printed out at www.vitality101.com. I would use this list as a record of your treatments and have it with you for follow-up/phone visits. Put a line through the number in front of any treatment you stop and note the reason stopped and date. Put the date started in front of the other treatments. Although it can take six weeks to see a treatment's benefits, most of the medications' side effects will usually occur within the first few days of starting a treatment. Except for treatments #1 through 10, which can all be started in the first one to three days, add in one new treatment each one to three days. If a side effect occurs, stop the last two or three treatments for a few days and see if it goes away. If the side effect is acute and worrisome, call your family doctor (or go to the ER) immediately. Do not get pregnant on treatment or drive if sedated. It is normal for a woman's periods to be irregular during the first three to four months of treatment. On average, it takes three months to start feeling better. You can begin to slowly taper off most treatments when you feel well for six months. Stop things one at a time (e.g., one pill every one to two weeks) so you can see if you still need it. If needed, however, most of these can be used long term, although this is usually not necessary. Some prescriptions can be obtained at a much lower cost from Consumers Discount Drug Company (323-461-3606). Another good source for generic prescription drugs is www.costco.com—click on "Pharmacy." Do not take any treatments below that you are allergic to or that have caused prohibitive side effects. Prescription items have "Rx" after their names. If a recommended (i.e., checked off) treatment has a double asterisk (**) by the number, it is a "most important" treatment; if it has a single asterisk (*), it is an important treatment; and no asterisk means the treatment is helpful but not critical. If you choose to simplify your program, you can begin taking just the double-asterisked items followed by the single-asterisked items and then no asterisked items that are checked off.

We have listed natural/over-the-counter alternatives for most prescription therapies that can be substituted for and/or added to the prescription ones. We often recommend products made by Enzymatic Therapy, Ultraceuticals, or Integrative Therapeutics (ITI), as these have excellent potency and purity. *Dr. Teitelbaum does not accept money from any pharmaceutical or natural products companies whose products he recommends. He has directed that all his royalties for products he makes be donated to charity.* Only the items that have been checked off as you read this book are the ones recommended for you.

Nutritional Treatments

_____1.   **Energy Revitalization System—Powder (by Enzymatic Therapy and Integrative Therapeutics): Half to one scoop a day (as feels best) blended with milk, water, or yogurt with one capsule of the included Daily Energy B-Complex (also available separately). This gives a solid foundation for nutritional support, and replaces more than thirty-five tablets' worth of supplements. If gas or diarrhea occurs, mix the powder with milk and/or start with a lower dose and work your way up to the dose that feels best, or divide the daily dose into smaller doses and take two to three times a day (½ a scoop a day is often adequate; use the dose that feels best to you). Be sure to take #10 (ribose) with it for optimal support.

_____2. *Complete GEST Enzymes (Enzymatic Therapy)/Similase (ITI): Two capsules with each meal to help digest your food properly. If you have ulcers or if the GEST enzymes irritate your stomach, begin with GS Similase.

_____3. **Vitamin B$_{12}$—1 I.M. injection (1 cc = 3,000 micrograms) three to seven times weekly for fifteen doses, then as needed (e.g., one to twelve times a month). This needs to be made by a compounding (holistic) pharmacy (e.g., ITC Pharmacy; 303-663-4224). If unable to get injections, take 5 milligrams (5,000 micrograms) a day by mouth for three months.

_____4. *NAC (N-Acetyl-L-Cysteine): 500 to 650 milligrams a day for two to three months. Makes glutathione.

_____5. **Iron (e.g., Chelated Iron by Ultraceuticals—29 milligrams plus 100 milligrams vitamin C): one tablet a day. Do not take within six hours of thyroid hormone preparations or Cipro (antibiotic), as this can prevent their absorption. Take on an empty stomach (i.e., take between 2 and 6 p.m. on an empty stomach). It is okay to miss up to three doses a week. Stop in four to six months or when your ferritin blood test is over 40. If afternoon fatigue or hair loss are problems, consider continuing iron supplements until your ferritin level is over 100. Iron may turn your stool black. If nausea is a problem, Floradix iron is much easier on the stomach and is not constipating (supplies 10 milligrams of highly absorbable iron per dose of 2 teaspoons).

_____6. *Eskimo-3 fish oil (Enzymatic Therapy) or Omega-3 fish oil (Ultraceuticals): 1 to 2 teaspoons (or three to six capsules) a day for three to nine months until the dry eyes and mouth resolve, and then as needed. Use these brands, as most others are rancid and often contain mercury, lead, or other toxins. Dry eyes and mouth, pain, inflammation, depression, or excessive hard earwax suggest a need for this.

For Anxiety—Natural treatments

____7.   **Calming Balance from Health Freedom Nutrition, or Tranquility from Ultraceuticals, or similar products containing 500 milligrams vitamin B_1, passionflower, theanine, magnolia, B vitamins, and magnesium: one to three capsules one to three times a day is outstanding for anxiety (the effect increases with one to four weeks of use). Both are also available from www.vitality101.com.

Mitochondrial Energy Treatments

Use these for four to nine months. Then drop the dose to the lowest dose that maintains the effect (or stop it if no benefit).

____8.   *Acetyl-L-carnitine: 500 milligrams, one capsule once or twice a day for three months. Then 250 to 500 milligrams a day or stop it. Although important in CFS/FMS, it is even more important to take this if you also have mitral valve prolapse, MS, and/or elevated blood triglycerides. This helps with weight loss.

____9.   Coenzyme Q_{10}: 200 milligrams once a day. Especially important if taking cholesterol-lowering prescriptions (e.g., Mevacor). Take it with vitamin E, with a meal that has fat, with oil supplements, or in an oil-based form to improve absorption. Vitaline/Enzymatic Therapy makes the best form, and this is the one I recommend. It also already contains vitamin E to enhance absorption.

____10.   ***D-ribose** (CORvalen): One scoop (5 grams) of powder three times a day for three weeks, then two times a day. If too energizing, take with milk or food or lower the dose. Effects are usually seen within two to three weeks. This is a key treatment. Take it with #1 (the vitamin powder). Can be found at www.vitality101.com.

**Sleeping Aids for Fibromyalgia

You can try these in the order listed or as you prefer based on your history. Adjust dose as needed to get eight to nine hours of solid sleep without waking or hangover. If unable to find a combination from the treatments below that does this, see the extensive treatment protocol at www .vitality101.com for many more options. No going to the bathroom if you wake up unless you still have to go five minutes later. Mixing low doses of several treatments is more likely to help you sleep without a hangover than a high dose of one medication. You can take up to the maximum dose of all checked-off treatments simultaneously. Do not drive if you have next-day sedation (adjust your treatment to avoid this). If you're not sleeping eight to nine hours a night without waking on the checked-off treatments, do not wait until your next appointment to contact your physician. Ambien and Klonopin are considered potentially addictive, but in the dose and form that we use this is rarely a problem. If you have next-day sedation, try taking the medications (except the Ambien) a few hours before bedtime. You can try the natural products in combination first to see if they give you eight hours of sleep a night. Add them in this order: #12, 16, 23, 15. If you have restless leg syndrome or pain that keeps you up at night, I would add treatments in the order #11, 12, 14, and 17. Otherwise, I would use the order #12, 11, 13, 16, 17, 23, 15, 14, 18, 20, 21, and 24.

_____ 11.   **Ambien (zolpidem): 10 milligrams—half to one and a half at bedtime. If you tend to wake during the night, leave an extra half to one tablet at bedside and you can take it as needed to help you sleep through the night, or use the Ambien CR sustained-release form.

_____ 12.   **Revitalizing Sleep Formula (by Enzymatic Therapy, Integrative Therapeutics): 200 milligrams valerian, 90 milligrams passionflower, 50 milligrams L-theanine, 30 milligrams hops, 12 milligrams piscidia, and 28 milligrams wild lettuce. Take two to four capsules each night thirty to ninety minutes before bedtime. It can also be used during the day for muscle pain and/or anxiety (up to four capsules three times a day). If valerian energizes you (occurs in 5 to 10 percent of people) use the other components for sleep. Do not take more than twelve capsules a day. Or use a similar herbal mix.

_____13.   *Desyrel (Rx; trazodone): 50 milligrams—half to six at bedtime. Although sedating, it can be used (50 to 250 milligrams at a time) for anxiety. Do not take more than 450 milligrams a day (or 150 milligrams a day if on other antidepressants).

_____14.   *Klonopin (Rx; clonazepam): ½ milligram—begin slowly and work your way up as sedation allows. Take half a tablet at bedtime, increasing up to six tablets at bedtime as needed. Can be very effective for sleep, pain, and restless leg syndrome. Klonopin may be addictive. Taking one-quarter to one-half tablet in the morning (not more) can actually decrease brain fog in some CFS patients.

_____15.   *5-HTP (5-Hydroxy-L-Tryptophan): 200 to 400 milligrams at night. Naturally stimulates serotonin. Don't take more than 200 milligrams a day if you are on Prozac, Paxil, Zoloft, Desyrel, or Celexa. Can help with pain and weight loss at 300 milligrams a day for at least three months.

_____16.   Calcium (500 to 1,000 milligrams) and magnesium (100 to 200 milligrams) at bedtime help sleep.

_____17.   *Neurontin (Rx; gabapentin): 300 milligrams—one to two capsules at bedtime. Also helps pain and restless leg syndrome.

_____18.   *Zanaflex (Rx; tizanidine): 4 milligrams—Take half to two at bedtime. For pain and sleep. If it causes nightmares, stop taking it. Do not take while on Cipro (raises blood levels of Zanaflex too high).

_____19.   Sonata (Rx; zaleplon): 10 milligrams—Take one to two capsules during the night if you wake after 3 a.m. or if you only have trouble falling (versus staying) asleep. Its sedation lasts only three to four hours.

_____20.   *Flexeril (Rx; cyclobenzaprine): 10 milligrams—half to two at bedtime. A muscle relaxant, it can cause dry mouth.

_____21.   *Sinequan (Rx; doxepin): 5 to 10 milligrams, one to three capsules at bedtime or doxepin liquid, 10 milligrams/cc. If a lower dose is needed you can start with one to three drops at night. A powerful antihistamine. Some people get the greatest benefit with the least next-day sedation with a dose of less than 5 milligrams a night.

_____22. Elavil (Rx; amitriptyline): 10 milligrams—half to five tablets at bedtime. May cause weight gain or dry mouth. Good for nerve pain and vulvodynia.

_____23. Melatonin: ½ to 1 milligram at bedtime. If you feel wide awake at bedtime, try 5 milligrams taken three to five hours before bedtime. Don't use a higher dose unless you find it more effective (0.5 milligrams is usually as effective as 5 milligrams and may be safer).

_____24. Gabitril (Rx; tiagabine): 2 to 6 milligrams at bedtime. The main side effects are sedation, dizziness, and gastric upset.

Hormonal Treatments

Several studies show that thyroid therapies can be helpful in CFIDS/FMS, even if your blood tests are normal. Thyroid supplementation is, however, controversial, even though it's usually safe. All treatments (even aspirin) can cause problems in some people, though. The main risks of thyroid treatment are:

- Triggering caffeinelike anxiety or palpitations. If this happens, cut back the dose and increase by half to one tablet each six to eight weeks (as is comfortable) or slower. Sometimes taking 500 milligrams vitamin B_1 (thiamine) one to three times a day will also help after about one to three weeks. If you have severe, persistent racing heart, call your family doctor and/or go to the emergency room.

- Triggering heart attack. For those who are already at high risk of having a heart attack or severe "racing heart" (atrial fibrillation), thyroid hormone can trigger a cardiac episode. In the long run, though, I suspect thyroid may decrease the risk of heart disease. If you have chest pain, go to the emergency room and/or call your family doctor. It will likely be chest muscle pain (not dangerous), but with heart attacks, it is *always* better to be safe than sorry. To put it in perspective, I've never seen this happen despite treating many thousands of patients with thyroid hormones. Increasing your thyroid dose to levels above the upper limit of the normal range may accelerate osteoporosis (which is already common in CFIDS/FMS). Because of this, you need to check your thyroid (free T4—not TSH) levels after four to eight weeks on your optimum dose of thyroid hormone. All this having been said, we find treatment with thyroid hormones to be safer than aspirin and Motrin. If you have risk factors for angina, do an exercise stress test to make sure your heart is healthy before beginning thyroid treatment. These risk factors include: diabetes; elevated cholesterol; hypertension; smoking; personal or family history of angina; gout; and age over fifty.

There are several forms of thyroid hormone, and one kind will often work when another does not. A compounded mix of T_4 and T_3 hormone may be best if your doctor is familiar with these. Do not take thyroid hormone within six hours of iron or calcium supplements or you won't absorb the hormone. It can take three to twelve months to see the thyroid's full benefit.

_____25.   **Armour Thyroid or a compounded T_4/T_3 combination (Rx): 30 milligrams (1/2 grain = 30 milligrams) (natural thyroid glandular). If Cortef is checked, begin the Cortef and/or adrenal support one to seven days before starting the thyroid. See paragraph below and thyroid information above.

Take half a tablet each morning on an empty stomach for one week and then one tablet each morning. Increase by half to one tablet each one to six weeks (until you're on three tablets or the dose that feels best). Check a repeat free T_4 blood level when you're on three tablets a day (or your optimum dose) for four weeks. If okay, you can continue to raise the dose by half to one tablet each morning each six to nine weeks to a maximum of five a day and then recheck the free T_4 four weeks later. Adjust it to the dose that feels the best (lower the dose if shaky or if your resting pulse is regularly over 88/minute). Do not go over five tablets a day without discussing it with your doctor (although it may take as many as ten a day to see the optimal effect). When on your optimum dose, you can often get a single tablet or capsule at that strength. If your energy wanes too early in the day, you can also take part of your thyroid dose between 11 a.m. and 3 p.m. Some people find that taking part of their thyroid dose at night feels better. You can divide your thyroid dose through the day to see what feels best.

_____26.   Iodine: 1,000 to 2,000 micrograms a day for two to four months if you have daytime body temperatures under 98.3°F or breast cysts or tenderness. Consider Iodoral, which contains 12.5 milligrams (5 milligrams iodine and 7.5 milligrams iodide). May flare Hashimoto's thyroiditis and rarely suppresses thyroid function (with long-term use).

_____27.   *Cytomel (pure active T_3) or compounded sustained-release T_3 (Rx): In fibromyalgia, resistance to normal thyroid doses may occur, and patients often need high levels of T_3 thyroid to improve. Dr. John Lowe's research group feels that the average dose needed in FMS is 75 to 125 micrograms each morning, much higher than your body's normal production. In the absence of resistance, 5 to 25 micrograms is often optimal. Because we are often going above normal levels with T_3, the risks/side effects noted above increase. Because of this, if you have risk factors, it is more important to consider an exercise stress test to make sure your heart is healthy (i.e., no underlying angina) before beginning this protocol. Also, consider a DEXA (osteoporosis) bone density scan every six to eighteen months while on treatment. There may be initial bone loss the first year, then increased bone density. This having been said, in our experience this treatment has been quite safe and, in some FMS patients, dramatically effective. Begin with 5 micrograms each morning and continue to increase by 5 micrograms every three days until you feel well, you feel shaky, or you're at 75 micrograms a day (whichever comes first) and then increase by 5 micrograms a day every one to six weeks until (whichever comes first):

1. You reach 125 micrograms each morning (or 60 micrograms if you're over fifty, unless approved by your physician).
2. You feel healthy.
3. You get shakiness, worsening significant palpitations (occasional "flip-flops" are common), anxiety, racing heart, sweating, or other uncomfortable side effects. If this happens, lower the dose a bit for two to four weeks and then try raising it again until you note significant improvement *without* uncomfortable side effects or you tried to raise it three times and still became shaky/hyper.

Blood tests for thyroid hormone or TSH are not reliable or useful on this regimen. If you feel no better even on the maximum dose, taper off (decrease by 5 micrograms each three days until you're at 15 micrograms a day. Take 15 micrograms a day for three weeks and then drop to 5 micrograms a day for three weeks, then stop.).

Some people do better on the timed-release form of T_3 (Cytomel is immediate release). Because there is marked variation in potency from many pharmacies, I strongly recommend that you use ITC Pharmacy; 303-663-4224.

After being on treatment for three to six months, some patients can lower the T_3 dose or stop taking it. Feel free to try dropping the dose. If you feel better initially and then worse (beginning more than four weeks after starting a new dose), you probably need to lower the dose. If you lose too much weight, try to eat more (and discuss this with your physician) and lower the dose.

ADRENAL HORMONES (GLANDULARS AND SUPPORT)

Helps your body deal with stress and maintains blood pressure.

_____28.   **Cortef (Rx; hydrocortisone): 5-milligram tablets—half to two and a half tablet(s) at breakfast, half to one and a half tablet(s) at lunch, and none to half a tablet at 4 p.m. Use the lowest dose that feels the best. Most patients find that one to one and a half tablets in the morning and half to one tablet at noon is optimal. Take it with food if it causes an acid stomach. Do not take more than four tablets a day without discussing the risks with your physician. Take calcium if on Cortef. If taken too late in the day, Cortef can keep you up at night. You can double the dose for up to one to three weeks (to maximum seven tablets a day) during periods of severe stress (e.g., infections—see or call your doctor for the infection and let him or her know that you're raising the dose). If routinely taking more than four tablets a day (at your doctor's direction), wear a Med-Alert bracelet that says "on chronic cortisol treatment." After nine to eighteen months, you can try to wean off the Cortef (decrease by half a tablet a day every two weeks) if you feel okay (or no worse) without it. Compounded sustained-release hydrocortisone is even better (available from ITC Pharmacy; 303-663-4224) if your energy drops in the afternoon.

_____29. **Adrenal Stress End (from Enzymatic Therapy or Integrative Therapeutics): One to two capsules each morning (or one to two in the morning and one at noon). If it upsets your stomach, take less or take with food.

_____30. *Increase your salt and water intake a lot. If your mouth and lips are dry (and you're not on Elavil), you're dehydrated—drink more water (or herbal tea or lemonade sweetened with stevia; see #37), not sodas or coffee. Celtic Sea Salt is an excellent form to use (800-867-7258).

OTHER HORMONES

_____31. *Biest 2.5 milligrams, plus progesterone 30 to 100 milligrams, plus testosterone 0 to 5 milligrams all in 1 gram of cream (Rx): Apply 1 gram of skin cream at bedtime. Available from ITC Pharmacy; 303-663-4224). Vaginal preparations may be more effective.

_____32. *Testosterone (Rx): Males 25 to 50 milligrams (order 100 milligrams/gram of cream) one to two times a day (less if acne occurs). Rub the cream into an area of thin skin on the abdomen or inner thigh. The cream is available by prescription from ITC Pharmacy; 303-663-4224) and can be mailed to you. Or Testim 1 percent 25 or 50 milligrams; apply gel one to two times a day. Consider also checking estrogen and DHT levels when you check your testosterone blood levels. If the DHT goes too high it can cause hair loss, which can be prevented by Proscar (Rx) or saw palmetto, 160 milligrams two times a day. If estrogen goes too high, this can be blocked by Arimidex (Rx) 0.5 milligram a day. If you are taking thyroid tablets, be aware that adding testosterone can increase your thyroid blood levels. If you get moody or anxious, or your heart races, check a blood level for your thyroid and consider lowering the dose.

Antiviral Agents

See also the article "Treating Respiratory Infections Without Antibiotics" in Chapter 5.

_____33.   Colloidal silver (Argentyn 23, available at www.vitality101.com, or wholesale from www.natural-immunogenics.com or 888-328-8840): For acute infections or aggressive treatment, take 2 tablespoons by mouth in the morning, 1 tablespoon before lunch, and 1 tablespoon twenty minutes before dinner. Silver should be taken on an empty stomach (at least ten minutes before eating or drinking). If you get a die-off reaction (flaring up of symptoms) as the infection is killed, lower the dose to 1 teaspoon a day and increase more slowly. Although the higher dose (a 240-ounce bottle is an eight-day course) can be taken safely for at least a year, 1 teaspoon a day is a good maintenance dose (a 240-ounce bottle lasts forty-eight days) after the infection resolves.

_____34.   Valcyte (Rx): 450 milligrams, two a day for six months. See "Infections" (Chapter 5) for more detailed information.

_____35.   *Anti-Viral (by Ultraceuticals): Three to six capsules twice a day. This contains a mix of milk thistle extract (80 percent silymarin), phylanthus amarius, phylanthus uraria, monoammonium glycyrrhizinate, L-lysine, N-Acetyl-L-Cysteine, astragalus herb powder, lactoferrin, olive leaf extract, dionea (Venus flytrap extract), and selenium (Selenomethionine).

_____35A.   Monolaurin (Rx): 300-milligram capsules: Nine capsules once a day on an empty stomach for one week, followed by six capsules once a day for twenty days. Take lysine 1,500 milligrams twice a day while on Monolaurin.

Anti-Yeast Treatments

For a nonprescription approach, use #36, 38, and 40.

_____36.   **Avoid sweets—this includes sucrose, glucose, fructose, corn syrup, or any other sweets—until your doctor says that it is okay to include them in your diet again. Also, avoid fruit juices, which are naturally sweet. Having one to two fruits a day (the whole fruit as opposed to the juice) is okay. Stevia is a great sugar substitute.

_____37. Stevia is an excellent herbal sweetener. A great-tasting one is by Body Ecology (800-478-3842). Use all you want.

_____38. **Acidophilus milk bacteria—Acidophilus Pearls form (by Enzymatic Therapy/Integrative Therapeutics): Take two twice a day for five months. Then consider one a day to help maintain a healthy bowel. Do not take within six hours of taking an antibiotic (i.e., take it midday, if you take the antibiotic morning and night). The Enzymatic Therapy/ITI Acidophilus or Probiotic Pearls form contains about 2.4 billion units per pearl even though the box says only 1 billion.

_____40. **Anti-yeast (Ultraceuticals) or Phytostan (ITI) are excellent natural antifungal mixes. Take 1 to 2 twice a day for three to five months.

_____41. Mycelex oral lozenges (Rx, for thrush and/or painful "in the mouth" sores): Suck on one lozenge five times a day for one to four days (as needed). After sucking on the lozenge for a while (i.e., ten minutes), put pieces of the lozenge up against the sore(s) until you are tired of them being there.

_____42. *Nystatin (Rx): 500,000 units, two tablets two to four times a day. Begin with one a day and increase by one tablet a day until you are up to the total dose. Your symptoms may initially flare up as the yeast die off. If this occurs, raise the dose more slowly, or stop for a while if die-off is still severe. The Nystatin is usually taken for five to eight months. If nausea occurs, take two twice a day and/or switch to the Nystatin powder in capsules or mixed in water (available from Kronos Pharmacy; 800-723-7455, in 1-million-unit capsules, which are much less expensive and better tolerated but need to be refrigerated). Repeat Nystatin for four to six weeks anytime you take an antibiotic or have recurrent bowel symptoms.

_____43. **Diflucan (fluconazole): 200 milligrams a day, or, if not effective, Nizoral 200 milligrams a day. Take it for six weeks.

Important: Begin taking the Diflucan four weeks after starting the Anti-Yeast herbal or Nystatin. See the paragraph below.

Begin taking the Diflucan or Nizoral four weeks after beginning the Anti-Yeast herbal or Nystatin. If the symptoms have improved and then worsen when you stop the antifungal, refill the prescription for another six weeks. If your symptoms flared when you began the Nystatin, begin with one-quarter to one half of the above dose for the first week. Do not take Mevacor family medications with Diflucan or Nizoral. If you need to stay on these medications more than three months, check liver blood tests (ALT, AST) every three months. If you feel well and symptoms (especially bowel symptoms) recur over time, consider re-treating yourself with Acidophilus Pearls anti-yeast and Diflucan for six weeks as needed.

Immune Stimulants

____44.   **Thymic protein (Pro Boost): Dissolve the contents of one packet under your tongue—any that is swallowed is destroyed. Take it three times a day for twelve weeks, then one a day for six weeks. Also take it three times a day at the first sign of any infection until the infection resolves (it is approximately two dollars a packet). It's available from our office (800-333-5287 or www.vitality101.com) and works in the first twenty-four hours for acute infections but takes two to three months to work for chronic infections.

____44A.   *Leuko-Stim (by Ultraceuticals). This mix mostly stimulates immune function, but the olive leaf may also have antiviral properties. It contains olive leaf extract; Beta 1,3; glucan; maitake mushroom extract; and arabinogalactan (larch).

____44B.   Maitake D-Fraction 30: Take with 330 milligrams of maitake mushroom and extract—an excellent immune stimulant (by Ultraceuticals).

If a chronic viral infection is suspected, consider three months of Anti-Viral (#35), with Leuko-Stim or maitake, plus Pro Boost. Adding the silver solution (#33) may also help. These can be taken on their own or with the antivirals. For suspected bacterial infections, consider Leuko-Stim or maitake plus Pro Boost and perhaps the silver solution, again on their own or with the antibiotics. Though these are more expensive than many natural supplements, they can be helpful in fighting these infections and are well tolerated. It can take three months to see the effects.

Water Filters

____45. *Multi-Pure Water Filter: Most other filters except those that use reverse osmosis are not optimally effective. Available from Bren Jacobson (410-224-4877). Decreases the risk of reinfection and removes chemicals and contaminants from your water.

Treatment for Bacterial, Mycoplasma, Chlamydial, Bladder (E. coli), Sinusitis, Chronic Lyme, or Other Infections

These infections usually take months to years to eradicate. It is common for your symptoms to flare (from the infection die-off) the first two to six weeks of treatment. Take the antibiotics for six months and, if better, then repeat six-week cycles until your symptoms stay gone. Antidepressants, Neurontin, and/or codeine may block the antibiotics' effectiveness. Be sure to take anti-yeast or nystatin (two tablets twice a day) and acidophilus while on the antibiotics. If you have occasional low-grade fever (i.e., over 98.6°F), check your oral temperature occasionally to see if the antibiotics reduce or eliminate the fever. If so, stay on those antibiotics. See Dr. Nicholson's Web site (www.immed.org) for more information. *You can use #33 and 44 instead of or with antibiotics.*

____46. Cipro (ciprofloxacin): 500 milligrams twice a day for six months (adults only). Do not take magnesium products (e.g., FibroCare, some antacids, Energy Revitalization System) within six hours of Cipro or you won't absorb the Cipro.
    OR
____47. *Doxycycline (a tetracycline): 100 milligrams two times a day for six months (adults only). If symptoms recur when the doxy-

cycline is completed, keep repeating six-week courses until the symptoms stay resolved. Take anti-yeast or nystatin (at least two twice a day) while on the antibiotic. Birth control pills may not work while on doxycycline. Do not take any doxycycline tablets older than their expiration date (dangerous).

OR

_____48.   Zithromax (azithromycin): 250 to 600 milligrams, one tablet a day (take with food if it bothers your stomach). Don't take magnesium-containing products within six hours of the Zithromax.

CHRONIC AND ACUTE SINUSITIS

_____49.   **Sinusitis nose spray (Rx, by prescription from ITC Pharmacy, 303-663-4224). It contains Sporanox, xylitol, Bactroban, and beclamethasone. Use one to two sprays in each nostril twice a day for six to twelve weeks. If it irritates the nose, use nasal saline spray just before using the prescription. Use with silver spray below.

_____50.   Nasal silver spray: Five to ten sprays in each nostril three times a day for seven to fourteen days until the sinusitis resolves (from www.vitality101.com). Can be used with #49.

E. COLI BLADDER INFECTIONS

_____51.   D-mannose: 1 teaspoon (2 grams) stirred in water every two to three hours while awake for two to five days for acute bladder infections (may use up to one to two times a day long term if needed for chronic infections) caused by E. coli (this causes approximately 90 percent of bladder infections). If not much better in twenty-four to forty-eight hours, get a urine culture and consider an antibiotic. Continue taking D-mannose for two to three days after the last symptom resolves. Taking 1 teaspoon an hour before and immediately after intercourse can also prevent bladder infections. D-mannose is available from BioTech (800-345-1199) or from www.vitality101.com.

Other Treatments

Antidepressants may help treat NMH and decrease pain as well as helping energy.

Food and Other Sensitivities

____52. **NAET: Wonderful for elimination of sensitivities/allergies (see www.naet.com for more information). In Kona, Hawaii, you can contact Laurie Teitelbaum at 410-266-6958.

____53. Food Allergy Elimination Diet (instruction sheet is available at www.vitality101.com).

IV NUTRITIONAL SUPPORT

____54. **Myers cocktail: IV nutritional therapies (very helpful). They are called the Standard IVs at the Fibromyalgia & Fatigue Centers (see www.fibroandfatigue.com). In the D.C./Virginia/Maryland region, I recommend having them given by Rhonda Kidd (443-994-0126).

*DETOXIFICATION

There are several simple things you can do that are helpful:

____55. Sweating can remove toxins—especially if you shower immediately after—and can be very helpful for health. Many of the newer saunas are what are called "far infrared," and thirty to sixty minutes three to seven times a week can help detoxification. I use the one from High Tech Health at www.hightech health.com. Heating your body can also decrease pain.

____55A. Some of you may be more comfortable with hot baths, which help a lot with general muscle aches and pains. This is one recipe for a detox bath that was given to me by a wonderful practitioner, Anette Mnabhi, D.O. in Montgomery, Illinois: 2

cups Epsom Salt, 1 cup baking soda, and ⅓ cup hydrogen peroxide. Fill tub with hot water and add above ingredients. Soak for twenty to thirty minutes. You will sweat in the tub and lose toxins (which causes you to lose some water as well). It is important to drink plenty of water while you soak. You can squeeze fresh lemon juice and mix with water and drink, or drink plain water, but it is essential to drink while you take the bath. If you have a tendency to get light-headed easily, be cautious when getting out of the tub, or have someone nearby the first time you take a detox bath. Take a lukewarm to cool shower after getting out of the tub to rinse off the salts or you may itch. Rest for thirty minutes after the bath.

____56. **Bone Health (Ultraceuticals) for improving bone density. Bone Health has calcium, magnesium, strontium, boron, and many other key nutrients. Studies suggest that it is much more effective than Fosamax, without the toxicity.

NMH AND/OR ENERGY BOOSTERS AND ANTIDEPRESSANTS

____57. *Dexedrine (dextroamphetamine): 5 milligrams, one to two tablets in the morning, plus half to one and a half tablets at noon, as needed for energy. Dexedrine is an amphetamine-family stimulant similar to Ritalin and may be addictive. Take less if you have caffeinelike shakiness. Most patients use one to three tablets of Dexedrine in the morning and half to two at noon. If appetite suppression and/or weight loss is a problem you can add 4 milligrams Periactin (cyproheptadine; antihistamine and antiserotonin) up to five tablets a day.

____58. Happiness 1–2–3! from Health Freedom Nutrition, In Harmony from Ultraceuticals, or similar mixes are outstanding for depression (the effect increases with six weeks of use). Contains Hypericum (Saint-John's-wort), 5-HTP, magnolia, and more (takes six weeks to see the full antidepressant effect). Take one to three capsules one to three times a day. Do not take with other prescription antidepressants without your doctor's okay.

____59. Effexor (venlafaxine): 37½ to 75 milligrams one to three times a day.

____60.   Loss of libido and sexual dysfunction can be treated with Desire in women and Potency Plus in men (both from Ultraceuticals). Other helpful treatments for antidepressant-induced sexual dysfunction include ginkgo biloba 120 milligrams twice daily, Dexedrine 5 to 25 milligrams each morning, or Symmetrel (amantadine) 100 milligrams twice daily, or switching to Wellbutrin.

CONSTIPATION

Adjust these as needed to have one soft bowel movement a day. Increasing your water, fiber intake (e.g., 1 bowl of whole grain cereal in the morning), and magnesium intake is also helpful.

____61.   MiraLAX laxative (Rx): 1 heaping tablespoon a day in 8 ounces of water (comes in 14- and 26-ounce bottles).

____62.   Prunes and/or prune juice.

Pain Treatments

The natural treatments can be substituted for or added to the prescription pain medications. If side effects occur, they can often be avoided by starting with a low dose and raising it every three to seven days as your body gets used to the medication. It may take two to six weeks for a treatment to start working.

NATURAL PAIN THERAPIES

____63.   Rolfing, Trager, myofascial release, chiropractic, other bodywork and manipulation modalities, and/or acupuncture.

____64.   **End Pain or Pain Formula or similar products. Both contain willow bark, boswellia, and cherry. Take two to four tablets three times a day. It takes two to six weeks to see the full effect. At that time, you can often lower the dose to one tablet three times a day or two twice a day. From Enzymatic Therapy and ITI (available at www.vitality101.com).

_____65. NF Joint Gel (Integrative Therapeutics): Simply roll it on and rub it in. For best results, massage Joint Gel into your skin until absorbed. You can use Joint Gel up to three to four times daily (available at www.vitality101.com).

_____66. Lipoic acid: 200 milligrams three times a day for neuropathic pain. Benefit usually begins to be seen by two to three months. It has been shown to be helpful for diabetic neuropathy and burning mouth syndrome (200 milligrams three times a day for five months).

_____67. Glucosamine sulfate: 750 milligrams two times a day (for arthritis). Takes six weeks to see if it helps. When the maximum benefit is seen, you can decrease to the lowest dose that maintains the effect.

_____68. MSM (methyl sulfanyl methane): 3 grams a day for arthritis.

Osteoporosis or Osteopenia (Loss of Bone Density)

_____69. Bone Health (Ultraceuticals). Contains strontium, calcium, magnesium, silica, and more. Excellent. Do not take it within three hours of your thyroid dose (take it at dinner and bedtime).

PHARMACOLOGIC PAIN TREATMENTS

If you are not clear about the source/type of your pain, there are many sequences in which to try the medications. One reasonable order to try them in is the one listed below. It can take two to six weeks to see the full effect of the medication. When there are several medications with the same number (e.g., 73A, 73B, and 73C), if the first medication helped but was not tolerated because of side effects, go to the next medication of the same number. If it simply did not help significantly, go to the next number. If you get partial benefit from a medication, continue it and add the next medication as needed to get pain free. IV lidocaine or narcotics may be appropriate early on for severe pain while trying other therapies.

____70. **Ultram (Rx; tramadol): 50 milligrams, one to two tablets up to four times a day as needed for pain. Side effects are less with four or fewer tablets a day. May cause nausea/vomiting. **Caution:** May very rarely cause seizures or raise serotonin too high when combined with antidepressants.

TOPICAL PAIN TREATMENTS

____71. *Pain Formula Lotion (Rx): Rub a pea-size amount onto painful areas three times a day as needed (available from ITC Pharmacy; 303-663-4224). You can use this on up to three or four silver dollar–size areas at a time.

____72. *Lidoderm patches (Rx; lidocaine): Can be cut into pieces to put over different areas. Leave the patch on for twelve to eighteen hours, then take it off the rest of the day. It can help localized pain (i.e., it helps pain that is right under the patch). Up to four patches can be used at a time each day. It can take two to three weeks to see if it works.

GABA AGONISTS

____73A. *Neurontin (Rx; gabapentin): 300 to 900 milligrams one to four times a day times a day (to a maximum of 3,600 milligrams a day). Cut back and increase by 100 milligrams a day every four to five days if it causes any uncomfortable or unusual neurologic symptoms or excessive sedation. Begin with 100 to 300 milligrams at night, then slowly increase to 300 to 900 milligrams three times a day as is comfortable. In some, pain relief is immediate; in others, it can take a minimum of 1,200 milligrams a day. You can go up to 3,600 milligrams a day.

____73B. Gabitril (Rx; tiagabine): 2 to 4 milligrams two times a day and increase by a maximum of 4 milligrams daily, every three to seven days, to a maximum of 12 milligrams a day. Helps relieve pain and increase deep sleep. The main side effects are sedation, dizziness, and gastric upset.

____73C. Lyrica (Rx; pregabalin): 100 milligrams two to three times a day. Helpful for relieving pain and restless leg syndrome and increasing deep sleep. The main side effects are dizziness and drowsiness, which tend to decrease over time, and weight gain.

Muscle Relaxants

____74.   Flexeril (Rx; cyclobenzaprine): 10 milligrams, half to one tablet three times a day. A muscle relaxant, it can cause dry mouth and be fairly sedating at 10 milligrams but much less so at 5 milligrams, so the lower dose may be better during the day.

____75.   **Skelaxin (Rx; metaxolone): 800 milligrams, one tablet four times a day as needed for pain. This is usually nonsedating.

To Lower Cholesterol

__75A.   Chol-Less (Ultraceuticals): This natural mix of cholesterol-lowering herbs is excellent. Give it six weeks to see the effects. Take three capsules a day.

Follow-Up Testing and Recommendations

____76.   Stool O&P (ova & parasite) at the Institute of Parasitology in Arizona. Call 480-767-2522 to get a kit.

____77.   **Stool O&P, plus cultures and sensitivity, must be sent to Genova/Great Smokies Mountain Labs (800-522-4762).

____78.   Sleep apnea study (get insurance preauthorization; it costs two thousand dollars). Or videotape yourself while sleeping to see if you snore and stop breathing or if your legs jump at night.

____79.   Sleep apnea study (get insurance preauthorization; it costs two thousand dollars). Go to a sleep lab that can look for upper airway resistance syndrome (UARS) and be sure that they do.

____80.   HHV–6 and CMV IgG and IgM antibodies and EBV VCA antibody to be done at Focus Labs only (part of Quest Labs).

____81.   Do vision test (VCS) at www.chronicneurotoxins.com. If test is positive, consider neurotoxin treatment.

____82.   Transglutaminase antibody (IgA and IgG) blood tests for celiac disease (wheat allergy).

____83.   Read my book *Pain Free 1-2-3*.

Lab Testing

If you have any of these symptoms:	You have the right to have these tests done:
Fatigue	Complete blood count (CBC), erythrocyte sedimentation rate (ESR), and differential chemistry (for example, chemistry 16) and magnesium
Anemia	Iron (Fe), total iron binding capacity (TIBC), and ferritin (all three iron studies are necessary); vitamin B_{12}
Fatigue, constipation, or achiness	Thyroid studies including free or total T_3, free T_4, and thyroid-stimulating hormone (TSH) (all three tests are necessary)
Anemia, confusion, poor memory, fatigue, or paresthesia (numbness or tingling in the fingers)	Vitamin B_{12}
Increased thirst or urination	$HgbA_1C$ (diabetes screen) or glycosylated hemoglobin
Chronic diarrhea or abdominal cramps, gas, bloating, or other gastrointestinal complaints	Stool for ova and parasites, with antigen testing for amoeba, giardia, cryptosporidium, and Clostridium difficile
Chronic muscle aches or joint aches	Creatine phosphokinase (CPK), antinuclear antibody (ANA), latex fixation (rheumatoid factor)

Fatigue, recurrent infections, or fever	HHV-6 and EBV VCA viral IgG and IgM antibodies
Fatigue, achiness, joint pains, confusion, or poor memory	Lyme disease testing
Runny nose, recurrent respiratory infections, nasal congestion, rashes, wheezing	Allergy testing and immunoglobulin E (IgE)
Under- or overactive thyroid (often helpful in interpreting the significance of borderline results)	Thyroid antibodies test to check for Hashimoto's thyroiditis
Irregular or absent periods or hot flashes (check for menopause)	Follicle-stimulating hormone (FSH), luteinizing hormone (LH), estradiol level
Decreased libido (in male or female), decreased erections	Testosterone and free testosterone
Abnormal body-hair growth, fatigue, or infertility	Dehydroepiandrosterone-sulfate (DHEA-S)
Fatigue, hypotension, or recurrent infections	Morning cortisol
Fatigue with snoring, overweight, high blood pressure, or periods of apnea	Sleep study
Fever and sweats	HHV-6, mycoplasma, chlamydia PCR, and/or antibody tests

Recommended Reading

Books

Ali, M. *The Canary and Chronic Fatigue.* Denville, NJ: IPM Press, 1994. Focuses on the damage to enzyme systems by environmental stresses and nutritional-herbal-lifestyle therapeutics.

Bell, D. S. *The Doctor's Guide to Chronic Fatigue Syndrome.* Written by a very compassionate pediatric CFS expert.

Blatman, H. *Winners' Guide to Pain Relief* (available online at www. winoverpain.com). Dr. Blatman is president of the American Holistic Medical Association. The book is a complement to *From Fatigued to Fantastic!* While this book focuses on the metabolic and mind-body aspects of treatment, Dr. Blatman's book focuses on physical treatments, many of which you can do on your own for quick pain relief.

Crook, W. G. *The Yeast Connection and Women's Health.* Jackson, TN: Professional Books, 2005. An excellent book. From the original teacher on yeast problems in CFIDS.

Goldstein, J. *Tuning the Brain.* Binghamton, NY: Haworth Press, 2001.

Hicks, Jerry, and Esther Hicks. *The Law of Attraction*. Carlsbad, CA: Hay House, 2006. An excellent book on the power of positive thinking and creating what you want in life.

Ivker, R. S. *Sinus Survival*. New York: Jeremy P. Tarcher, 2000. Must-reading for patients with chronic sinusitis.

Jefferies, W. M. *Safe Uses of Cortisol*, 2nd edition. Springfield, IL: Charles C. Thomas, 1996. A landmark monograph on adrenal insufficiency. Written for physicians.

Kelly, J. W., M.S., R.N., and Rosalie Devonshire, MSW. *Taking Charge of Fibromyalgia: Everything You Need to Know to Manage Fibromyalgia* (2005 edition). This is a great and highly useful guide to self-managing your FM treatment program.

Pellegrino, M. J. *Fibromyalgia: Up Close & Personal*. Columbus, OH: Anadem Publishing, 2005. Dr. Pellegrino's tenth book on FM offers practical advice to readers about up-to-date drug and alternative treatments, diet and exercise, posttraumatic FM, and disability and personal injury issues.

Rogers, S. A. *Tired or Toxic*. Syracuse, NY: Prestige Publishing, 1990. An extensive review of chemical sensitivity problems.

Rosenbaum, M., and M. Susser. *Solving the Puzzle of Chronic Fatigue Syndrome*. Tacoma, WA: Life Sciences Press, 1992. A good review of CFS treatments and also of infectious problems.

Shomon, M. *Living Well with Chronic Fatigue Syndrome and Fibromyalgia*. New York: HarperCollins, 2004.
An excellent overview by one of my favorite patient advocates.

Teitelbaum, J. *Pain Free 1–2–3*. New York: McGraw-Hill, 2006. Reviews most types of pain and how to eliminate them.

Teitelbaum, J. *Three Steps to Happiness! Healing Through Joy*. Annapolis, MD: Deva Press, 2003. (Available at www.vitality101.com).

Travell, J. G., and D. G. Simons. *Myofascial Pain and Dysfunction: The Trigger Point Manual.* Baltimore, MD: Williams & Wilkins, 1983. A crucial text for anyone treating myofascial (muscle) pain. Chapter 4 discusses perpetuating factors, which are also important when treating fibromyalgia.

Journals and Newsletters

CFIDS Chronicle. A subscription comes with membership in the Chronic Fatigue and Immune Dysfunction Syndrome Association of America. Available from the Chronic Fatigue and Immune Dysfunction Syndrome Association of America, P.O. Box 220398, Charlotte, NC 28222-0398; 800-442-3437.

Fibromyalgia Network Newsletter. Available from the Fibromyalgia Network, P.O. Box 31750, Tucson, AZ 85751; 800-853-2929. From an excellent national FMS support group.

FM Aware by the NFA (National Fibromyalgia Association).

From Fatigued to Fantastic! newsletter. This is my free e-mail newsletter, which will keep you up to date on the newest developments in CFS, fibromyalgia, and pain management. I invite you to sign up for it at www.vitality101.com.

Herbalgram by the American Botanical Council. An excellent way to stay updated on herbs; 800-373-7105 or 512-331-8868.

Immune Support newsletter. This excellent newsletter is available from www.immunesupport.com.

Journal of Chronic Fatigue Syndrome. For physicians. Available from Haworth Press, 10 Alice St., Binghamton, NY 13904; 800-429-6784.

Journal of Musculoskeletal Pain. For physicians. Available from Haworth Press, 10 Alice St., Binghamton, NY 13904; 800-429-6784.

Resources

Physicians Specializing
in Chronic Fatigue Syndrome

Physician Organizations

Holistic physicians are often familiar with effective CFIDS/FMS therapies. The following are organizations of physicians who take a holistic approach to medicine.

American Board of Holistic Medicine
Certifies physicians as having advanced training in the use of natural therapies.
Web site lists more than 1,000 physicians.
www.holisticboard.org

American College for Advancement of Medicine
P.O. Box 3427
Laguna Hills, CA 92654
http://www.apma.net

American Holistic Medical Association (AHMA)
4101 Lake Boone Trail, Suite 201
Raleigh, NC 27607
919-787-5146
Provides speakers through its speakers bureau.

INDIVIDUAL PRACTITIONERS

Instead of trying to teach your doctor how to treat CFS/FMS, go to specialists. The Fibromyalgia & Fatigue Centers (see Chapter 12) have offices throughout the United States and see people from all over the world. Their physicians are excellent and, being the medical director, I get to be sure they stay on top of the newest information. To find the center nearest you, go to www.fibroandfatigue.com or call 866-443-4276. In addition, the educational computer program at www.vitality101.com will also analyze your medical history (and laboratory test results, if available) to make a thorough medical record, a list of the most likely underlying problems in your case, and a treatment protocol tailored to your case. This will allow you to begin the natural parts of the protocol on your own and will assist and support your doctor in giving you the best possible care.

Products and Services

All these resources are recommended. Those that are most noteworthy are marked with a single or double asterisk, depending on how commonly people tend to use or need them.

Amy Podd/A. P. Business Solutions
1109 Little Magothy View
Annapolis, MD 21401
410-757-7295
Sells therapeutic magnets.

Bio Brite
4340 East West Highway, Suite 401S
Bethesda, MD 20814
800-621-LITE (800-621-5483); 301-961-5940

Fax: 301-961-5943

www.biobrite.com

Sells light boxes and light visors for persons suffering from seasonal affective disorder.

**Bioenergy Life Science, Inc.

13840 Johnson Street NE

Ham Lake, MN 55304

866-267-8253

Fax: 763-757-0588

www.corvalen.com

E-mail: info@bioenergy.com

For D-ribose (CORvalen) or D-ribose with magnesium and malic acid (CORvalenM).

This company is to be especially commended for its commitment to quality, in both finished products and extensive patient-focused research.

Body Ecology

1266 West Paces Ferry Road, Suite 505

Atlanta, GA 30327

800-4-STEVIA (800-478-3842)

Stevia; stevia cookbooks.

*Brugh Joy, Inc.

P.O. Box 1059

Lucerne Valley, CA 92356

800-448-9187

For information on workshops that help people understand their deep psyches and learn to accept and understand more fully who they really are.

*Cape Apothecary

1384 Cape St. Claire Road

Annapolis, MD 21401

800-248-5978; 410-757-3522; 410-974-1788

Fax: 410-626-7226

www.rxstat.com/capedrug

An excellent holistic compounding pharmacy that fills mail orders.

*Consumers Discount Drug Company
323-461-3606
This mail-order pharmacy has the best prices I've found on mail-order prescriptions.

**Enzymatic Therapy
825 Challenger Drive
Green Bay, WI 54311
800-783-2286
www.enzy.com
Produces many excellent products, including the Fatigued to Fantastic! product line, which I developed. This line includes Fatigued to Fantastic! Energy Revitalization System vitamin powder and B complex; Fatigued to Fantastic! Daily Energy B Complex; End Pain; and Revitalizing Sleep Formula. Enzymatic Therapy products can be found in most health food stores, as well as at www.vitality101.com.

General Nutrition, Inc.
Customer Resources Department
300 Sixth Avenue
Pittsburgh, PA 15222
888-462-2548
www.gnc.com
Markets a good form of magnesium-potassium aspartate and DHEA. There are General Nutrition Centers (GNC) stores throughout North America. You can contact the company at the address above to find a store in your area.

*Genova (previously Great Smokies Diagnostic Laboratory)
63 Zillicoa Street
Asheville, NC 28801
800-522-4762
Fax: 828-252-9303
www.gsdl.com
Stool culture and sensitivity tests. Does an excellent job with stool testing for ova and parasites (O&P testing) and bacterial infections, as well as many other tests.

*Grove Self-help Kits
www.thegroveapproach.com
1-888-774-7007
One of my favorite self-help kits for those who want guidance on yoga, diet, and much more. Comes from Karen Grove of the Grove Approach. It contains: "Healthier Living with Fibromyalgia"; her products; her self-help book, *How to Lighten the Heavy Load of Fibromyalgia*; her cookbook, *Get to the Core of Healthy Fibromyalgia Cooking*; and valuable exercise therapy specifically designed for people with fibromyalgia (the Fibroga 1 exercise DVD).

G.Y. and N.
877-864-5112
Carries ingredients for Myers cocktails.

Harvard Drug Company
800-783-7103
Carries ingredients for Myers cocktails.

*Health Freedom Nutrition
800-980-8780
www.HFN-USA.com
This mail-order company has a good newsletter and also makes Calming Balance and Happiness 1-2-3! (also available at www.vitality 101.com).

Hemex Labs
2505 West Beryl Avenue
Phoenix, AZ 85021-1461
800-999-CLOT (800-999-2568)
www.hemex.com
Blood testing, including CFIDS coagulation blood profile/immune system activation of coagulation (ISAC) panel test and hereditary thrombotic panel to see if heparin therapy may help.

*High Tech Health Saunas
www.hightechhealth.com
Sweating can remove toxins, especially if you shower immediately after, and can be helpful for health. Many of the newer saunas are what are called

"far infrared," and a half hour three to seven times a week can help detoxification. I use and recommend the one from High Tech Health.

Institute for Molecular Medicine
15162 Triton Lane
Huntington Beach, CA 92649
714-903-2900
Fax: 714-379-2082
www.immed.com
For mycoplasma and chlamydia PCR testing, HHV–6 testing by Dr.
Garth Nicolson.

**Integrative Therapeutics, Inc (ITI)
Wilsonville, Oregon
800-931-1709
Cathy Leet, representative
920-737-8828
I feel that this is the best company in the United States making products for
health practitioners only, and I am so impressed with it that I asked it to
make my End Fatigue line of products. These include the Energy Revitalization System vitamin powder and B complex, which can replace more than
thirty-five different vitamin tablets a day; Daily Energy B Complex; Pain
Formula herbal mix; Adrenal Stress-End; and Revitalizing Sleep Formula.
ITI actually voluntarily registered with the FDA so that its products have to
go through the same testing for potency and purity as pharmaceuticals. ITI
has many excellent products, and Cathy Leet is excellent to work with.

**ITC Pharmacy
303-663-4224
This mail-order compounding pharmacy does a superb job of quality control, and makes a wide range of bioidentical hormones, topical pain formulas, the sinusitis nose spray, and much more. Although there are many
excellent compounding pharmacies, this is the one I recommend first.

**Bren Jacobson
Does excellent pastoral psychological counseling by phone ($95/hour) and
also consults on how to use the best of natural and prescription therapies
to treat difficult medical issues.

410-224-4877
bren.jacobson@gmail.com

Steven P. Krafchick
Krafchick Law Firm
2701 First Avenue, Suite 340
Seattle, WA 98121
206-374-7370
Fax: 206-374-7377
www.krafchick.com
E-mail: klf@krafchick.com
An attorney who specializes in CFS/FMS private (not Social Security) disability cases, Krafchick has a master's in public health from the University of Michigan and has practiced law since 1983. He represents people all over the United States in their long-term disability claims and has been doing Employee Retirement Income Security Act (ERISA) LTD claims for almost fifteen years. The good news is that he is an expert in CFS/FMS, so you will not need to explain the illnesses to him.

Metagenics
100 Avenida La Pata
San Clemente, CA 92673
800-692-9400; 949-366-0818
www.metagenics.com
www.ultrabalance.com
Manufacturer of the UltraBalance Medical Foods line of products, including UltraClean, a hypoallergenic powdered food to use with bowel detoxification and elimination diets. Developed by nutritional biochemist Dr. Jeffrey Bland, this product is expensive, but it can help determine food sensitivities.

Partnership for Prescription Assistance (PPA)
888-477-2669
www.pparx.org
For assistance to help pay for or get free medications, if your income is less than $19,000 a year for an individual or $32,000 for a family of three.

**Pure Water
www.purewatermd.tripod.com

410-224-4877
443-949-0409
Consultant on health and environmental concerns, especially water, and distributor of Multi-Pure water filters.

Sinus Survival by Dr. Robert Ivker
www.sinussurvival.com
Contains tools such as nasal steamers to help with chronic sinusitis. His Web site has many other helpful tools and resources.

**Jacob Teitelbaum, M.D.
466 Forelands Road
Annapolis, MD 21401
800-333-5287; 410-573-5389
www.vitality101.com
Many of the products recommended in this book, especially hard-to-find ones, are available through my Web site. Among them are delta wave sleep-inducing CDs and tapes; D-mannose; stevia; thymic protein (Pro Boost); Fatigued to Fantastic! Energy Revitalization System multivitamin, amino acid, and mineral formula; Daily Energy B Complex; Adrenal Stress-End, End Pain; and the Revitalizing Sleep Formula. It also carries many of the Ultraceutical products. At the Web site, you can sign up for free e-mail newsletters that will keep you on the cutting edge of developments in CFS/FMS and effective pain therapies and a second newsletter on general health. There is also a computer program that will tailor a treatment protocol to your case and an extensive list of CFIDS/FMS support groups.

A word about Fatigued to Fantastic! products: I direct any company making my formulas to donate to charity all of the royalties that I would have received. I also never accept any money from any natural or pharmaceutical product companies.

*To Your Health
800-801-1406
FMS products. Margy Squires and Dave Squires are sweethearts and a wonderful information resource as well.

**Ultraceutical Products
This line of natural products is used at the Fibromyalgia & Fatigue Centers, and is also available at www.vitality101.com.

SUPPORT GROUPS AND INFORMATION SOURCES

*American Botanical Council
P.O. Box 201660
Austin, TX 78720
800-373-7105; 512-331-8868
Supplies information on specific herbs and publishes *Herbalgram*, a magazine with information on helpful herbal remedies.

BioSET
P.O. Box 5356
Larkspur, CA 94977
877-927-0741; 415-927-0741
www.bioset.net
Offers an allergy desensitization technique that also employs detoxification and enzyme therapy.

Chronic Fatigue and Immune Dysfunction Syndrome
    Association of America
P.O. Box 220398
Charlotte, NC 28222-0398
800-442-3437; 704-365-2343
Fax: 704-365-9755
www.cfids.org

**Fibromyalgia Coalition International
913-384-4673
www.fibrocoalition.org
An excellent information and advocacy group formed by Yvonne Keeny.

*Fibromyalgia Network
P.O. Box 31750
Tucson, AZ 85751
800-853-2929
www.fmnetnews.com

Guild for Structural Integration
P.O. Box 1559

Boulder, CO 80306

800-447-0150

For practitioners of the Rolf method of structural integration.

International and American Association for Chronic Fatigue
    Syndrome (IACFS)

P.O. Box 895

Olney, MD 20830

www.AACFS.org

An umbrella organization focusing on scientific research.

**International Coalition for the Advancement of
    Fibromyalgia/CFIDS Treatment (ICAF)

www.icafcoalition.org

This group is dedicated to representing patient needs first. It is a new umbrella organization of patient, business, and practitioner groups that is directed by patients. Its goal is to evaluate new therapies and supply the most
accurate and useful information available to patients.

The organization also has excellent DVDs of lectures by me and other
excellent speakers.

Myalgic Encephalitis Association of Canada

246 Queen Street, Suite 400

Ottawa, Ontario K1P 5E4

Canada

613-563-1565

An excellent source of general information for CFIDS and fibromyalgia
patients, as well as a good source of important information for Canadian
patients.

**NAET

6714 Beach Boulevard

Buena Park, CA 90621

714-523-8900

Fax: 714-523-3068

www.naet.com

Supplies information about the Nambudripad allergy elimination techniques (NAET), including help with locating practitioners.

National CFIDS Foundation
103 Aletha Road
Needham, MA 02492
781-449-3535
Fax: 781-449-8606
www.ncf-net.org
An excellent national patient support group and educational resource.

**National Fibromyalgia Association
Lynne Matallana, director
2200 Glassell Street, Suite A
Orange, CA 92865
714-921-0150
www.fmaware.org
This is a must-join group for fibromyalgia patients. Along with ICAF, one of the two organizations I would consult first. Their magazine *FMAware* is also on the recommended list.

National Myalgic Encephalitis/Fibromyalgia Action Network
3836 Carling Avenue Highway, 17B
Nepean, Ontario K2H 7V2
Canada
613-829-6667

National Organization for Seasonal Affective Disorder
P.O. Box 40133
Washington, DC 20016
www.NOSAD.org

National Sanitation Foundation (NSF) International
P.O. Box 130140
789 North Dixboro Road
Ann Arbor, MI 48113-0140
800-NSF-MARK (800-673-6275); 734-769-8010
Fax: 734-769-0109
www.nsf.org
An independent, not-for-profit organization that tests and certifies drinking water treatment products.

Nightingale Research Foundation
383 Danforth Avenue
Ottawa, Ontario K2A OE3
Canada
www.nightingale.ca
An organization dedicated to the study of ME/CFS. Dr. Byron Hyde also offers expert legal counsel.

Qigong Research and Practice Center
P.O. Box 1727
Nederland, CO 80466
To receive information on qigong, send a self-addressed, stamped envelope.

Restless Leg Foundation
P.O. Box 314JH
514 Daniels Street
Raleigh, NC 27605
507-287-6465
www.RLS.org
For information on restless leg syndrome.

Rolf Institute
205 Canyon Boulevard
Boulder, CO 80302
303-449-5903; 800-530-8875
For information on and referrals to a Rolfing practitioner in your area.

Trager Institute
440-834-0308
www.trager-us.org
For referrals to Trager instructors, tutors, and practitioners.

Surviving the Disability Insurance Process

Although most of you will be able to recover enough to live a full life, some of you may have been too ill for your bodies to handle the stress of returning to the workplace—even if you are well enough to enjoy day-to-day life. Usually, I find that people try to return to work too early rather than too late, as this is a disease of overachievers.

Although many disability companies are reputable, some are not and will try to deny benefits for CFS/FMS. For those of you dealing with this problem or with Social Security disability, you'll find helpful articles at www.scottdavis.com. If you need assistance with a private disability insurer, I recommend Steven P. Krafchick, JD (see Appendix E: Resources). Below is an article he has written, which I think you'll find helpful. Check with your local CFS/FMS support group to find out which attorneys in your area are knowledgeable about the illnesses.

Long-Term Disability Claims Can Be Won, but Do Not Assume It Will Be Easy

Long-term disability insurance provides a safety net for anyone injured or sick and unable to work. Unfortunately, when people need to rely on this coverage to replace lost income, they often assume that a diagnosis and a statement from their doctor or doctors with copies of records will be sufficient. However, many people find that despite this unequivocal support for their disability, the long-term disability plan or the insurer handling the coverage denies the claim. Sometimes, even after granting benefits, the plan or insurer reexamines the claim at a later date and terminates benefits with little or no notice.

Denial or termination of long-term disability coverage can result in catastrophe for the unsuspecting claimant. Needless to say, it creates unwanted financial stress, leading to emotional stress, which often leads to worsening of physical symptoms. The downward spiral precipitated by the disability company's unfair decisions hits you when you are down and least able to mount a fight.

Facing denial or termination of benefits, you should find a knowledgeable attorney. Pick an attorney wisely because few attorneys understand the traps that long-term disability plans lay for the unsuspecting. In most cases, it is wise to consult an experienced long-term disability attorney early in your claim. Definitely seek legal help before a final decision is made on your claim. If your insurer wants to interview you or have you see one of its hired doctors, or you suspect for any reason that it's going to deny your claim, consult an experienced disability attorney. Get help with any appeal of a claim denial or termination. Do not go it alone. You may only have one appeal. Once a final denial with no claims appeal rights is made, the help an attorney can give will be limited, and your chances for a successful claim greatly diminished.

Claims can be terminated if your doctor incorrectly fills out a form or fails to fill out a form; if a new claims manager with something to prove comes on your claim; or if the economy shifts and insurers take measures to increase their bottom lines by rejecting and terminating claims. Nevertheless, disability claims can be won, but winning begins with what you do when you first apply for benefits and throughout your claim.

In making a claim for benefits, you need to follow some basic rules. First, get your doctor to recommend that you stop working and confirm that the doctor will continue to support your claim and is willing to fill out paperwork. Find out from Human Resources or the personnel department what your disability benefits include. Get a copy of your disability insurance policy or plan, as well as the initial paperwork that you, your doctor, and your employer will need to fill out to begin your claim.

Recognize, too, that while you are making a claim for long-term disability benefits, your life has not ended. At the time you make the claim, you are taking advantage of the coverage to give you an extended period of time to learn your true limits. You are not making an irrevocable decision that you will never work again.

If the basis for your claim is a diagnosis of chronic fatigue syndrome or fibromyalgia, there are some important considerations. Look at the limitations of benefits in the policy. There is usually a twenty-four-month limit to benefits based on a mental health condition. Insurers often try to wrongly classify CFS and FMS as mental health conditions. More recently, insurers and disability plans have added provisions limiting to twenty-four months benefits based on "self-reported" symptoms or conditions that are usually defined to include pain and fatigue. These can be overcome with some foresight and good claim preparation. In some plans and policies, insurers specifically limit coverage for disability benefits based on CFS or FMS to twenty-four months. These can only be overcome if a court finds them against public policy, or an insurance commissioner refuses to approve them. If there is such a draconian limit in your policy you will need to get your company to change it. The provisions are so broad that they provide illusory coverage. Most policies, if they grant benefits, will cover these conditions until you reach age sixty-five of the maximum normal Social Security retirement age, based on your date of birth.

So, how do you win a long-term disability claim? The law that governs your claim will have a significant effect on how to win. Figure out what law applies, state law or federal ERISA law. State law, which typically applies to insurance you find and buy on your own, affords a much wider range of damages for wrongful denial or termination of benefits. The law favors paying benefits and making sure insurers live up to their promises. However, most large employers will have long-term disability benefits that will be governed by federal law: the Employee Retirement Income Security Act (ERISA). ERISA is the reason many attorneys do not handle these cases, because it is a complicated area of law. You do not get a jury trial. You usually cannot call witnesses. You cannot get punitive or bad-faith damages. ERISA law emphasizes protecting the money rather than paying benefits. In the remainder of this chapter, I boil down for you a few basics in presenting a CFS or FMS claim under an ERISA plan. These basics will also help in making a claim under state law–governed policies.

More important than determining which law applies, get a copy of your policy or disability plan and make sure you understand the coverage that you have. The policy should tell you which law will govern the plan. Usually there is ERISA language in the back of the policy if it is an ERISA plan. Check for the definition of disability. Usually a policy will cover you for the inability to perform the material and substantial duties of your own occupation for the first twenty-four months. This is typically not just the inability to do your job, but also to do a job in your occupation for *any* employer with a similar job. After the first twenty-four months the definition often changes to the inability to do the material and substantial duties of any occupation. The limits previously discussed often take effect at the same time the disability definition changes. Look particularly for the mental-health-condition limit. If it contains a limit to benefits "caused or contributed by" a mental health condition, be wary. Make sure you make very clear that your depression, for example, is not the *basis for* the disability but the *result of* your disability. Without FMS or CFS and the pain, fatigue, cognitive problems, and other physical problems, you would be able to work.

Prepare your claim and application with an eye to what will happen if your claim is terminated or denied. In addition to your attending physician statement, your own statement, and your employer's statement, you should seriously consider submitting more supporting documentation. This can include statements from family members, friends, and coworkers; statements from your primary physicians and other treating health-care providers; applicable medical literature; and further expert evaluations.

You need to assume that if your claim is wrongly denied or terminated and you have to go to court, you will not be permitted to call any witnesses or submit any additional information for the court to consider. It must all be submitted for consideration by the disability insurer before it makes its final decision. Evaluation of the decision to deny or terminate your benefits will be based solely on what is in the claim file at the time of final denial of your claim.

Statements from family, friends, and coworkers can be helpful if they address the right issues. The statements need to share observations and anecdotes that demonstrate the problems you have that interfere with your ability to work. "We went to the movies, but you were unable to sit through the movie." "We went out for a day of shopping, but had to call it quits after an hour." When they see you they notice a slow gait and that you move as if you are in pain or fatigued (because you are). The light has gone out of your eyes. They notice that you take much longer to accomplish tasks you used to do without any problem. They notice problems with memory (missing appointments, forgetting instructions or directions) or concentration (easily distracted or missing instructions). In addition, they should state who they are, how they know you, and how often they see you.

Treating health-care providers, in addition to your primary physician or rheumatologist, can help your claim. Your primary treating physician is perhaps the most important, as that doctor will need to fill out regular attending-physician statements and certify your disability. If the claim becomes more contentious, that physician will need to provide more detailed information on your behalf reviewing the knowledge he or she has of you, your symptoms, and why you are unable to work. Physical therapists, massage therapists, chiropractors—anyone who sees you more than just a couple times per year, especially people who can talk about feeling muscle spasms when they examine you, or who can report the consistency of symptoms despite their best efforts, can help.

Not only do you need to get statements, you need to check your medical records because they will be requested by your disability insurer. These companies can omit or misstate important history or they can tend to be overly optimistic: "patient feeling better"; "showing improvement"; "hasn't felt this good in years." Hired medical evaluators for the insurers will tend to cherry-pick your records for entries that support their predictable opinions that you can work. It is important to look at the symptoms recorded regularly. This means it is important that you tell your treating health-care providers about your symptoms when they ask you. Carry a list to remind yourself.

All written statements need to be able to stand on their own, as health-care providers will not get a chance to explain themselves. A common problem arises when your doctor says you have FMS or CFS and you cannot work but does not add any additional information. The disability insurer will not ask them for more. However, your doctor needs to describe the symptoms arising from your diagnoses and why those symptoms interfere with your ability to work. They need to set out their experience with you and other CFS and FMS patients.

So what interferes with your ability to perform the material duties of your own or any occupation? An important material duty is the ability to show up for work consistently and continuously. For people with FMS or CFS, one of the most common problems is showing up for work eight hours per day, five days per week, week after week. Even when you are able to get to work, you may have impaired productivity. Specific limiting problems include pain, fatigue, and cognitive problems. Doctors who are reluctant to label you "disabled" may be much more willing to say you cannot be expected to show up consistently for forty hours of work every week because of your symptoms.

Other expert evaluations can also help win CFS and FMS disability claims. While expensive, they also can provide powerful evidence to support your claim. These include physical capacity evaluations (PCEs or FCEs); neuropsychological evaluations; vocational evaluations; and psychological and psychiatric evaluations. However, beware of an important caveat: not all physical capacity evaluators, neuropsychologists, vocational counselors, psychologists, or psychiatrists will understand the types of problems people with CFS and FMS typically experience that interfere with their ability to work. If you believe such evaluations are necessary, then get a referral from your doctor or a knowledgeable attorney. An evaluator who has no experience with patients with CFS and FMS will likely be of little value. The benefit of an attorney referral is the ability to bury the evaluation if it is not supportive. It is difficult to predict whether or not a PCE or neuropsychological evaluation will be supportive until you do it. Most times they are supportive, but sometimes they are not.

In addition to these experts, if the economics of your claim justify the expense, it is useful to get an expert evaluation from one of the top CFS or FMS doctors you can find. Ideally these are health-care providers who dedicate their practices to helping people with CFS and FMS. One of these doctors can provide a good background about the medical condition that many treating doctors cannot. They can offer opinions based on seeing hundreds if not thousands of patients with FMS and CFS. They can help explain the relevant medical knowledge, including helpful published studies, regarding the disabling effects of CFS and FMS, as well as relate the studies done that show that these are legitimate medical conditions recognized by the Social Security Administration, the Veterans Administration, the Centers for Disease Control, and the National Institutes of Health.

Reading this chapter, you could be feeling a little overwhelmed with all that you may need to manage simply to get disability benefits owed you. The unremitting effects of FMS and CFS never make applying for disability benefits easy. The strong skills that previously served you well now fail you. But that is the very reason you have to seek and keep the benefits in the first place. A good doctor and a skillful lawyer can help make the process more bearable and contribute greatly to a successful claim. Until insurer attitudes toward CFS and FMS change, you must be prepared to fight for your benefits and seek and accept help from others.

For Physicians

**Effective Treatment of Chronic Fatigue Syndrome, Fatigue,
Fibromyalgia, and Muscle/Myofascial Pain—
Using a Comprehensive Medicine Approach**

*Jacob Teitelbaum, M.D., medical director of the Fibromyalgia & Fatigue
Centers and senior author of the landmark study "Effective Treatment
of Chronic Fatigue Syndrome and Fibromyalgia—a Placebo-Controlled
Study" and the recently published study "Effective Treatment of CFS and
Fibromyalgia with D-Ribose." See www.vitality101.com for the full text.
He is also the author of* Three Steps to Happiness! Healing Through Joy
and Pain Free 1-2-3: A Proven Program to Get YOU Pain Free Now.

Thank you for your interest in these syndromes. This section will give you
an overview of how to apply our treatment protocol, which resulted in an
average 91 percent improvement of symptoms and helped 91 percent of patients with CFS and fibromyalgia (p<.0001 versus placebo). I can also be
reached through the Q&A section of my Web site at www.vitality101.com.

Chronic fatigue syndrome (CFS) and fibromyalgia (FMS) are two common names for overlapping and disabling syndromes. It is estimated that
FMS alone affects more than 6 million Americans, causing more disability
than rheumatoid arthritis.[1] Myofascial pain syndrome (MPS) affects many

millions more. Although we still have much to learn, effective treatment is now available for the large majority of patients with these illnesses.[2, 3]

CFS/FMS/MPS represents a spectrum of processes with a common end point. Because the syndromes affect major control systems in the body, there are myriad symptoms that initially do not seem to be related. Recent research has implicated mitochondrial and hypothalamic dysfunction as common denominators in these syndromes.[4–7] Dysfunction of hormonal, sleep, and autonomic control (all centered in the hypothalamus) and energy production centers can explain the large number of symptoms and why most patients have a similar set of complaints.

To make it easier to explain to patients, we use the model of a circuit breaker in a house. If the energy demands on their body are more than it can meet, their body "blows a fuse." The ensuing fatigue forces the person to use less energy, protecting them from harm. On the other hand, although a circuit breaker may protect the circuitry in the home, it does little good if you do not know how to turn it back on or even that it exists.

This analogy actually reflects what occurs. Research in genetic mitochondrial diseases shows not simply myopathic changes, but also marked hypothalamic disruption. Since the hypothalamus controls sleep, the hormonal and autonomic systems, and temperature regulation, it has higher energy needs for its size than other areas. Because of this, as energy stores are depleted, hypothalamic dysfunction occurs early on, resulting in the disordered sleep, autonomic dysfunction, low body temperatures, and hormonal dysfunctions commonly seen in these syndromes. In addition, inadequate energy stores in muscles result in muscle shortening (think of rigor mortis or writer's cramp) and pain that is further accentuated by the loss of deep sleep. Reductions in stages 3 and 4 of deep sleep result in secondary drops in growth hormone and tissue repair. As discussed below, disrupted sleep causes pain. Therefore, restoring adequate energy production through nutritional, hormonal, and sleep support, and eliminating the stresses that overutilize energy (e.g., infections, situational stresses) restore function in the hypothalamic "circuit breaker" and also allows muscles to release, thus allowing pain to resolve. Our placebo-controlled study showed that when this is done, 91 percent of patients improve, with an average 90 percent improvement in quality of life, and the majority of patients no longer qualified as having FMS by the end of three months (p<.0001 versus placebo).[3]

CFS, fibromyalgia, and to some degree myofascial pain syndrome reflect an energy crisis in the body. It is similar to blowing a fuse in your home. There can be many causes. This "fuse blowing" protects the body from further harm, but it dramatically reduces function. Causes include infections, disrupted sleep, pregnancy, hormonal deficiencies, toxins, and other physical and/or situational stresses. The "blown fuse" is the dysfunctional hypothalamus—resulting in poor sleep, and hormonal, autonomic, and temperature dysregulation.

Diagnosis

The criteria for diagnosing CFS are readily available elsewhere. What is important is that these criteria were meant to be used for research and therefore have stringent exclusion criteria to create a "pure" research cohort. These exclusionary criteria eliminate approximately 80 to 90 percent of patients who clinically have CFS, and therefore I do not recommend them for clinical use. For example, anyone who was significantly depressed in the past, even thirty years earlier, can technically never develop CFS. The American College of Rheumatology (ACR) criteria for fibromyalgia are more useful clinically. According to the ACR, a person can be classified as having fibromyalgia if he or she has:

- A history of widespread pain. The patient must have experienced pain or achiness, steady or intermittent, for at least three months. At times, the pain must have been present:
  - on both the right and left sides of the body.
  - both above and below the waist.
  - midbody—for example, in the neck, midchest, or midback, including a headache.
- Pain on pressing at least eleven of the eighteen spots on the body that are known as tender points.

The presence of another clinical disorder, such as arthritis, does not rule out a diagnosis of fibromyalgia.[8]

Although the tender point exam takes a good bit of time to master, it clinically adds little and will likely be eliminated in the future. Relative to the time they take to learn, the 11/18 tender points offer little predictive value to whether the person will respond to the treatment approach described in this appendix. In fact, patients with 6/18 points were often also found to have FMS, but the 11/18 level was chosen to increase specificity (at the expense of sensitivity). There is a simpler approach that is effective clinically. If the patient has the paradox of severe fatigue combined with insomnia (if one is exhausted, one should sleep all night), does not have severe primary depression, and these symptoms do not go away with rest, the patient likely has a CFS-related process. If he or she also has widespread pain, fibromyalgia is probably present as well. Both respond well to proper treatment as discussed below. In addition, clinicians may wish to ask the patient if he or she has the following symptoms:

- Severe fatigue lasting more than four months.
- Feeling worse the day after exercise. Patients may even describe this as feeling as if they'd been "hit by a truck."
- Diffuse, often migratory, achiness.
- Disordered sleep. Is the patient able to get seven to eight hours of uninterrupted sleep a night?
- Difficulty with word finding and substitution, poor short-term memory, and poor concentration, often described as "brain fog."
- Bowel dysfunction. Many people diagnosed with irritable bowel syndrome (IBS) or spastic colon have CFS/FMS, and their IBS resolves along with the FMS.
- Recurrent infections such as sore throats, nasal congestion, or sinusitis.
- Chemical/medication sensitivities.

In addition to helping diagnose CFS/FMS, questions about the above symptoms show the patient that their health-care provider understands their illness.

Fibromyalgia may be secondary to other causes. Secondary causes may be suggested by laboratory findings such as an elevated erythrocyte sedimentation rate (ESR), alkaline phosphatase, creatine kinase (CPK), or thyroid-stimulating hormone (TSH). Depression is less likely to be a secondary cause of fibromyalgia and CFS symptoms in patients who express frustration over not having the energy to do the things they want to do as opposed to having a lack of interests. These patients likely are simply frustrated secondary to their illness and not depressed. MPS shares many of the metabolic features seen in FMS, and often resolves with the treatments discussed in this appendix, but evaluation for structural problems should also be done for this more localized process.

Current research and clinical experience show that these patients have a mix of disordered sleep, hormonal insufficiencies, low body temperature, and autonomic dysfunction with low blood pressure and neurally mediated hypotension (NMH). This mix makes sense when you recognize that the hypothalamus is the major control center for all four of these functions.

Simple Diagnostic Approach

If the patient has the paradox of severe fatigue combined with insomnia (if one is exhausted, one should sleep all night), does not have severe primary depression, and these symptoms do not go away with vacation, he or she likely has a CFS-related process. If he or she also has widespread pain, fibromyalgia is probably present as well. Both respond well to proper treatment as discussed below.

Anything that results in inadequate energy production or energy needs greater than the body's production ability can trigger hypothalamic dysfunction. This includes infections, disrupted sleep, pregnancy, hormonal deficiencies, and other physical and/or situational stresses. Although still controversial, a large body of research also strongly suggests mitochondrial dysfunction as a unifying theory in CFS/FMS.[7] Some viral infections have been shown to suppress both mitochondrial and hypothalamic function. As noted on page 330, in several genetic mitochondrial diseases, severe hypothalamic damage is seen. This is likely because the hypothalamus has high energy needs. The mitochondrial dysfunction, combined with secondary hypothalamic suppression, can cause the poor function seen in many tissues with high energy needs. This includes dysfunction of the immune system aggravated by glutathione deficiency, dysfunction of the liver with medication/chemical sensitivities secondary to a decreased ability to detoxify, irritability of the gastrointestinal tract (from opportunistic infections and autonomic dysfunction), muscle pain, and dysfunction of the central nervous system (CNS) neurotransmitter production and blood flow with secondary brain fog.

Integrative Therapy

Fortunately, two studies (including our recent RCT)[2, 3] showed an average 90 percent improvement rate when using the SHIN protocol. SHIN stands for treating Sleep, Hormonal dysfunction, and Infections, and optimizing Nutritional support. When patients have fatigue and insomnia coupled with widespread pain, see them as having a bodywide "energy crisis." Treating with the SHIN approach can help them. An editorial in the *Journal of the American Academy of Pain Management* notes that "this study by Dr. Teitelbaum et al confirms what years of clinical success have shown—that the treatment approach described in Chapter 4 of *The Trigger Point Manual* is effective, that subclinical abnormalities are important, and that the comprehensive and aggressive metabolic approach to treatment in Teitelbaum's study is highly successful and makes fibromyalgia a very treatable disorder. The study by Dr. Teitelbaum et al and years of clinical experience make this approach an excellent and powerfully effective part of the standard of practice for treatment of people who suffer from FMS and MPS—both of which are common and devastating syndromes."[9]

Two studies (including our RCT) showed an average 90 percent improvement rate when using the SHIN protocol for treating CFS and fibromyalgia. SHIN stands for treating Sleep, Hormonal dysfunction, and Infections, and optimizing Nutritional support.

As discussed above, using the acronym SHIN will simplify treatment of these patients. Because of this, we will structure our treatment recommendations using this model. Let's begin with *S* for sleep.

DISORDERED SLEEP

A foundation of CFS/FMS is the sleep disorder.[10] Many patients can only sleep solidly for three to five hours a night with multiple wakings. Even more problematic is the loss of deep-stage three and four "restorative" sleep. Using natural therapies and/or medications that increase deep restorative sleep, so that patients get eight to nine hours of solid sleep without waking or hangover, is critical. If using medications, the next-day sedation that some patients experience often resolves in two to three weeks. Meanwhile, have patients take the medication earlier in the evening so that it wears off earlier the next day, or switch to shorter-acting agents such as Ambien, Sonata, and/or Xanax. Continue to adjust the medications each night until patients are sleeping eight hours a night without a hangover.

Most addictive sleep remedies, except for clonazepam (Klonopin) and alprazolam (Xanax), actually decrease the time that is spent in deep sleep and can worsen fibromyalgia. Therefore, they are not recommended. There are more than twenty natural and prescription sleep aids that can be tried safely and effectively in fibromyalgia and CFS. For the complete list, I am happy to e-mail you my free "long-form" treatment protocol (discussed below).

The natural sleep remedies that I recommend you begin with include the following:

1. Herbal preparations containing (per capsule):

   Valerian (200 milligrams)
   Passionflower (90 milligrams)
   L-theanine (50 milligrams)
   Hops (30 milligrams)
   Wild lettuce (18 milligrams)
   Jamaican dogwood (12 milligrams)

   These are all combined in an excellent product called the Revital- izing Sleep Formula by Integrative Therapeutics. Patients (and anyone with poor sleep) can take one to four capsules at bedtime. These six herbs can help muscle pain and libido as well as improving sleep.[11–15] Patients can take one to four capsules TID for anxiety and/or muscle pain. The effectiveness of valerian increases with continued use, but 5 to 10 percent of patients will actually find it stimulating and not be able to use it for sleep. I would note as an aside that, although I am very picky about what products I recommend, I have a policy of not taking money from any natural products or pharmaceutical compa- nies, and 100 percent of the royalties for my products goes to charity.

2. Melatonin: 0.5 to 1 milligram at bedtime. All it takes to bring low levels to the mid-normal range is 0.5 milligram. The data show that in most patients the 0.5-milligram dose is as effective for sleep as 3, 5, and 10 mil- ligrams. As we do not know the long-term effect of pharmacologic

dosing of this critical hormone, I recommend that you don't use a higher dose unless the patient finds it to be more effective. Having said this, many excellent practitioners use higher doses for "life-extension" purposes.

3. 5-HTP (5-Hydroxy-L-Tryptophan): 200 to 400 milligrams at night. This naturally stimulates serotonin, but may take six to twelve weeks to be fully effective. Don't give more than 200 milligrams a day if the patient is on antidepressants, as it theoretically could drive serotonin too high. 5-HTP can also help with pain and weight loss at 300 milligrams a day for at least three months.

4. Give calcium and magnesium at bedtime, as these can help sleep.

5. Cuddle Ewe mattress pad: Lying on this sheepskin pad can help if pain interferes with sleep (800-328-9493).

If natural remedies are not adequate to result in at least eight hours a night of sleep, consider these medications:

- Zolpidem (Ambien): 5 or 10 milligrams. Use 5 to 20 milligrams at bedtime. This medication has fewer side effects than most other sleep medications. It is helpful for most CFS/FMS patients and is my first choice among the sleep medications. Experience shows that extended use is appropriate and safe in CFS/FMS. Patients can take an extra 5 to 10 milligrams in the middle of the night if they wake or switch to the sustained-release Ambien CR (6.25 to 12.5 milligrams). Neurontin (gabapentin), 100 to 900 milligrams, and/or Klonopin (clonazepam), 0.5 to 2 milligrams at bedtime, can help sleep, pain, and restless leg syndrome as well.

- Cyclobenzaprine (Flexeril), 10 milligrams, and/or carisoprodol (Soma), 350 milligrams. Use half to two tablets at bedtime. These medications are often sedating but can be helpful if pain during the night is a major problem.

- Trazodone (Desyrel): 50 milligrams. Take half to six tablets at bedtime. Use this medication first if anxiety is a major problem. Warn patients to call immediately if priapism (an erection that won't go away) occurs.

- Amitriptyline (Elavil) or doxepin: 10 milligrams. Use half to five tablets at bedtime. Elavil causes weight gain, and can worsen neurally mediated hypotension and restless leg syndrome.

- Doxylamine (Unisom for Sleep): 25 milligrams at bedtime.

Some patients will sleep well with the Revitalizing Sleep Formula herbal and/or 5 to 10 milligrams of Ambien, while others will require all of the above treatments combined. Because the malfunctioning hypothalamus controls sleep, and muscle pain also interferes with sleep, it is often necessary, and appropriate to use multiple sleep aids. Zanaflex, Gabatril, and many other nonbenzodiazepines can also help sleep, and many other options are listed on the available treatment protocol. Because of next-day sedation and each medication having its own independent half-life, CFS/FMS patients do better with combining low doses of several medications than with a high dose of one.

It is critical that these patients get at least eight hours of deep sleep a night. Because of the hypothalamic dysfunction, they often need aggressive assistance to treat their insomnia. Begin with herbal mixes such as the Revitalizing Sleep Formula, and then add in calcium, magnesium, 5-HTP, and melatonin at bedtime as needed. If additional pharmaceutical support is needed, I recommend beginning with Ambien, Desyrel, Klonopin, and/or Neurontin.

Although less common, three other sleep disturbances must be considered and, if present, treated. The first is sleep apnea. This should especially be suspected if the patient snores and is overweight and/or hypertensive. If two of these three conditions are present and the patient does not improve with our treatment, I would consider a sleep apnea study. Ask the sleep lab to also look for upper airway resistance syndrome (UARS), which mimics CFS and is associated with snoring, decreased airflow in the nose or throat, low blood pressure, and autonomic dysfunction. I would get preapproval from the patient's insurance company, as the sleep testing usually costs about two thousand dollars. Some patients prefer to do their own inexpensive screening by videotaping themselves one night during sleep. This will screen for apnea and the third sleep disturbance, restless leg syndrome (RLS), but, unfortunately, will not pick up UARS. If there is no snoring at night, then both UARS and obstructive sleep apnea are unlikely.

Sleep apnea and UARS are treated with nasal C-pap or dental appliances that move the lower jaw forward during sleep. A sleep study or having patients videotape themselves while sleeping will also detect RLS, which is also fairly common in fibromyalgia.[16] Asking the patient if the bedsheets are scattered about when he or she awakes and/or if the patient kicks his or her spouse during the night will often let you know RLS is present. It is treated with supplemental magnesium and Ambien, Klonopin, and/or Neurontin and by keeping ferritin levels over 50.

Evaluation and Treatment of Associated Hormonal Dysfunction

Hormonal imbalance is associated with FMS. Sources of this imbalance include hypothalamic dysfunction and autoimmune processes such as Hashimoto's thyroiditis. When the hypothalamus is not able to efficiently regulate hormone balance, medical management can do so until hypothalamic function is restored. When focusing on achieving hormonal balance, the standard laboratory testing aimed at identifying a single hormone deficiency is not effective. For example, increased hormone binding to carrier proteins is often present in CFS/FMS. Because of this, total hormone levels are often normal while the active hormone levels are low. This creates a functional deficiency in the patient. Also, most blood tests use two standard deviations to define blood test norms. By definition, only the lowest or highest 2.5 percent of the population is in the abnormal (treatment) range. This does not work well if more than 2.5 percent of the population has a problem. For example, it is estimated that as many as 20 percent of women over sixty have positive anti-TPO antibodies and may be hypothyroid. Other tests use late signs of deficiency such as anemia for iron or B_{12} levels to define an abnormal lab value.

The goal in CFS/FMS management is to restore optimal function while keeping labs in the normal range for safety. One way to convey the difference between the "normal" range based on two standard deviations and the optimal range that patients would maintain if they did not have CFS/FMS is as follows.

Pretend your lab test uses two standard deviations to diagnose a "shoe problem." If you accidentally put on someone else's shoes and had on a size 12 when you wore a size 5, the normal range derived from the standard deviation would indicate you had absolutely no problem. You would insist the shoes did not fit, although your shoe size would be in the normal range. Similarly, if you lost your shoes, the doctor would pick any shoes out of the "normal range pile" and expect them to fit you.

Thyroid Function

Suboptimal thyroid function is common and important in CFS/FMS. Because thyroid-binding globulin function and conversion of T_4 to T_3 may be altered in CFS/FMS, it is important to check a free T_4. It is also important to treat all chronic myalgia patients with thyroid-hormone replacement if their T_4 blood levels are below even the 50th percentile of normal (Janet Travell—personal communication). Many CFS/FMS patients also have difficulty converting T_4, which is fairly inactive, to T_3, the active hormone. Additionally, T_3 receptor resistance may be present, requiring higher levels.[17–18]

Synthroid has only inactive T_4, while Armour Thyroid has both inactive T_4 and active T_3. Many clinicians will give an empiric trial of Armour Thyroid, half to three grains every morning, adjusted to the dose that feels best to the patient as long as the free T_4 is not above the upper limit of normal. I am likely to try an empiric trial of thyroid-hormone therapy in patients who feel poorly if one or more of the following is true:

- The patient has fibromyalgia, and/or
- The patient's oral temperature is generally less than 98.0°F, and/or
- The patient has symptoms and signs suggestive of hypothyroidism, and/or
- The patient's TSH test result is less than 0.95 or greater than 3.0, and/or
- The patient's T_3 or T_4 is below the 50th percentile of normal.

Physicians generally interpret a low-normal TSH—that is, 0.5 to 0.95—as confirmation of euthyroidism. The rules, however, are different with CFS/FMS. In this setting, hypothalamic hypothyroidism is common, and the patient's TSH can be low, normal, or high.[19] This is why I recommend an empiric therapeutic trial of thyroid-hormone treatment even if the TSH and T_4 are both low normal. Also, if subclinical hypothyroidism is missed, the patient's fatigue and fibromyalgia/MPS simply will not resolve. The inadequacy of thyroid testing is further suggested by studies that show:

- That most patients with suspected thyroid problems have normal blood studies.[20, 21]
- That when patients with symptoms of hypothyroidism and normal labs were treated with thyroid (in this study, Synthroid at an average dose of 120 micrograms per day) a large majority improved significantly.[20]

In addition, I recommend adding the following:

- If the patient does not respond to Synthroid, switch to Armour Thyroid, and vice versa. For every 50 micrograms of Synthroid, have the patient take half a grain (30 milligrams) of Armour Thyroid. If the free or total T_3 result is low or low normal, begin with Armour Thyroid, which has both T_3 and T_4, instead of Synthroid, which has only T_4. In most patients, however, I usually recommend beginning with Armour Thyroid.
- Adjust the thyroid dose clinically using the dose that feels the best to the patient, as long as the free T_4 test does not show hyperthyroidism. Do not use TSH or T_3 levels to monitor thyroid replacement.[21] Because of the hypothalamic suppression, TSH may be low despite inadequate hormonal dosing. As T_3 is largely produced and functions intracellularly, we do not have normal ranges for exogenously given T_3. Therefore, I predominantly use free T_4 levels to monitor therapy.
- Make sure that the patient does not take any iron supplements within six hours or calcium within two to four hours of the morning thyroid dose or the thyroid hormone will not be absorbed. Have the patient take the iron between 2 and 6 p.m.—on an empty stomach and away from any hormone treatments.
- Thyroid supplementation can increase patients' cortisol metabolism and unmask subclinical adrenal insufficiency. If patients feel worse on low-dose thyroid replacement, they may need adrenal support as well.

> Because of the hypothalamic dysfunction, hormonal deficiencies are common in CFS/FMS despite normal blood tests. If symptoms suggest deficiencies, treat hypothyroidism with Armour Thyroid (a therapeutic trial is warranted in most of these patients), adrenal insufficiency (suggested by low blood pressure, irritability when hungry/hypoglycemia, and recurrent respiratory infections and sore throats) with Cortef, and natural adrenal support (e.g., Adrenal Stress-End, by ITI) and low estrogen/testosterone with bioidentical hormones.

Adrenal Insufficiency

The hypothalamic-pituitary-adrenal (HPA) axis does not function well in CFS/FMS.[4, 22, 23] This and adrenal exhaustion from chronic/severe stress are two key causes of inadequate adrenal function. Because early researchers studying adrenal insufficiency and cortisol did not know the optimal physiologic doses for cortisol, they treated with high doses and their patients developed severe complications. These side effects are not seen with adrenal glandular/herbal/nutritional support or with physiologic dosing of hydrocortisone (Cortef), that is, up to 20 milligrams a day.[24] Twenty milligrams of Cortef is approximately equivalent in potency to 4 to 5 milligrams of prednisone.

To put it in perspective, if the early thyroid researchers had given ten times the physiologic dose of thyroid hormone (for example, 1,000 to 2,000 micrograms daily instead of 100 to 200 micrograms), a situation analogous to early adrenal research, most people would have had severe complications. Thyroid hormone would be viewed as very dangerous, and we would only be treating hypothyroid patients on the verge of myxedema and coma. In adrenal insufficiency, this is what occurs now. Many hypoadrenal patients are only treated when they are ready to go into Addisonian crisis. Research and clinical experience show that this approach misses many hypoadrenal patients.[2, 3, 24, 25]

Symptoms of underactive adrenal glands include weakness, hypotension, dizziness, sugar cravings with irritability when hungry, and recurrent infections—all of which are common in CFS/FMS. I recommend natural adrenal support for most patients with CFS/FMS—especially if they have any of the above symptoms. The needed natural therapies include:

- Adrenal glandulars, which contain most of the "building blocks" needed for adrenal repair.
- Licorice extract, which contains glycyrrhizin, a compound that raises adrenal hormone levels. Licorice also protects against stomach irritation, which can occur with Cortef and occasionally even with glandulars.
- Pantothenic acid, vitamin C, vitamin B_6, betaine, and tyrosine, nutrients that are critical for adrenal function and energy, and high doses are often needed.

All of these are present in an excellent glandular/herbal for adrenal support called Adrenal Stress-End (from Integrative Therapeutics), which is safe and effective. I usually prescribe one to two capsules each morning (or one to two in the morning and one at noon), and they can be taken along with Cortef. This helps both symptoms and with adrenal repair.

In addition, you can evaluate CFS/FMS patients' adrenal function with an adrenocorticotropic hormone (ACTH) stimulation test to determine whether Cortef should be added, although I consider it appropriate to use adrenal support based simply on symptoms and/or a morning cortisol < 16 mcg/dl (up to 20 milligrams a day of Cortef). The test must be begun between 7 a.m. and 9 a.m. The patient should be NPO and have had no caffeine for twenty-four hours before the test. Check a baseline cortisol level and then give ACTH (Cortrosyn) 25 units or one unit IM (current data suggest that the one-unit Cortrosyn test is more reliable) and recheck cortisol levels at thirty minutes and at one hour. Although a baseline cortisol of 6 mcg/dl is often considered "normal," most healthy people run approximately 16 to 24 mcg/dl at 8 a.m.

My treatment guidelines are that if the baseline cortisol is less than 16 mcg/dl or the cortisol level does not increase by at least 7 mcg/dl at thirty minutes and 11 mcg/dl at one hour, or does not double by one hour and is less than 35 mcg/dl, I treat with a therapeutic trial of 5 to 15 milligrams Cortef in the morning, 2.5 to 10 milligrams at lunchtime, and 0 to 2.5 milligrams at 4 p.m. (maximum of 20 milligrams a day). Most patients find 5 to 7.5 milligrams of Cortef each morning plus 2.5 to 5 milligrams at noon to be optimal (the equivalent of 1.5 to 3 milligrams prednisone daily). Cortef is much more effective than prednisone in CFS/FMS.

After keeping the patient on the initial dose for two to four weeks, adjust the dose up to a maximum of 20 milligrams daily or, if no benefit has been evident, taper it off. Adjust the Cortef to the lowest dose that feels the best. Give most of the Cortef in the morning and at lunchtime. I often tell my patients to take the last dose, 2.5 to 5 milligrams, no later than 4 p.m. Otherwise, the Cortef may keep the patient up at night.

After nine to eighteen months, taper the Cortef off over a period of one to four months. If the other physiologic stresses, such as infections or fibromyalgia, have been eliminated, the patient's adrenal function may be adequate or normalized. If symptoms recur off the Cortef, continue treatment with the lowest optimal dose.

Improvement is often dramatic, and is usually seen within two to four weeks. The Cortef should be doubled during periods of acute stress and raised even higher during periods of severe stress, such as surgery. Consider also giving the patient 1,000 milligrams of calcium and 400+ international units (IU) of vitamin D daily with the Cortef if the patient is at high risk for osteoporosis.

There are different approaches to treatment and more is not necessarily better. High-dose cortisol taken at night will worsen already disrupted sleep patterns. A study by Mckenzie et al administered patients a high dose (25 to 35 milligrams) of Cortef daily, which disrupted patients' sleep (p≤.02).[26] Although they did not treat the disrupted sleep, most patients still felt somewhat better on treatment. A small percentage of the patients had significantly suppressed posttreatment Cortrosyn tests, without complications, and McKenzie et al therefore, I believe incorrectly, recommend against using any dose of Cortef in CFS/FMS.[27] Our study did not show adrenal suppression using lower Cortef dosing.[3] Dr. Jefferies, with thousands of patient-years' experience in using low-dose Cortef, recommends an empiric trial of 20 milligrams a day of Cortef in all patients with severe, unexplained fatigue, and has found this to be quite safe for long-term use.[24, 25] Our research and clinical experience suggest that using Cortef at 20 milligrams a day or less in CFS and fibromyalgia patients is safe and often very helpful.

DHEA

Dehydroepiandrosterone (DHEA) is a major adrenal hormone that has recently been getting a lot of attention in the press for its role as a "fountain-of-youth" hormone.[28] DHEA is stored as DHEA-sulfate (DHEA-S), and levels of free DHEA fluctuate markedly throughout the day. Because of this, I recommend checking DHEA-S levels and not DHEA levels.

Many CFS/FMS patients have suboptimal DHEA-S levels, and the benefit of treatment is sometimes dramatic. Most women need 5 to 25 milligrams a day and most men 25 to 50 milligrams a day. I use the middle of the normal range for a twenty-nine-year-old, keeping the DHEA-S level at 150 to 180 mcg/dl in women and 350 to 480 mcg/dl in men. Too high a dose can cause acne or darkening of facial hair in women.

Low Estrogen and Testosterone

Although we are trained to diagnose menopause by cessation of periods, hot flashes, and elevated FSH and LH, these are late findings. Estrogen deficiency often begins many years earlier, and may coincide with the onset of fibromyalgia.[29] To compound the problem, research done by Sarrel shows that the majority of women who have a hysterectomy, even with the ovaries left in, develop estrogen deficiency within six months to two years after their surgery.[29] Some physicians suspect that this may also occur in women who have had a tubal ligation, which, like a TAH, may also disrupt the ovarian blood supply.

In her book on estrogen and testosterone deficiency, Dr. Elizabeth Vliet gives a well-referenced, in-depth foundation for evaluation and treatment of these problems.[29] To summarize, the initial symptoms of estrogen deficiency are poor sleep, poor libido, brain fog, achiness, PMS, and decreased neurotransmitter function. Dr. Vliet feels that estradiol levels at midcycle should be at least 100 pg/ml. If a woman's CFS/FMS symptoms are worse at ovulation and the ten days before her period (times when estrogen levels are dropping), then a trial of estrogen is warranted. While a birth control pill can be used, side effects of bleeding and fluid retention are common for the first three to four months. Bioidentical hormones are better tolerated and likely safer. Therefore natural 17-B-estradiol as Climara patches or Estrace may be preferable. The usual dose of Climara is one 0.05- to 0.1-milligram patch a week, and the usual dose of Estrace is 0.5 to 2 milligrams a day, adjusted to what feels best to the patient. I prefer to use Biest, a compounded natural estrogen that combines estriol with estradiol, which is usually dosed at 1.25 to 2.5 milligrams a day.

Unlike estradiol, early data on estriol suggest that it does not raise breast cancer risk and may actually lower it (see article at end of Chapter 4). In addition, estriol also has immune-modulating effects and other properties that can be beneficial in FMS. In the absence of a hysterectomy, progesterone must be added to prevent uterine cancer. Since progesterone is essential for GABA function, sleep, and the prevention of anxiety, and not only prevention of uterine cancer, I add natural progesterone to the estrogen even if the patient has had a hysterectomy. Natural progesterone is available from most pharmacies as Prometrium 100 milligrams and is better tolerated than Provera. The dose is 100 milligrams at bedtime, instead of Provera 2.5 milligrams, or 200 milligrams a day for ten to fourteen days a month, instead of Provera 10 milligrams. If you are prescribing the Bi-Est cream, have the compounding pharmacist (e.g., ITC Pharmacy; 303-663-4224) make a combination of Bi-Est 2.5 milligrams, plus progesterone 30 to 100 milligrams, plus testosterone 2 to 5 milligrams, all in 1 gram of cream (which can be applied to the skin). If estrogen levels drop after two to three years, it suggests dermal absorption is decreasing. Have the compounding pharmacist make a cream that can be applied to the mucosal surface of the labia or intravaginally each evening. If the creams are applied to the skin instead of mucosal surfaces, patients may stop absorbing the cream after a few years of use. Overall, patients respond best to Bi-Est applied intravaginally.

Testosterone Deficiency

Testosterone deficiency is important in both men and women. It is important to check a free testosterone level rather than total testosterone, since free testosterone is a better measure of testosterone function. If the age-adjusted free testosterone is low or low normal (lowest quartile), a trial of treatment is often very helpful. Among my CFS/FMS patients, seventy percent of men and many women have free testosterone levels in the lowest quartile while their total testosterone levels are usually normal. A recently completed study found that treating low testosterone in women decreases FMS pain. Be sure the free testosterone normal range is age-adjusted using ten-year age groups, since a normal range that includes both twenty- and eighty-year-olds is not clinically meaningful.

Only treat with natural testosterone. In men, the new prescription medication topical Testim 1% actually works fairly well. Applying 25 to 100 milligrams of testosterone once daily keeps testosterone levels around 600 to 750 ng/dl throughout the day. In women, compounded creams should be used. For those without prescription insurance, compounded testosterone creams are much less expensive than standard prescriptions.

In women, acne, intense dreams, or darkening of facial hair suggests that the dose is too high. An elevated testosterone level in women can also increase insulin resistance. Symptoms are generally reversible. These side effects can also be caused by low estrogen relative to the testosterone level, and may be avoided in women by supplementing both together. As noted above, this can be done easily by adding 2 to 5 milligrams of testosterone to the estrogen (Bi-Est) cream.

In men, acne suggests that the dose is too high. Monitor levels because elevated levels of testosterone can cause elevated blood counts, liver inflammation, reversibly decreased sperm counts with transient infertility, and elevated cholesterol with increased risk of heart disease. These are the symptoms seen in athletes given many times the recommended physiologic dose to enhance sports performance. Because of this, in men it may be reasonable to monitor CBC, cholesterol, and liver enzymes intermittently. Testosterone supplementation can also cause elevated thyroid hormone levels in men taking thyroid supplements. If a patient is on thyroid supplements, recheck thyroid hormone levels after six to twelve weeks or sooner if he gets palpitations or anxious or hyper feelings. Despite the concerns about athletes using very high levels of synthetic testosterone, it is important to remember that research shows that raising low testosterone levels in men using natural testosterone actually results in lower cholesterol, decreased angina and depression, and improved diabetes.[30]

In addition, low testosterone is associated with increased mortality.[30A] Studies to date also suggest that testosterone therapy does not affect prostate tissue significantly,[30B] and that there is no increase in prostate cancer in those taking testosterone therapy.

Immune Dysfunction and Infections

Immune dysfunction is part of the CFS/FMS process. In fact, CFIDS, the other name for CFS, stands for chronic fatigue and immune dysfunction syndrome. Opportunistic infections present in CFIDS/FMS include chronic URIs and sinusitis, bowel infections, and chronic, low-grade prostatitis. These need to be treated.

Chronic sinusitis responds poorly to antibiotics but well to antifungals. Conservative measures such as saline nasal rinsing and avoiding refined carbohydrates are more appropriate than chronic antibiotics.[31] Our experience has shown, as does research at the Mayo Clinic, that chronic sinusitis is predominantly caused by a sensitivity reaction to yeast, with secondary bacterial infections due to swelling and obstruction. Most of our patients find that their chronic sinusitis goes away on the yeast protocol discussed below. Avoiding antibiotics also decreases the risk of secondary fungal overgrowth in the sinuses and GI tract.

When initially treating the sinusitis and for acute flares, our patients find that a compounded nose spray containing a combination of Sporanox, xylitol, Bactroban, and cortisone can be very helpful. This is available from some compounding pharmacies (e.g., ITC Pharmacy; 303-663-4224). If the spray is irritating, patients can dilute it with a little bit of normal saline. The dose is one to two sprays in each nostril twice a day for two to six weeks. Ordering one bottle is adequate for most patients. Although the chronic sinusitis often resolves after six weeks of Diflucan and the sinus spray, patients can use the spray on an as-needed basis if symptoms recur. If sinusitis or spastic colon symptoms recur, however, patients are likely also having regrowth of candida in the gut, and if other CFS symptoms are recurring, you should consider a six-week retreatment with Diflucan.

In addition to sinusitis, bowel infections with fungal overgrowth, parasitic infections, and alterations of normal bacterial flora are generally present. These are reflected by the patient's bowel symptoms. Because of the lack of a definitive test for yeast overgrowth, little research is published in this area, and treatment is controversial. Treatment is empiric, and based on the patient's history. Yeast vaginitis, onchomycosis, sinusitis, a history of frequent antibiotic use such as tetracycline for acne, sinusitis, gas, bloating, diarrhea, or constipation warrants an empiric therapeutic antifungal trial. Many CFIDS/FMS patients who have failed other therapies for spastic colon or sinusitis have responded dramatically to antifungal treatments, though some also require treatment for small intestinal bacterial overgrowth (SIBO) and/or parasites.

Treatment for yeast in CFS/FMS patients consists of:

- Acidophilus bacteria, 4 to 8 billion units per day, can also help restore normal bowel flora. I recommend the Probiotic Pearls form from Integrative Therapeutics, two pearls twice a day for five months, as many other products do not have viable acidophilus bacteria. In addition, it is critical that patients avoid sugar, as yeast grows by fermenting sugar. This includes fruit juices, which have as much sugar as sodas. To improve compliance (and show compassion), I do allow patients to have chocolate but recommend an excellent-tasting sugar-free line made by Russell Stover.

- Anti-Yeast (an excellent mix of natural antifungals by Ultraceuticals), or nystatin (two 500,000-IU tablets two to three times a day) for five months. The patient's symptoms, especially fibromyalgia pain, may flare up initially as the yeast dies off. Therefore, begin with a low dose and work up as tolerated.

After four weeks on Anti-Yeast or nystatin, add 200 milligrams of fluconazole (Diflucan) every day for six weeks. Rare and mild liver enzyme elevations are sometimes seen with Diflucan, but taking lipoic acid (already present in Anti-Yeast) 200 milligrams per day seems to decrease this side effect. If symptoms are only partially relieved or recur after the first six weeks on Diflucan, I recommend repeating the 200 milligrams per day for another six weeks. If no benefit is derived from the first course, the candida may be Diflucan resistant. Switch to Nizoral (which may lower cortisol levels) 200 milligrams per day for another six weeks. Patients should continue the Anti-Yeast herbal mix or nystatin for a total of five to eight months. I recommend patients be on these drugs while they are taking Nizoral or Diflucan not only for their antifungal activity but also to avoid development of resistant organisms.

Because of the immune suppression, most CFS/FMS patients need to be treated empirically for yeast/fungal/candida overgrowth. Nasal congestion/sinusitis and spastic colon are also often caused by the candida, and resolve with the treatments discussed above.

Parasitic infections, often with nonpathogenic or normally self-limiting organisms, are also common in CFS/FMS. Stool samples can be sent to your local lab for antigenic and chemical testing for giardia, cryptosporidium, and especially clostridium difficile. One-sixth of our study patients had a positive O&P. Most labs do a poor job of microscope testing for parasites, and I only have my O&P testing done (by mail) at the Genova/Great Smokies Diagnostic Labs (800-522-4762). If patients have parasites, even if usually nonpathogenic, treat them, as these patients should be considered immune suppressed.

In patients with low-grade fevers and/or chronic lung congestion, occult infections such as chlamydia and mycoplasma Incognitus are being found. Empiric therapy with doxycycline, 100 milligrams twice a day, or azithromycin (Zithromax), 250 to 600 milligrams a day for six months to two years, while on Anti-Yeast or nystatin, can be very helpful. Recent research is showing that HHV-6, CMV, and EBV are also sometimes active in CFS/FMS and that in select populations (see Chapter 5) treatment with Valcyte for six months can be very helpful.

An outstanding immune stimulant is Pro Boost (by Klabin Marketing; 800-933-9440). This thymulin mimic is taken sublingually three times a day at the first sign of any infection, and dramatically decreases the duration of the infection. I recommend that most of my patients keep it in their medicine cabinet for themselves and their family. This product is very popular with my patients.

Nutritional Deficiencies

CFS/FMS patients are often nutritionally deficient. This occurs because of (1) malabsorption from bowel infections, (2) increased needs because of the illness, and (3) inadequate diet. B vitamins, ribose, magnesium, iron, coenzyme Q_{10}, malic acid, and carnitine are essential for mitochondrial function.[7, 32] These nutrients are also critical for many other processes. Although blood testing is not reliable or necessary for most nutrients, I do recommend that you check B_{12}, Fe, total iron-binding capacity (TIBC), and ferritin levels.

I begin CFS/FMS patients on the following nutritional regimen:

1. A quality multivitamin suited to their needs. It should contain at least 50 milligrams of B complex, 200 milligrams of magnesium glycinate, 900 milligrams of malic acid, 1,000 units of vitamin D, 500 milligrams of vitamin C, 15 milligrams of zinc, 200 micrograms of selenium, 200 micrograms of chromium, and amino acids. A powdered vitamin is generally better tolerated, better absorbed, and less expensive. The one I use in my practice for most of my patients is called the Energy Revitalization System, by Integrative Therapeutics; 800-931-1709. A single good-tasting drink plus one capsule contains more than fifty nutrients

and replaces more than thirty-five tablets of nutritional supplements each day. This should be taken long term, and would be an outstanding daily multivitamin for most people. It should be given as a basic nutritional foundation in all fatigue and pain patients.

2. D-ribose (CORvalen, by Bioenergy Life Science, Inc.; 866-267-8253; www.corvalen.com). As CFS/FMS represents an energy crisis, it is critical that patients have what is needed for optimal mitochondrial function. Although most of these are present in the Energy Revitalization System vitamin powder discussed above, a critical rate-limiting nutrient in the production of energy is called ribose. If you remember your biochemistry training on the Krebs Citric Acid Cycle, your key energy molecules are ATP, FADH, and NADH. These molecules are predominantly made up of ribose plus B vitamins and adenine. Some of our patients improved markedly with improved energy and decreased pain when given one scoop (5 grams) of ribose three times a day for three weeks, followed by one scoop twice a day. This effect was marked enough that we conducted a study on this nutrient in our research center, which showed an astounding average 44.7 percent increase in energy and 30 percent increase in overall quality of life after less than three weeks. In addition, the ribose significantly decreased pain while improving sleep and mental clarity (see the study abstract in Appendix A). One 280-gram container is a fair therapeutic trial. Ribose has also been shown to be dramatically effective in treating cardiac problems, including congestive heart failure (CHF). For example, one of the patients in our ribose study also had atrial fibrillation. After being on ribose for less than three weeks his arrhythmia resolved and he was able to stop taking his arrhythmia medications. For a review of research on ribose in both energy production and heart disease, I invite you to read Chapter 2. Ribose is an outstanding new addition to our therapeutic

---

Widespread nutritional deficiencies are common, and no single tablet will take care of them all. The Energy Revitalization System vitamin powder replaces thirty-five tablets of supplements daily with one drink and one capsule and should be used long term. In addition, add 5 grams ribose (CORvalen) three (later two) times daily in all patients. Some patients may also benefit from 200 milligrams of coenzyme Q_{10}, and 1,000 milligrams of acetyl-L-carnitine daily for about four months.

armamentarium for treating fatigue, pain, and cardiac dysfunction, and I use it in all of these patients. Proper dosing is critical, so it is important to follow the dosing instructions above.

D-ribose (CORvalen) is natural and quite safe, tastes good (sweet like sugar but healthy—comes as a powder) and is low in side effects. Rarely, it can cause a mild drop in blood sugar as it gets energy production moving. If patients feel dizzy or hungry when they take it, simply have them take it with a meal or lower the dose.

3. Iron. If the iron percent saturation is under 22 percent or the ferritin is under 40 mg/ml, supplement with iron. I recommend Chromagen Forte, one a day for four months. It should be taken on an empty stomach, since food decreases iron absorption by more than 60 percent. It should not be taken within six hours of thyroid hormone, since iron blocks thyroid absorption. Caution should be taken in supplementing with iron because continuing supplementation beyond what is needed can result in excess body iron stores, and iron is very pro-oxidative. Check levels before supplementing, as even one dose of iron can be harmful in persons with primary hemochromatosis. Continue treatment until the ferritin level is between 50 and 100 and the iron percent saturation is over 22 percent. If hair thinning is a problem, continue Chromagen for a target ferritin of 70 to 100.

4. If the B_{12} level is under 540 pg/ml, I recommend B_{12} injections, 3,000 micrograms IM three times a week for fifteen injections, then as needed based on the patient's clinical response. Studies in CFS show absent or near-absent CSF B_{12} levels despite normal serum B_{12} levels.[33] Metabolic evidence of B_{12} deficiency is seen even at levels of 540 pg/ml or more.[34] Severe neuropsychiatric changes are also seen from B_{12} deficiency even at levels of 300 pg/ml (a level over 209 is technically normal).[35] As an editorial in the *New England Journal of Medicine* suggests, the old-time doctors may have been right about giving B_{12} shots.[36] Compounding pharmacies can make B_{12} at 3,000 mcg/cc concentrations. I use hydroxycobalamin, although methylcobalamin may be more effective, though also somewhat more expensive. The Energy Revitalization System multivitamin also contains 500 micrograms of B_{12} daily for ongoing use.

5. Coenzyme Q_{10}, 200 milligrams a day. This is a conditionally essential nutrient that improves energy production in patients with CFS/FMS. It is especially critical in patients on Mevacor-family cholesterol treatments (which can actually cause fibromyalgia pain). I use the Vitaline

form made by ITI (which is the one used in many studies), as quality control is especially important with this nutrient.

6. Potassium-magnesium aspartate. This can be very helpful in fatigue states.[7] The dose is 500 milligrams, twice a day for three months.

7. Treating with acetyl-L-carnitine, 500 milligrams twice daily for four months is strongly recommended. Biopsies show CFS patients' intracellular levels to be routinely low. This not only causes weakness, but also contributes to the average thirty-two-pound weight gain seen in CFS/FMS.

8. Vitamin D insufficiency is associated with seasonal affective disorder symptoms, deep muscle pain, and compromised immunity. It can exacerbate these symptoms, which are already present in persons with CFS/FMS. Supplemental vitamin D at 600 to 1,000 IU daily (present in the vitamin powder) is recommended. Vitamin D deficiency is estimated to cause more than 85,000 cancer deaths a year in the United States.

9. Diet. There is no one diet that is best for everyone. I recommend that patients eat those things that leave them feeling the best (which is not always the same as what they crave). Having said this, however, the majority of CFS patients find that they do best with a high-protein, low-carbohydrate diet. Patients should avoid sugar, as well as excessive caffeine (which is a loan shark for energy) and excess alcohol. Warn patients that there may be a seven- to ten-day withdrawal period when coming off sugar and caffeine. If they have low blood pressure and/or orthostatic dizziness, they should also consider markedly increasing their salt intake.

General Pain Relief

Although pain will often resolve within three months of simply treating SHIN as discussed above, it is also critical to eliminate pain directly. Many studies show a marked analgesic and anti-inflammatory effect from optimal doses (the effect is very dose dependent) of two herbals, willow bark (containing at least 240 milligrams of salicin) and Boswellia (900+ milligrams), which have been shown to be as effective as or more effective than NSAIDs and COX-2 inhibitors but without the GI or other toxicity.[37–54] These herbals are excellent for arthritic, inflammatory, and other pain. They can be found in optimal doses combined with cherry (which is high in antioxidants and also has COX-2-inhibiting effects) in an excellent pain herbal called the Pain Formula by Integrative Therapeutics. Have the patient begin with two to four tablets three times a day as needed. Although it can be helpful for acute pain, it is especially helpful when taken on a regular basis for six weeks, as the effect continues to increase over time. Once pain is controlled, the dose can be lowered or it can simply be taken as needed.

In addition to anti-inflammatory herbals, the herbs in the Revitalizing Sleep Formula (discussed above under Sleep) can also be very helpful for muscle pain. Other natural remedies that help pain include 5-HTP (300 milligrams at bedtime), high-dose curcumin, and ginger. The medications Neurontin, Lyrica, Ultram, and Skelaxin are also far more effective for fibromyalgia pain than NSAIDs.

Treating the underlying metabolic problems will often eliminate the pain. In addition, the Pain Formula herbal mix and the medications Neurontin, Lyrica, Ultram, and Skelaxin are also far more effective for fibromyalgia pain than NSAIDs.

Autonomic Dysfunction

This is especially important to treat in patients under eighteen years of age. Low blood pressure and dizziness, increased thirst, polyuria, cold extremities, and night sweats are a few of the symptoms that reflect autonomic dysfunction in CFS/FMS. A study at Johns Hopkins Hospital showed that a majority of CFS patients had neurally mediated hypotension (NMH) on tilt-table testing.[55] This means that the blood pressure of CFS/FMS patients can severely drop with standing or minimal exertion. If the patient has low blood pressure, dizziness, or a positive tilt-table test, a treatment trial is appropriate. Treatment consists of markedly increasing salt and water intake. In children, fludrocortisone (Florinef), 1/10-milligram tablets, one to two daily, can be helpful, although it is usually not helpful in adults. Florinef helped only 14 percent of adult CFS patients in an NIH study, versus 10 percent of placebo patients. Fluoxetine (Prozac), sertraline (Zoloft), and especially dextroamphetamine (Dexedrine) are clinically much more effective in treating NMH in CFIDS patients, and I rarely use Florinef in anyone over twenty. Dexedrine also has many other benefits in CFS/FMS. I think it is overused in ADHD and underused in CFS/FMS.

Psychological Well-Being

Many illnesses are associated with various psychological profiles. In CFS/FMS, a common profile is a mega-type-A overachiever who, because of childhood low self-esteem, overachieves to get approval. These patients tend to be perfectionists and have difficulties protecting their boundaries—that is, they say yes to requests when they feel like saying no. Instead of responding to their bodies' signal of fatigue by resting, they redouble their efforts. Taking time to rest, and getting and staying out of abusive personal and work environments, is critical. As they start to feel better, they need to be instructed to take it slowly and not to go back to the toxic environment or level of over-functioning that made them sick in the first place. They especially need to be instructed not to make up for lost time by trying to do too much. A simplified approach to helping these patients overcome an unhealthy psychodynamic can be found in my book *Three Steps to Happiness! Healing Through Joy.*

Although it is important to treat the underlying metabolic problems in CFS/FMS, most chronic illnesses will not fully resolve unless mind-body issues are also treated. In CFS and FMS this means patients must stop seeking approval, and learn to say no when they feel like it. Teach patients to keep their attention on what feels good from a centered place. In summary, follow your bliss!

Treating Anxiety and Depression Naturally

Anxiety and depression can be seen in chronic illness of any sort, including CFS and fibromyalgia. Fortunately, natural treatments for these can be effective. For anxiety, it is important that patients get adequate amounts of B vitamins and magnesium. In addition, clinical experience has shown that very high-dose vitamin B_1 (thiamine) at a level of 500 milligrams one to three times daily can be helpful in decreasing anxiety after several weeks of use. Passionflower, theanine (from green tea), and magnolia can also be helpful and can work quickly, calming the patient without being sedating. An excellent product for the treatment of anxiety in general (which contains all of the above) is called Calming Balance (available from Health Freedom Nutrition; 800-980-8780).

For depression, nutritional support including B vitamins, magnesium, tyrosine, and 5-HTP can be helpful. In addition, Saint John's wort at 900 to 1,800 milligrams daily and magnolia can also be effective for mild to moderate depression. All of the above are combined in a formula called Happiness 1–2–3! (also available from Health Freedom Nutrition; 800-980-8780). Although some of its components work fairly quickly, the Saint John's wort can take six weeks to be optimally effective, so patients should know to give the herbal an adequate amount of time. Because this product can be so effective at raising serotonin, I would not use the maximal dose in those on high levels of antidepressants (e.g., Prozac at 40 milligrams a day or higher) to avoid excess serotonin levels. In addition, making sure that you do not miss subclinical hypothyroidism (regardless of the blood tests' levels) and adding a mercury-free fish oil (such as Eskimo-3) can also be helpful.

Treatment Review

Although this chapter and the summary below will give you an excellent start in treating fibromyalgia, CFS, and myofascial pain syndrome metabolically, the treatment protocol at www.vitality101.com has more than 270 useful natural and prescription therapies with resources and far more detailed instructions for use (organized by category). For example, dozens of sleep and pain therapies are reviewed, and the information on each treatment is given in far more clinical detail. I will be happy to e-mail you this free file, plus long- and short-form patient questionnaires that you can modify for use in your office, as they can dramatically simplify the care of these patients. Simply e-mail me at Endfatigue@aol.com or in the Q&A section at www.vitality101.com. This book (*From Fatigued to Fantastic!*), and the recently released *Pain Free 1–2–3: A Proven Program to Get YOU Pain Free!* also contain more detailed information, including more than five hundred references related to our treatment recommendations.

Treat CFS, fibromyalgia, and myofascial pain syndrome by restoring energy levels metabolically. Do this by using the SHIN protocol. SHIN stands for Sleep, Hormonal support, Infections, and Nutritional support. In addition, give pain support when needed. It is almost never acceptable to leave somebody in pain. Below I have listed some of the key parts of the protocol. The most important and commonly used treatments are indicated with two asterisks and in bold. Almost all of the treatments can be stopped after three to twelve months, except for the Energy Revitalization System vitamin powder plus something for sleep, which should both be taken long term. Many patients also prefer to stay on ribose long term.

NUTRITIONAL TREATMENTS

1. ****Energy Revitalization System vitamin powder.** Half to one scoop a day (as feels best). If diarrhea occurs, mix the powder with milk and/or start with a lower dose and work your way up to the dose that feels best, or divide the daily dose into smaller doses and take two to three times a day. These products are made by Integrative Therapeutics/ITI and are also available retail at www.vitality101.com and most health food stores. One drink and one capsule replace more than thirty-five tablets of supplements daily and give outstanding overall nutritional support for almost everyone.

2. Vitamin B_{12}: If blood levels are less than 540, give 3,000 micrograms IM three to seven times weekly for fifteen doses, then as needed.

3. Chromagen Forte (iron): One tablet a day if ferritin is under 40.

Take on an empty stomach and not within six hours of taking thyroid hormones.

MITOCHONDRIAL ENERGY TREATMENTS

Use these for four to nine months. Then drop the dose to the lowest dose that maintains the effect (or stop it if no benefit).

4. ****D-ribose** (CORvalen, from Bioenergy; 866-267-8253; www .corvalen.com): One scoop of powder three times a day for three weeks, then two times a day.

5. Coenzyme Q_{10}: 200 milligrams a day. Vitaline makes the best form.

6. *Acetyl-L-carnitine: 500 milligrams twice a day for three months.

SLEEP AIDS

Adjust dose as needed to get eight to nine hours of solid sleep without waking or hangover.

7. **Revitalizing Sleep Formula** (by Integrative Therapeutics/ITI): 200 milligrams valerian, 90 milligrams passionflower, 50 milligrams L-theanine, 30 milligrams hops, 12 milligrams piscidia, and 28 milligrams wild lettuce. Take two to four capsules each night thirty to ninety minutes before bedtime. It can also be used during the day for anxiety. If valerian energizes you (occurs in 5 to 10 percent of people), use the other components.

8. 5-HTP (5-Hydroxy-L-Tryptophan): 200 to 400 milligrams at night.

9. Calcium: 500 to 600 milligrams; magnesium: 100 to 200 milligrams at bedtime.

10. Melatonin; 0.5 milligram at bedtime.

11. **Ambien (zolpidem): 10 milligrams, half to one and a half at bedtime.

12. Desyrel (trazodone): 50 milligrams, half to six at bedtime.

13. Klonopin (clonazepam): 0.5 milligrams. Begin slowly and work your way up as sedation allows. Take half a tablet at bedtime, increasing to six tablets at bedtime as needed. Can be effective for sleep, pain, and restless leg syndrome. Klonopin may be addictive.

14. Doxylamine (Unisom for Sleep) or Benadryl: 25 milligrams at night (antihistamines). May also help pain.

15. Neurontin (gabapentin): 300 milligrams, one to two capsules at bedtime. Also helps pain and restless leg syndrome.

HORMONAL TREATMENTS

THYROID SUPPLEMENTATION

The main side effect of thyroid treatment is triggering benign caffeinelike anxiety or palpitations. Although rare, as also seen with exercise (e.g., climbing steps), if one is on the edge of having a heart attack or severe "racing heart" (atrial fibrillation), thyroid hormone can trigger it. In the long run, though, I suspect that thyroid may decrease the risk of heart disease. To put it in perspective, I've never seen angina in treating thousands of patients with thyroid. Increasing the thyroid dose to levels above the upper limit of the normal range may accelerate osteoporosis (which is already common in CFS/FMS). Because of this, check the thyroid (free T_4—not TSH) levels after four to eight weeks on the optimum dose of thyroid hormone. Do not take thyroid within six hours of iron or calcium supplements or you won't absorb the thyroid.

16. **Armour Thyroid: 30 milligrams (½ grain = 30 milligrams) (natural thyroid glandular). If Cortef is checked, begin the Cortef and/or adrenal support one to seven days before starting the thyroid. Take half a tablet each morning on an empty stomach for one week and then one tablet each morning. Increase by half to one tablet every one to six weeks (until the patient is on three tablets or the dose that feels best). Check a repeat free T_4 blood level when on three tablets a day (or the optimum dose) for four weeks. If okay, you can continue to raise the dose by half to one tablet each morning every six to nine weeks to a maximum of five grains (300 milligrams) a day and then recheck the free T_4 four weeks later. Adjust it to the dose that feels the best (lower the dose if shaky or if your resting pulse is regularly over 88/minute).

ADRENAL HORMONES (GLANDULARS AND SUPPORT)
Helps the body deal with stress and maintains blood pressure.

17. *Cortef: 5-milligram tablets, half to two and a half tablet(s) at breakfast, half to one and a half tablet(s) at lunch, and 0 to half a tablet at 4 p.m. Use the lowest dose that feels the best. Most patients find that one to one and a half tablets in the morning and half to one tablet at noon is optimal. Take it with food if it causes an acid stomach. Do not take more than four tablets a day.

18. Adrenal Stress-End (from Integrative Therapeutics or www .vitality101.com): Take one to two capsules each morning (or one to two in the morning and one at noon). Take less or take with food if it upsets your stomach.

19. Isocort (adrenal glandular): Contains approximately 2.5 milligrams cortisol (Cortef) per pellet (do not give more than six a day). Order from 800-743-2256.

20. *DHEA: 5 to 25 milligrams each morning or twice daily (lower the dose if acne or darkening of facial hair occurs). Some experts recommend that the entire dose be taken in the morning. Keep DHEA levels between 140 and 180 micrograms/dL for females and 300 and 500

micrograms/dL for males. If the patient has breast cancer, do not use DHEA. See information sheet for dosing.

21. Increase your salt and water intake substantially. If your mouth and lips are dry (and you're not on Elavil), you're dehydrated; drink more water (or herbal tea or lemonade sweetened with stevia—not sodas or coffee). Celtic sea salt is an excellent form to use (800-867-7258).

OTHER HORMONES

22. Biest, 2.5 milligrams, plus 30 to 100 milligrams progesterone, plus 2 to 5 milligrams testosterone, all in 1 gram of cream. Apply 1 gram of cream to your abdomen at bedtime. (I recommend ITC Pharmacy for my compounded medications; 303-663-4224.)

23. Testosterone: Males Testim 1 percent 25 to 100 milligrams daily. Consider checking total estrogen and DHT levels when you check the testosterone blood levels. If the DHT goes too high it can cause hair loss—which can be prevented by Proscar or saw palmetto, 160 milligrams two times a day. If estrogen goes too high, this can be blocked by Arimidex, 1 milligram every other day. If taking thyroid tablets, be aware that adding testosterone can increase thyroid blood levels. If the patient gets moody or anxious, or has a racing heart, check a blood level for thyroid and consider lowering the dose.

INFECTIONS

ANTI-YEAST TREATMENTS

24. **Avoid sweets—this includes sucrose, glucose, fructose, corn syrup, and any other sweets until the doctor says that it is okay to include them in your diet again. Avoid fruit juices, which are naturally sweet. Having one to two fruits a day (the whole fruit as opposed to the juice) is okay. Stevia is a great sugar substitute. Inositol (helps anxiety and depression) and xylitol (helps osteoporosis) are also excellent and healthy sugar substitutes that look and taste just like sugar.

25. Stevia is a wonderful herbal sweetener. A great-tasting one is by Body Ecology; 800-478-3842. Use all you want.

26. *Acidophilus milk bacteria: Use the Probiotic Pearls form (by ITI). Take two twice a day for five months. Then consider one a day to help maintain a healthy bowel.

27. *Anti-Yeast (Ultraceuticals) is an excellent natural antifungal mix. Take for three to five months.

28. Citricidal: 100 milligrams (use the tablets) two twice a day.

29. Nystatin: 500,000 units, two tablets two to four times a day. Begin with one a day and increase by one tablet a day until you are up to the total dose. Symptoms may initially flare as the yeast die off.

30. **Diflucan (fluconazole): 200 milligrams a day for six to twelve weeks. Begin taking the Diflucan four weeks after starting Phytostan or nystatin.

IMMUNE STIMULANT

31. Thymic Protein (Pro Boost): Dissolve the contents of one packet under your tongue—any that is swallowed is destroyed. Take it three times a day for twelve weeks, then once a day for six weeks. Also take it three times a day at the first sign of any infection until the infection resolves (it is approximately two dollars a packet). Available from www.vitality101.com or wholesale from Klabin Marketing (800-933-9440). Works in the first twenty-four hours for acute infections but takes two to three months to work for chronic infections.

CHRONIC AND ACUTE SINUSITIS

32. **Sinusitis Nose Spray: By prescription from ITC Pharmacy (303-663-4224). Contains Sporanox, xylitol, Bactroban, and Beclamethasone. Use one to two sprays in each nostril twice a day for six to twelve weeks. If it irritates the nose, dilute with nasal saline spray.

OTHER TREATMENTS

FOOD AND OTHER SENSITIVITIES

35. **NAET: Wonderful for elimination of sensitivities/allergies (see www.naet.com for more information).

36. Food Allergy Elimination Diet (instruction sheet is available at www.vitality101.com).

IV NUTRITIONAL SUPPORT

37. **Myers cocktail—IV nutritional therapies (very helpful). See further information on contents on page 364.

*DETOXIFICATION

There are several simple things that you can do that can be helpful:

38. Sweating can remove toxins—especially if you shower immediately after—and can be beneficial for health. Many of the newer saunas are what are called "far infrared," and a half hour three to seven times a week can help detoxification. I use the one from High Tech Health (800-794-5355).

PAIN TREATMENTS

NATURAL PAIN THERAPIES
Dozens more are discussed at length in *Pain Free 1–2–3.*

39. Rolfing, Trager, myofascial release, chiropractic, other bodywork and manipulation modalities, and/or acupuncture.

40. **Pain Formula:** Contains willow bark, Boswellia, and cherry. Take two to four tablets three times a day. It takes two to six weeks to see the full effect. At that time, you can often lower the dose to one tablet three times a day or two tablets twice a day. From ITI (Integrative Therapeutics).

PHARMACOLOGIC PAIN TREATMENTS
See my book *Pain Free 1–2–3* for dozens more options and details for use.

41. **Ultram (Rx: tramadol): 50 milligrams, one to two tablets up to four times a day as needed for pain. Fewer side effects are seen with four or fewer tablets a day. May cause nausea/vomiting. **Caution:** May very rarely cause seizures or raise serotonin too high when combined with antidepressants.

TOPICAL PAIN TREATMENTS
42. **Topical Pain Formula cream or lotion (Rx): Contains a mix of prescription pain medications. Rub a pea-size amount onto painful areas three times a day as needed. Available by prescription from ITC Pharmacy (303-663-4224). You can use this on up to three or four silver-dollar-size areas at a time.

43. *Lidoderm Patches (Rx; lidoderm): Can be cut into pieces to put over different areas. Leave the patch on for twelve to eighteen hours, then off the rest of the day. It can help localized pain (i.e., it helps pain that is right under the patch). Up to four patches can be used at a time each day. It can take two to three weeks to see if it works.

GABA Agonists

44. Neurontin (gabapentin): 300 to 900 milligrams one to four times a day (to a maximum of 3,600 milligrams a day). Cut back and increase by 100 milligrams a day every four to five days if it causes any uncomfortable or unusual neurologic symptoms or excessive sedation. Begin with 100 to 300 milligrams at night, then slowly increase to 300 to 900 milligrams three times a day as is comfortable. In some, pain relief is immediate; in others, it can take a minimum of 1,200 milligrams a day.

45. Lyrica (pregabalin): 50 to 150 milligrams three times a day. The main side effects are sedation and weight gain.

Muscle Relaxants

46. Flexeril (cyclobenzaprine): 10 milligrams, half to two at bedtime. Muscle relaxant; can cause dry mouth.

47. *Skelaxin (Rx; metaxolone): 800 milligrams, 1 tablet four times a day as needed for pain. This is usually nonsedating.

Anxiety

48. Calming Balance: One to three capsules three times a day as needed. A unique mix of eleven herbs and nutrients. Some effect is immediate and the rest builds over two weeks (available retail at www.vitality101 .com and wholesale from Health Freedom Nutrition at 800-980-8780).

Depression

49. Happiness 1–2–3: One to two capsules three times a day. A unique mix of twelve herbs and nutrients that may help depression. The effect builds over six weeks (available retail at www.vitality101.com and wholesale from Health Freedom Nutrition at 800-980-8780).

Wholesale Sources

The following companies can provide some of the more important supplements used in the protocol (most can be obtained retail at www.vitality101 .com). As an aside, I note that I take NO money from any company whose products I recommend, and 100 percent of the royalties for my products go to charity.

- Integrative Therapeutics Inc. (ITI). This is the company that I respect most in the natural supplements industry. It actually voluntarily registered with the FDA as a pharmaceutical company, and therefore has to go through all the quality-control testing done by drug companies. It did this so that customers can be assured of both the purity and potency of its products. As would be expected, the science the goes into making its products is also outstanding. ITI carries the Energy Revitalization System vitamin powder and B complex, Revitalizing Sleep Formula, Adrenal Stress-End, Pain Formula, Probiotic Pearls, Vitaline coenzyme Q_{10}, and Eskimo-3 fish oils. For ordering and product information, I recommend that you call Cathy Leet at 920-737-8828 or call 800-931-1709.
- Bioenergy Life Sciences, Inc. For D-ribose (CORvalen); 866-267-8253; www.corvalen.com
- Klabin Marketing. Carries the wonderful immune stimulant Pro Boost (800-933-9440).
- Health Freedom Nutrition. Makes Happiness 1–2–3! supplement for depression and Calming Balance for anxiety (800-980-8780).
- Body Ecology brand of stevia (1-800-4-STEVIA). Many brands of stevia are bitter but this brand is excellent-tasting and well accepted by patients as a sugar substitute.
- ITC Pharmacy. An excellent source for bioidentical hormones, concentrated injectable B_{12}, pain creams, and the sinusitis nose spray; ships worldwide (303-663-4224).
- www.vitality101.com. This is my Web site, and I invite you and your patients to sign up for my free e-mail newsletters. In addition, copies of all my books (*From Fatigued to Fantastic!*, *Three Steps to Happiness: Healing Through Joy*, and *Pain Free 1–2–3*) and information on getting our two- and three-day conference CDs are available. Our computer-

ized online program is a resource that will make treatment of these patients much easier. Patients can do the online program at www .vitality101.com. The online program will analyze their labs and symptoms to create a complete medical record of their case. This will create a complete H&P with assessment and recommendations for your chart. Another option that many doctors prefer is to have patients go to a data-collecting site that looks like your site and enter their symptoms. Only the doctor's office can enter the labs (which are optional) and get a printout. A short form that creates only the assessment and recommendations is also available. For more information on these www.medicalwebrecord.com options, e-mail us at the Q&A section at www.vitality101.com.

Myers Cocktail

For further information about sources of the products and services mentioned in this section, see Appendix E: Resources.

1. The following are instructions for making and administering the slow IV Myers Push (MP).

Supplies Needed	Amount
1. Bacteriostatic water	7 cc
2. Ascorbic acid (500 mg/ml), preservative-free	1 to 10 cc
(I often give 20 to 40 cc vitamin C over thirty to forty minutes— see next page)	
3. Magnesium sulfate (MgSO4), 50 percent (0.5 mg/ml)	2 to 4 cc
4. Pyridoxine (100 mg/ml), preservative-free	1 cc
5. Methylcobalamin (3,000 mcg/ml)	1 cc
6. B complex 100	0.5 to 1 cc
7. Dexpanthenol (250 mg/ml)	0.5 cc
8. Glutathione, 200 milligrams per cc (optional)	2 to 5 cc
(Push in separately—do not mix in the same syringe with other nutrients)	
9. 20-cc or 25-cc syringes	
10. 18-gauge, 1- to 1½-inch needles	
11. 25-gauge, I-inch butterfly sets	
12. Calcium gluconate, 10 percent, preservative-free (optional)	4 to 10 cc

Items 1 through 3 and 6 through 12 can be ordered (among other sources) from Harvard Drug Company (800-783-7103). Item 4 is available from compounding pharmacies, including Pathways and Wellness and Health Pharmaceuticals. Item 5 may be purchased from G.Y. and N. Most of the above items are also available from McGuff.

To make the Myers Push (MP), draw up each ingredient using a separate syringe/needle and squirt it into the mouth of a 20-cc to 25-cc syringe. Attach the 25-gauge butterfly to the large syringe, pushing fluid through the butterfly tubing until the entire tubing and needle are filled. Now the mixture is ready for venipuncture and a slow IV push. The glutathione should be kept in the initial syringe (not mixed with other nutrients) and pushed in over one to ten minutes (1 cc every one to two minutes).

The dose of $MgSO_4$ typically begins at 2 cc. If the patient feels comfortable, without dizziness, nausea, or hypotension (warmth in the neck, face, chest, abdomen, groin, and/or extremities is normal, and is a sign of physiological action of the magnesium as a vasodilator), I usually increase the $MgSO_4$ to 4 cc and give it over ten to forty minutes. Alternately, all these nutrients can be added in an IV bag and allowed to drip in over thirty to sixty minutes.

The desired result is to inject at a rate at which the patient feels comfortable warmth without excessive flushing or feeling ill—that is, dizziness, nausea, and headache, symptoms that are rare.

Prior to the injection, it is important for the patient to be instructed to give frequent feedback about any developing warm feeling early on, so that the injection may be slowed down, or even temporarily stopped, before excessive, uncomfortable flushing occurs. Likewise, feedback by the patient needs to be given when the warm feeling has mostly subsided so that the injection may be resumed at a reduced rate. Eventually, the infusion will find the "happy medium" rate of injection, which maintains the "comfortable warmth" (see above).

Also, prior to the first few MP injections, explain that a taste of B vitamins usually appears during the infusion, often early in the push.

The physician needs to consider one major option, which has become routine in many quarters—the possible addition of calcium gluconate, 10 percent injectable. Some of the major reasons for deciding to include calcium are:

- If the patient feels consistently unwell for any reason after the MP (weakness, fatigue, sleepiness, palpitations—all rare and mild, if present).

- If the patient has a history, or laboratory evidence, of calcium deficit.
- If the physician's clinical judgment dictates it for any reason.

The dose of calcium gluconate 10 percent injectable varies from 4 cc to 10 cc, depending on the clinician's judgment. The key is to maintain balance without diluting the magnesium's positive effects.

A final caveat is that one needs to keep in mind the third of the troika—oral potassium. Over a period of time, IV magnesium may deplete potassium; the danger is that one may be tempted to increase the dose of magnesium, only to aggravate the low potassium picture. Always keep in mind that a potassium deficit may prevent magnesium repletion and vice versa.

It is also, of course, possible to create calcium deficit by the MP. However, potassium depletion, in my experience, is clinically more frequent and more symptom provoking, and at times alarming. (If needed, give the potassium by mouth—**not IV, as an IV push potassium is fatal.** I use Micro K Extentabs, 10 MEQ, one to two times a day if potassium levels are under 4.0.)

2. Intravenous Vitamin C (IVC)

The following are instructions for making and administering the intravenous vitamin C (IVC.)

Supplies Needed		Amount
1.	.45 percent NS infusion bag	150–500 cc
2.	Ascorbic acid (500mg/ml), preservative-free	30 cc
3.	Sodium bicarbonate, 8.4 percent	3 cc
4.	20-cc to 25-cc syringes	
5.	18-gauge, 1- to 1½-inch needles	
6.	3-cc syringes	
7.	IV tubing	
8.	23-gauge, I-inch butterfly infusion sets	
9.	Hypoallergenic tape	
10.	Xylocaine, 1 to 2 percent (optional)	3 cc

All of the above supplies can be obtained from Harvard Drug Company.

To make the IVC, add the ascorbic acid and the sodium bicarbonate to the IV bag. This infusion can be mixed one to two days before administration and stored in the refrigerator. It is best to bring the IV bag to room temperature before starting the infusion. This can be accomplished by taking the IV bag out of the refrigerator one to two hours ahead of time. Also, protect the IV bag from light.

The infusion is usually given over a period of forty-five to sixty minutes. It is best to select a large vein for the IV (that is, antecubital region) because the vitamin C can irritate the vessel wall. The 3 cc of sodium bicarbonate helps with the irritation problem. If the patient experiences pain or discomfort, slow down the infusion and apply a warm heating pad to the area. Also, squeezing and releasing the fist of the infused arm helps any discomfort.

It is rare for any patient not to tolerate the IVC. However, if discomfort continues and is unbearable, remove the needle and select a different vein. Another option is to add some IV procaine or lidocaine 2 percent to the infusion bag, starting with 3 cc (don't give more than 5 cc of 2 percent lidocaine per hour). Always make certain the patient is not sensitive to any of the "-caine" products, that the procaine or lidacaine is for IV use, and that it does not contain epinephrine.

Notes

Introduction

1. J. E. Teitelbaum and B. Bird, "Effective Treatment of Severe Chronic Fatigue: A Report of a Series of 64 Patients," *Journal of Musculoskeletal Pain* 3 (4) (1995): 91–110.

2. J. E. Teitelbaum, B. Bird, R. M. Greenfield, et al., "Effective Treatment of CFS and FMS: A Randomized, Double-Blind Placebo Controlled Study," *Journal of Chronic Fatigue Syndrome* 8 (2) (2001).

3. J. E. Teitelbaum, C. Johnson, and J. St. Cyr, "The use of D-ribose in chronic fatigue syndrome and fibromyalgia: A pilot study." *J Alt Comp Med* 2006; 12 (9): 857–862.

4. H. Blatman, "Effective Treatment of Fibromyalgia and Myofascial Pain Syndrome." Editorial: *American Journal of Pain Management*, April 2002.

Chapter 1. What Are Chronic Fatigue Syndrome and Fibromyalgia?

1. G. P. Holmes, J. E. Kaplan, N. M. Gantz, et al., "Chronic Fatigue Syndrome: A Working Case Definition," *Annals of Internal Medicine* 108 (1988): 387–389.

2. R. K. Price, C. S. North, S. Wessely, et al., "Estimating the Presence of Chronic Fatigue Syndrome in the Community," *Public Health Reports* 107 (September-October 1992): 514–522.

3. R. B. Marchesani, "Critical Antiviral Pathway Deficient in Chronic Fatigue Syndrome Patients." *Infectious Disease News*, August 1993, p. 4.

4. L. A. Jason, J. A. Richman, A. W. Rademaker, et al., "A Community-Based Study of Chronic Fatigue Syndrome," *Archives of Internal Medicine* 159 (18) (11 October 1999): 2129–2137.

5. D. L. Goldenberg, "Fibromyalgia Syndrome: A Decade Later," *Journal of the American Medical Association* 159 (1999): 777–785.

6. S. E. Straus, S. Fritz, J. K. Dale, et al., "Lymphocyte Phenotype and Function in the Chronic Fatigue Syndrome," *Journal of Clinical Immunology* 13 (1) (January 1993): 30–40.

7. J. E. Teitelbaum and B. Bird, "Effective Treatment of Severe Chronic Fatigue: A Report of a Series of 64 Patients," *Journal of Musculoskeletal Pain* 3 (4) (1995): 91–110.

8. F. Wolfe et al., "The American College of Rheumatology 1990 Criteria for the Classification of Fibromyalgia: Report of the Multicenter Criteria Committee," *Arthritis and Rheumatology* 33 (1990): 160–172.

9. J. E. Teitelbaum, B. Bird, A. Weiss, et al., "Effective Treatment of CFS and FMS: A Randomized, Double-Blind Placebo Controlled Study," *Journal of Chronic Fatigue Syndrome* 8 (2) (2001): 3–24.

10. J. G. Travell and D. G. Simons, *Myofascial Pain and Dysfunction: The Trigger Point Manual*, Vol. 1 (Baltimore, MD: Williams & Wilkins, 1983), pp. 103–164.

11. M. A. Demitrack, K. Dale, S. E. Straus, et al., "Evidence for Impaired Activation of the Hypothalamic-Pituitary-Adrenal Axis in Patients with Chronic Fatigue Syndrome." *Journal of Clinical Endocrinology and Metabolism* 73 (6) (December 1991): 1223–1234.

12. J. E. Teitelbaum, "Estrogen and Testosterone in CFIDS/FMS," *From Fatigued to Fantastic!* newsletter, February 1997.

13. P. O. Behan, "Post-Viral Fatigue Syndrome Research," in *The Clinical and Scientific Basis of Myalgic Encephalitis and Chronic Fatigue Syndrome*, ed. Byron Hyde, Jay Goldstein, and Paul Levine (Ottawa, Ontario, Canada: Nightingale Research Foundation, 1992), p. 238.

14. J. E. Teitelbaum, "Mitochondrial Dysfunction [in CFS/FMS]," *From Fatigued to Fantastic!* newsletter 1 (2) (1997).

15. T. Brockow et al., "A Randomized Controlled Trial on the Effectiveness of Mild Water-filtered Near Infrared Whole-body Hyperthermia as an Adjunct to a Standard Multimodal Rehabilitation in the Treatment of Fibromyalgia," *Clin J Pain*, January 1, 2007; 23 (1): 67–75.

16. D. Halpin and S. Wessely, "VP-1 Antigen in Chronic Postviral Fatigue Syndrome," *The Lancet* 1 (8645) (6 May 1989): 1028–1029.

17. G. E. Yousef, E. J. Bell, G. F. Mann, et al., "Chronic Enterovirus Infection in Patients with Postviral Fatigue Syndrome," *The Lancet* 1 (8578) (23 January 1988): 146–147.

18. L. E. Archard, N. E. Bowles, P. O. Behan, et al., "Postviral Fatigue Syndrome Persistence of Enterovirus RNA in Muscle and Elevated Creatine Kinase," *Journal of the Royal Society of Medicine* 81 (6) (June 1988): 326–329.

19. A. Martin Lerner, M. Zervos, and H. J. Dworkin, "New Cardiomyopathy: Pilot Study of Intravenous Ganciclovir in a Subset of the Chronic Fatigue Syndrome," *Infectious Diseases in Clinical Practice* 6 (1997): 110–117.

20. G. L. Nicolson, "Considerations When Undergoing Treatment for Chronic Infections Found in Chronic Fatigue Syndrome, Fibromyalgia, and Gulf War Illness," *Journal of Internal Medicine* 1 (1988): 115–117, 123–128.

21. G. L. Nicolson, M. Y. Nasralla, J. Haier, et al., "Mycoplasmal Infections in Chronic Illness: Fibromyalgia and Chronic Fatigue Syndrome, Gulf War Illness, Human Immunodeficiency Virus, and Rheumatoid Arthritis," *Medical Sentinel* 4 (1999): 172–176.

22. J. Brewer, K. K. Knox, and D. R. Carrigan, "Longitudinal Study of Chronic Active HHV-6 Viremia in Patients with CFS," paper presented at IDSA Conference, Philadelphia, PA, November 1999.

23. D. Wakefield, A. Lloyd, J. Dwyer, et al., "Human Herpesvirus 6 and Myalgic Encephalomyelitis," *The Lancet* 1 (8593) (7 May 1988): 1059.

24. Byron Hyde, Jay Goldstein, and Paul Levine, eds., *The Clinical and Scientific Basis of Myalgic Encephalitis and Chronic Fatigue Syndrome* (Ottawa, Ontario, Canada: Nightingale Research Foundation, 1992).

25. W. Jefferies, Safe Uses of Cortisol, monograph (Springfield, IL: Charles C. Thomas, 1981).

26. C. A. Everson, "Sustained Sleep Deprivation Impairs Host Defense," *American Journal of Physiology* 265 (5 Part 2) (November 1993): R1148–1154.

27. S. Pillemer, L. A. Bradley, L. J. Crofford, et al., "The Neuroscience and Endocrinology of FMS—[An NIH] Conference Summary," *Arthritis and Rheumatism* 40 (11) (November 1997): 1928–1939.

28. H. Moldofsky, "Sleep and Chronic Fatigue Syndrome," in *Chronic Fatigue Syndrome*, ed. D. Dawson and S. Sabin (Boston, MA: Little, Brown and Company, 1993).

29. F. Wolfe, K. Ross, J. Anderson, I. J. Russell, and L. Hebert, "The Prevalence and Characteristics of Fibromyalgia in the General Population," *Arthritis Rheum* 1995 January; 38 (1): 19–28.

30. L. Lindell, S. Bergman, I. F. Petersson, L. T. Jacobsson, and P. Herrstrom, "Prevalence of Fibromyalgia and Chronic Widespread Pain." *Scand J Prim Health Care* 2000 September; 18 (3): 149–153.

31. M. Matucci Cerinic, M. Zoppi, C. Taieb, J. Caubere, G. Hamelin, and C. Schmitt, "Prevalence of Fibromyalgia in Italy: Updated Results," *Annals of the Rheumatic Diseases* 2006; 65 (supplement 2): 555.

32. M. Guermazi, S. Ghroubi, M. Sellami, M. Elleuch, E. André, C. Schmitt, C. Taieb, J. Damak, and M. Elleuch, "Epidemiology of Fibromyalgia in Tunisia," *Annals of the Rheumatic Diseases* 2006; 65 (supplement 2): 553.

33. V. Cobankara, Ö. Ünal, M. Öztürk, and A. Bozkurt, "The Prevalence of Fibromyalgia Among Textile Workers in the City of Denizli in Turkey," *Annals of the Rheumatic Diseases* 2006; 65 (supplement 2): 554.

34. C. Schmitt, M. Spaeth, E. André, J. Caubere, and C. Taieb, "Fibromyalgia Syndrome: A German Epidemiological Survey," *Annals of the Rheumatic Diseases* 2006; 65 (supplement 2): 554.

Chapter 2. Create Your Individual Treatment Protocol— Beginning with Ribose for Energy Production

1. J. E. Teitelbaum and B. Bird, "Effective Treatment of Severe Chronic Fatigue: A Report of a Series of 64 Patients," *Journal of Musculoskeletal Pain* 3 (4) (1995): 91–110.

2. Ibid.

3. D. C. Vernon et al., "Preliminary Evidence of Mitochondrial Dysfunction Associated with Postinfective Fatigue After Acute Infection with Epstein-Barr Virus," *BMC Infectious Diseases* 2006, 6;15 doi:10.1186/1471–2334–6–15, 31 January 2006, http://www.biomedcentral.com/1471–2334/6/15/abstract.

4. J. Eisinger, A. Plantamura, and T. Ayavou, "Glycolysis Abnormalities in Fibromyalgia," *Journal of the American College of Nutrition* 1994; 13 (2): 144–148.

5. A. Bengtsson, and K. G. Henriksson, "The Muscle in Fibromyalgia—A Review of Swedish Studies," *Journal of Rheumatology Supplement* 1989; 19: 144–149.

6. N. Lund, A. Bengtsson, and P. Thorborg, "Muscle Tissue Oxygen in Primary Fibromyalgia," *Scandinavian Journal of Rheumatology* 1986; 15 (2): 165–173.

7. E. S. Strobl, M. Krapf, M. Suckfull, W. Bruckle, W. Fleckenstein, and W. Muller, "Tissue Oxygen Measurement and 31P Magnetic Resonance Spectroscopy in Patients with Muscle Tension and Fibromyalgia," *Rheumatology International* 1997; 16 (5): 175–180.

8. F. Douche-Aourik, W. Berlier, L. Feasson, T. Bourlet, R. Harrath, S. Omar, F. Grattard, C. Denis, and B. Pozzetto, "Detection of Enterovirus in Human Muscle from Patients with Chronic Inflammatory Muscle Disease or Fibromyalgia and Healthy Subjects," *Journal of Medical Virology* 2003; 71 (4): 540–547.

9. J. H. Park, P. Phothimat, C. T. Oates, M. Hernanz-Schulman, N. J. Olson, "Use of P-31 Magnetic Resonance Spectroscopy to Detect Metabolic Abnormalities in Muscles of Patients with Fibromyalgia," *Arthritis and Rheumatology* 1998; 41 (3): 406–413.

10. M. J. Kushmerick, "Muscle Energy Metabolism, Nuclear Magnetic Resonance Spectroscopy and Their Potential in the Study of Fibromyalgia," *Journal of Rheumatology* [supplement] 1989; 19: 40–46.

11. A. Bengtsson, K. G. Henriksson, and J. Larsson, "Reduced High-Energy Phosphate Levels in the Painful Muscles of Patients with Primary Fibromyalgia," *Arthritis and Rheumatology* 1986; 29 (7): 817–821.

12. E. Lund, S. A. Kendall, B. Janerot-Sjoberg, and A. Bengtsson, "Muscle Metabolism in Fibromyalgia Studied by P-31 Magnetic Resonance Spectroscopy During Aerobic and Anaerobic Exercise," *Scandinavian Journal of Rheumatology* 2003; 32 (3): 138–145.

13. J. Eisinger, D. Bagneres, P. Arroyo, A. Plantamura, and T. Ayavou, "Effects of Magnesium, High-Energy Phosphates, Piracetam and Thiamin on Erythrocyte Transketolase," *Magnetic Research* 1994; 7 (1): 59–61.

14. S. Jacobsen, K. E. Jensen, C. Thomsen, B. Danneskiold-Samsoe, and O. Henriksen, "Magnetic Resonance Spectroscopy in Fibromyalgia: A Study of Phosphate-31 Spectra from Skeletal Muscles During Rest and After Exercise," *Ugeskr Laeger* 1994; 156 (46): 6841–6844.

15. N. J. Olson and J. H. Park, "Skeletal Muscle Abnormalities in Patients with Fibromyalgia," *American Journal of Medical Science* 1998; 315 (6): 351–358.

16. K. G. Henriksson, "Muscle Pain in Neuromuscular Disorders and Primary Fibromyalgia," *Neurologija* 1989; 38 (3): 213–221.

17. M. W. Krapf, S. Muller, P. Mennet, T. Stratz, W. Samborski, and W. Muller, "Recording Muscle Spasms in the Erector Spinae Using in Vivo 31P Magnetic Resonance Spectroscopy in Patients with Chronic Lumbalgia and Generalized Tendomyopathies," *Z Rheumatology* 1992; 51 (5): 229–237.

18. P. O. Behan, "Post-Viral Fatigue Syndrome Research," in *The Clinical and Scientific Basis of Myalgic Encephalitis and Chronic Fatigue Syndrome*, eds. Byron Hyde, Jay Goldstein, and Paul Levine (Ottawa, Ontario, Canada: Nightingale Research Foundation, 1992), p. 238.

19. J. E. Teitelbaum, J. A. St. Cyr, and C. Johnson, "The Use of D-ribose in Chronic Fatigue Syndrome and Fibromyalgia: A Pilot Study," *J Alternative and Complementary Medicine* 2006; 12 (9): 857–862.

20. Y. Hellsten, L. Skadgauge, and J. Bangsbo, "Effect of Ribose Supplementation on Resynthesis of Adenine Nucleotides After Intense Intermittent Training in Humans," *American Journal of Physiology* 2004; 286 (1): R182–R188.

21. P. C. Tullson and R. L. Terjung, "Adenine Nucleotide Synthesis in Exercising and Endurance-Trained Skeletal Muscle," *American Journal of Physiology* 1991; 261: C342–C347.

22. J. J. Brault and R. L. Terjung, "Purine Salvage to Adenine Nucleotides in Different Skeletal Muscle Fiber Types," *Journal of Applied Physiology* 2001; 91: 231–238.

23. B. Gebhart and J. A. Jorgenson, "Benefit of Ribose in a Patient with Fibromyalgia," *Pharmacotherapy* 2004; 24 (11): 1146–1648.

24. J. S. Ingwall, *ATP and the Heart* (Boston, MA: Kluwer Academic Publishers).

25. D. Reibel and M. Rovetto, "Myocardial ATP Synthesis and Mechanical Function Following Oxygen Deficiency," *American Journal of Physiology* 1978; 234 (5): H620–H624.

26. H. G. Zimmer, H. Ibel, and U. Suchner, "Ribose Intervention in the Cardiac Pentose Phosphate Pathway Is Not Species-Specific," *Science* 1984; 223: 712–714.

27. H. Omran, S. Illien, D. MacCarter, J. A. St. Cyr, and B. Luderitz, "D-Ribose Improves Diastolic Function and Quality of Life in Congestive Heart Failure Patients: A Prospective Feasibility Study," *European Journal of Heart Failure* 2003; 5: 615–619.

28. N. Vijay, D. MacCarter, M. Washam, and J. St. Cyr, "Ventilatory Efficiency Improves with D-Ribose in Congestive Heart Failure Patients," *Journal of Molecular and Cellular Cardiology* 2005; 38 (5): 820.

29. O. Carter, D. MacCarter, S. Mannebach, J. Biskupiak, G. Stoddard, E. M. Gilbert, and M. A. Munger, "D-Ribose Improves Peak Exercise Capacity and Ventilatory Efficiency in Heart Failure Patients," *Journal of the American College of Cardiology* 2005; 45 (3 supplement A): 185A.

30. J. C. Griffiths, J. F. Borzelleca, and J. St. Cyr, "Lack of Oral Embryotoxicity/Teratogenicity with D-Ribose in Wistar Rats," *Journal of Food and Chemical Toxicology* 2007; 45 (3): 388–395.

31. J. C. Griffiths, J. F. Borzelleca, and J. St. Cyr, "Sub-Chronic (13-Week) Oral Toxicity Study with D-Ribose in Wistar Rats," *Journal of Food and Chemical Toxicology* 2007; 45 (1): 144–152.

32. M. Gross, B. Dormann, and N. Zollner, "Ribose Administration During Exercise: Effects on Substrates and Products of Energy Metabolism in Healthy Subjects and a Patient with Myoadenylate Deaminase Deficiency," *Klin Wochenschr* 1991; 69: 151–155.

33. D. R. Wagner, U. Gresser, and N. Zollner, "Effects of Oral Ribose on Muscle Metabolism During Bicycle Ergometer in AMPD-Deficient Patients," *Annals of Nutrition and Metabolism* 1991; 35: 297–302.

34. M. Gross, S. Reiter, and N. Zollner, "Metabolism of D-Ribose Administered to Healthy Persons and to Patients with Myoadenylate Deaminase Deficiency," *Klin Wochenschr* 1989; 67: 1205–1213.

35. E. K. Guymer and K. J. Clauw, "Treatment of Fatigue in Fibromyalgia," *Rheum Dis Clin North Am* 2002; 28 (2): 67–78.

36. D. S. Rooks, C. B. Silverman, and F. G. Kantrowitz, "The Effects of Progressive Strength Training and Aerobic Exercise on Muscle Strength and Cardiovascular Fitness in Women with Fibromyalgia: A Pilot Study," *Arthritis Rheum* 2002; 47 (1): 22–28.

37. R. Geenen, J. W. Jacobs, and J. W. Bijlsma, "Evaluation and Management of Endocrine Dysfunction in Fibromyalgia," *Rheum Dis Clin North Am* 2002; 28 (2): 389–404.

38. C. L. Schachter, A. J. Busch, P. M. Peloso, and M. S. Shepard, "Effects of Short Versus Long Bouts of Aerobic Exercise in Sedentary Women with Fibromyalgia: A Randomized Controlled Trial," *Phys Ther* 2003; 83 (4): 340–358.

39. D. L. Williamson, P. M. Gallagher, M. P. Goddard, and S. W. Trappe, "Effects of Ribose Supplementation on Adenine Nucleotide Concentration in Skeletal Muscle Following High-Intensity Exercise," *Med Sci Sport Exc* 2001; 33 (5 supplement).

40. N. Zollner, S. Reiter, M. Gross, D. Pongratz, C. D. Reimers, K. Gerbitz, I. Paetzke, T. Deufel, and G. Hubner, "Myoadenylate Deaminase Deficiency: Successful Symptomatic Therapy by High-Dose Oral Administration of Ribose," *Klin Wochenschr* 1986; 64: 1281–1290.

41. B. M. Patton, "Beneficial Effect of D-ribose in Patients with Myoadenylate Deaminase Deficiency," *The Lancet* May 1982; 1701.

42. C. Salerno, P. D'Eufemia, R. Finocchiaro, M. Celli, A. Spalice, C. Crifo, and O. Giardini, "Effect of D-ribose on Purine Synthesis and Neurological Symptoms in a Patient with Adenylsuccinase Deficiency," *Biochim Biophys Acta* 1999; 1453: 135–140.

43. C. Salerno, M. Celli, R. Finocchiaro, P. D'Eufemia, P. Iannetti, C. Crifo, and O. Giardini, *Effect of D-ribose Administration to a Patient with Inherited Defect of Adenylosuccinase. Purine Metabolism in Man IX* (New York: Plenum Press, 1998).

44. D. Pauly and C. Pepine, "D-Ribose as a Supplement for Cardiac Energy Metabolism," *J Cardiovasc Pharmacol Ther* 2000; 5 (4): 249–258.

45. D. Pauly, C. Johnson, and J. A. St. Cyr, "The Benefits of Ribose in Cardiovascular Disease," *Med Hypoth* 2003; 60 (2): 149–151.

46. D. F. Pauly and C. J. Pepine, "Ischemic Heart Disease: Metabolic Approaches to Management," *Clin Cardiol* 2004; 27 (8): 439–441.

47. S. L. Dodd, C. A. Johnson, K. Fernholz, and J. A. St. Cyr. "The Role of Ribose in Human Skeletal Muscle Metabolism," *Med Hypoth* 2004; 62 (5): 819–824.

48. R. Zarzeczny, J. J. Brault, K. A. Abraham, C. R. Hancock, and R. L. Terjung, "Influence of Ribose on Adenine Salvage After Intense Muscle Contractions," *J Appl Physiol* 2001; 91: 1775–1781.

49. J. W. Wallen, M. P. Belanger, and C. Wittnich, "Preischemic Administration of Ribose to Delay the Onset of Irreversible Ischemic Injury and Improve Function: Studies in Normal and Hypertrophied Hearts," *Can J Physiol Pharmacol* 2003; 81: 40–47.

50. R. Wilson, D. MacCarter, and J. St. Cyr, "D-ribose Enhances the Identification of Hibernating Myocardium," *Heart Drug* 2003: 3: 61–62.

51. D. Van Gammeren, D. Faulk, and J. Antonio, "The Effects of Four Weeks of Ribose Supplementation on Body Composition and Exercise Performance in Healthy, Young Male Recreational Bodybuilders: A Double-Blind, Placebo-Controlled Trial," *Curr Ther Res* 2002; 63 (8): 486–495.

52. R. Sharma, M. Munger, S. Litwin, O. Vardeny, D. MacCarter, and J. A. St. Cyr, "D-ribose Improves Doppler TEI Myocardial Performance Index and Maximal Exercise Capacity in Stage C Heart Failure," *J Mol Cell Cardiol* 2005; 38 (5): 853.

53. W. Pliml, T. von Arnim, A. Stablein, H. Hofmann, H. G. Zimmer, and E. Erdmann, "Effects of Ribose on Exercise-Induced Ischaemia in Stable Coronary Artery Disease," *The Lancet* 1992; 340: 507–510.

54. D. Perkowski, S. Wagner, A. Marcus, and J. St. Cyr, "D-ribose Improves Cardiac Indices in Patients Undergoing "Off" Pump Coronary Arterial Revascularization," *J Surg Res* 2007; 173 (2): 295.

55. C. Muller, H. Zimmer, M. Gross, U. Gresser, I. Brotsack, M. Wehling, and W. Pliml, "Effect of Ribose on Cardiac Adenine Nucleotides in a Donor Model for Heart Transplantation," *Eur J Med Res* 1998; 3: 554–558.

56. G. F. Grant and R. W. Gracey, "Therapeutic Nutraceutical Treatments for Osteoarthritis and Ischemia," *Exp Opin Ther Patent*s 2000; 10 (1): 1–10.

57. A. V. Plioplys and S. Plioplys, "Amantadine and L-carnitine Treatment of Chronic Fatigue Syndrome," *Neuropsychobiology* 35 (1) (1997): 16–23.

58. H. Kuratsune, K. Yamaguti, M. Takahashi, et al., "Acylcarnitine Deficiency in Chronic Fatigue Syndrome," *Clinical Infectious Disease* 18 (3 supplement 1) (January 1994): S62–S67.

59. http://www.hsrmagazine.com/hotnews/66h21048207977.html)

60. P. R. Palan, K. Connell, et al., "Effects of Menopause and Hormone Replacement Therapy on Serum Levels of Coenzyme Q_{10} and Other Lipid-Soluble Antioxidants," *Biofactors*, 2005; 25 (1–4): 61–66.

61. H. K. Berthold, A. Naini, et al., "Effect of Ezetimibe and/or Simvastatin on Coenzyme Q_{10} Levels in Plasma: A Randomized Trial," *Drug Saf*, 2006; 29 (8): 703–712.

62. S. Sander, S. I. Coleman, et al., "The Impact of Coenzyme Q_{10} on Systolic Function in Patients with Chronic Heart Failure," *Journal of Cardiac Failure*, 2006; 12 (6): 464–472.

63. K. A. Weant and K. M. Smith, "The Role of Coenzyme Q_{10} in Heart Failure," *Ann Pharmacother*, 2005; 39 (9): 1522–1526.

64. K. Folkers, S. Shizukuishi, K. Takemura, et al., "Increase in Levels of IgG in Serum of Patients Treated with Coenzyme Q_{10}," *Research Communications in Chemical Pathology and Pharmacology* 38 (2) (1982): 335–338.

65. K. Folkers, P. Langsjoen, Y. Nara, et al., "Biochemical Deficiencies of Coenzyme Q_{10} in HIV Infection and Exploratory Treatment," *Biochemical and Biophysical Research Communications* 153 (2) (1988): 888–896.

66. K. Lockwood, S. Moesgaad, T. Hanoike, et al., "Apparent Partial Remission of Breast Cancer in High-Risk Patients Supplemented with Nutritional Antioxidants, Essential Fatty Acids and Coenzyme Q_{10}," *Molecular Aspects of Medicine* 15 (supplement) (1994): S231–S240.

67. K. Lockwood, S. Moesgaard, T. Yamamoto, et al., "Progress on Therapy of Breast Cancer with Coenzyme Q_{10} and the Regression of Metastases," *Biochemical and Biophysical Research Communications* 212 (1) (6 July 1995): 172–177.

67A. L. Rusciani, I. Proietti, et al., "Low Plasma Coenzyme Q_{10} Levels as an Independent Prognostic Factor for Melanoma Progression," *J Am Acad Dermatol*, 2006; 54 (2): 234–241.

68. P. Mayer, H. Hamberger, and J. Drew, "Differential Effects of Ubiquinone Q7 and Ubiquinone Analogs on Macrophage Activation and Experimental Infections in Granulocytopenic Mice," *Infection* 8 (1980): 256–261.

69. E. Bliznakov, A. Casey, and E. Premuzic, "Coenzymes Q: Stimulants of Phagocytic Activity in Rats and Immune Response in Mice," *Experientia* 26 (1970): 953–954.

70. L. Van Gaal, I. D. de Leeuw, S. Vadhanavikit, et al., "Exploratory Study of Coenzyme Q_{10} in Obesity," in K. Folkers and Y. Yamamura, eds., *Biomedical and Clinical Aspects of Coenzyme Q*, Vol. 4 (New York, NY: Elsevier Publishers, 1984), pp. 235–373.

71. P. S. Sandor, L. Di Clemente, et al., "Efficacy of Coenzyme Q_{10} in Migraine Prophylaxis: A Randomized Controlled Trial," *Neurology*, 2005; 64 (4): 713–715.

72. A. Gaby, "The Role of Coenzyme Q_{10} in Clinical Medicine. Part I," *Alternative Medicine Review* 1 (1) (1996): 11–17.

73. Y. Ishihara, Y. Uchida, S. Kitamura, et al., "Effect of Coenzyme Q_{10}, a Quinone Derivative, on Guinea Pig Lung and Tracheal Tissue," *Arzneimittelforschung* 35 (1985): 929–933.

Chapter 3. S—Sleep: The Foundation of Getting Well

1. A. Theadom, M. Cropley, and K. L. Humphrey, "Exploring the Role of Sleep and Coping in Quality of Life in Fibromyalgia," *J Psychosom Res*, February 1, 2007; 62 (2): 145–151.

2. C. A. Everson, "Sustained Sleep Deprivation Impairs Host Defense," *American Journal of Physiology* 265 (5 Part 2) (November 1993): R1148–R1154.

3. S. Pillemer, L. A. Bradley, L. J. Crofford, et al., "The Neuroscience and Endocrinology of FMS—[An NIH] Conference Summary," *Arthritis and Rheumatism* 40 (11) (November 1997): 1928–1939.

4. H. Moldofsky and P. Scarisbrick, "Induction of Neuresthenic Musculoskeletal Pain Syndrome by Selective Sleep Stage Deprivation," *Psychosomatic Medicine* 38 (1) (January-February 1976): 35–44.

5. A. M. Drewes, K. D. Nielson, S. J. Taagholt, et al., "Slow Wave Sleep in FMS," abstract, *Journal of Musculoskeletal Pain* 3 (supplement 1) (1995): 29.

6. S. R. Patel, et al., Associated Professional Sleep Societies (APSS) 2006 Annual Meeting: Abstract 349. Presented June 19, 2006 annual meeting, held in Salt Lake City, Utah.

7. T. Fleming, ed., "Jamaican Dogwood," *PDR* for herbal medicines, 1998, pp. 428–429.

8. "Humulus Lupus," Monograph, *Alternative Medicine Review*, 8 (2) 2003; 190–192.

9. J. R. Cronin, "Passionflower—Reigniting Male Libido and Other Potential Uses," *Alternative and Complementary Therapies*, April 2003; pp. 89–92.

10. K. Dhawan et al., "Reversal of Morphine Tolerance and Dependence by Passiflora Incarnata," *Pharmaceutical Biology*, 2002; 40 (8): 576–580.

11. S. Hadley et al., "Valerian," *American Family Physician*, 2003; 67 (8): 1755–1758.

12. Kobayashi et al., *Nippon Nogeikagaku Kaishi*, 1998; 72: 153–157.

13. Yagyu et al., *Neuropsychobiol*, 1997; 35: 46–50.

14. Juneja et al., *Trends in Food Sci Tech*, 1999; 199–204.

15. G. Zheng, K. Sayama, T. Okubo, L. R. Juneja, and I. Oguni, "Anti-obesity Effects of Three Major Components of Green Tea, Catechins, Caffeine and Theanine, in Mice." *In Vivo*, 2004 January-February; 18 (1): 55–62.

16. J. E. Teitelbaum, C. Johnson, and J. St. Cyr. "The Use of D-ribose in Chronic Fatigue Syndrome and Fibromyalgia: A Pilot Study," *J Alt Comp Med* 2006; 12 (9): 857–862.

17. H. Dressing and D. Riemann, "Insomnia: Are Valerian/Melissa Combinations of Equal Value to Benzodiazepine?" *Therapiewoche* 42 (1992): 726–736.

18. I. Caruso, P. Sarzi Puttini, M. Cazzola, and V. Azzolini, "Double-Blind Study of 5-Hydroxy-L-Tryptophan Versus Placebo in the Treatment of Primary Fibromyalgia Syndrome," *J Int Med Res.* (1990) 18 (3): 201–209.

19. R. Cluydt, "Insomnia Treatment: A Postgraduate Medicine Special Report," 114–123.

20. B. P. Grubb, D. A. Wolfe, D. Samoil, et al., "Usefulness of Fluoxetine HCL for Prevention of Resistant Upright Tilt Induced Syncope," *Pacing and Clinical Electrophysiology* 16 (1993): 458–464.

21. D. Germanowicz, M. S. Lumertz, D. Martinez, and A. F. Margarites, "Sleep-Disordered Breathing Concomitant with Fibromyalgia Syndrome," *J Bras Pneumol*, July 1, 2006; 32 (4): 333–338.

22. C. Guilleminault and A. Bassiri, "Clinical Features and Evaluation of Obstructive Sleep Apnea-Hypopnea Syndrome and the Upper Airway Resistance Syndrome," In *Principles and Practice of Sleep Medicine*, edition 4, M. H. Kriger, T. Roth, and W. C. Dement, eds., Philadelphia: W. B. Saunders; 2004.

23. C. Guilleminault, L. Palombini, D. Poyares, et al., "Chronic Insomnia, Post-menopausal Women, and SDB, Part 2: Comparison of Nondrug Treatment Trials in Normal Breathing and UARS Postmenopausal Women Complaining of Insomnia," *J Psychosom Res* 2002; 53: 617–623.

24. C. Guilleminault, J. L. Faul, and R. Stoohs, "Sleep-Disordered Breathing and Hypotension," *Am J Respir Crit Care Med* 2001; 164: 1242–1247.

25. C. Guilleminault, A. Khramtsov, R. A. Stoohs, et al., "Abnormal Blood Pressure in Prepubertal Children with Sleep-Disordered Breathing," *Pediatr Res* 2004; 55: 76–84.

26. P. E. Peppard, T. Young, M. Palta, et al., "Prospective Study of the Association Between Sleep-Disordered Breathing and Hypertension," *New England Journal of Medicine* 2000; 342: 1378–1384.

27. A. R. Gold, F. Dipalo, M. S. Gold, et al., "The Symptoms and Signs of Upper Airway Resistance Syndrome: A Link to the Functional Somatic Syndromes," *Chest* 2003, 123: 87–95.

28. C. Guilleminault, R. Winkle, R. Korobkin, et al., "Children and Nocturnal Snoring: Evaluation of the Effects of Sleep-Related Respiratory Resistive Load and Daytime Functioning," *Eur J Pediatr* 1982, 139: 165–171.

29. Ibid.

30. C. Guilleminault and A. Bassiri, "Clinical Features and Evaluation of Obstructive Sleep Apnea-Hypopnea Syndrome and the Upper Airway Resistance Syndrome," In *Principles and Practice of Sleep Medicine*, edition 4, M. H. Kriger, T. Roth, W. C. Dement, eds. Philadelphia, PA: W. B. Saunders, 2004. Clinical presentation of OSAS and UARS with examples of craniofacial presentations and clinical scales to define patients.

31. N. C. Netzer, R. A. Stoohs, C. M. Netzer, et al., "Using the Berlin Questionnaire to Identify Patients at Risk for Sleep Apnea Syndrome," *Annals of Internal Medicine* 131 (7) (5 October 1999): 485–491.

32. D. Buchwald, R. Pascualy, and C. Bombardier, et al., "Sleep Disorders in Patients with Chronic Fatigue," *Clin Infect Dis* 1994; 18 (supplement 1): S68–S72.

33. R. P. Millman, "Do You Ever Take a Sleep History?" *Annals of Internal Medicine* 131 (7) (October 1999): 535–536.

34. E. G. Lutz, "Restless Legs, Anxiety and Caffeinism," *Journal of Clinical Psychiatry* 39 (9) (September 1978): 693–698.

35. H. J. Roberts, "Spontaneous Leg Cramps and Restless Legs Due to Diabetogenic (Functional) Hyperinsulinism: A Basis For Natural Therapy," *Journal of the Florida Medical Association* 60 (5) (1973): 29–31.

36. K. A. Ekbom, "Restless Leg Syndrome," *Neurology* 10 (1960): 868–873.

37. S. Ayres and R. Michan, "Restless Leg Syndrome: Response to Vitamin E," *Journal of Applied Nutrition* 25 (1973): 8–15.

38. M. I. Boutez et al., "Neuropsychological Correlates of Folic Acid Deficiency: Facts and Hypothesis," *Folic Acid and Neurology, Psychiatry and Internal Medicine*, ed. M. I. Boutez and E. K. Reynolds (New York, NY: Raven Press, 1979).

Chapter 4. H—Hormonal Support: Optimizing Adrenal, Thyroid, Testosterone, and Estrogen Function

1. O. N. Pamuk and N. Cakir, "The Frequency of Thyroid Antibodies in Fibromyalgia Patients and Their Relationship with Symptoms." *Clin Rheumatol*, 2006 March 16; [Epub ahead of print].

2. W. K. Jerjes, S. Wessely, A. J. Cleare, et al., "Urinary Cortisol and Cortisol Metabolite Excretion," *Chronic Fatigue Syndrome Psychosomatic Medicine*, Vol. 68, July/August 2006, #4, 578–582.

3. M. A. Demitrack and L. J. Crofford, "Evidence for and Pathophysiologic Implications of Hypothalamic-Pituitary-Adrenal Axis Dysregulation in Fibromyalgia and Chronic Fatigue Syndrome," *Ann N Y Acad Sci* 1998 May 1; 840: 684–697.

4. J. E. Teitelbaum and B. Bird, "Effective Treatment of Severe Chronic Fatigue: A Report of a Series of 64 Patients," *Journal of Musculoskeletal Pain* 3 (4) (1995): 91–110.

5. W. M. Jefferies, "Safe Uses of Cortisol," 2nd ed., monograph (Springfield, IL: Charles C. Thomas, 1996).

6. M. A. Demitrack, J. K. Dale, S. E. Straus, L. Laue, S. J. Listwak, and M. J. P. Kruesi, et al., "Evidence for Impaired Activation of the Hypothalamic-Pituitary-Adrenal Axis in Patients with Chronic Fatigue Syndrome," *J Clin Endocrinol Metab* 1991; 73: 1224–1234.

7. D. J. Torpy et al., "Responses of the Sympathetic Nervous System and the Hypothalamic-Pituitary-Adrenal Axis to Interleukin-6 in Fibromyalgia," *Arthritis and Rheumatism* 2000; 43: 872–880.

8. G. Neeck and W. Riedel, "Thyroid Function in Patients with Fibromyalgia Syndrome," *Journal of Rheumatology* 1992; 19–7: 1120–1122.

9. M. Calis and C. Gokce, "Investigation of the Hypothalamo-Pituitary-Adrenal Axis (HPA) by 1ug ACTH Test and Metyrapone Test in Patients with Primary Fibromyalgia Syndrome," *J Endocrinol Invest* 2004; 27: 42–46.

10. M. Kirnap, R. Colak, C. Eser, O. Ozsoy, A. Tutus, and F. Kelestimur, "A Comparison Between Low-Dose (1 microg), Standard-Dose (250 microg) ACTH Stimulation Tests and Insulin Tolerance Test in the Evaluation of Hypothalamo-Pituitary-Adrenal Axis in Primary Fibromyalgia Syndrome," *Clin Endocrinol* (Oxf). 2001 October; 55 (4): 455–459.

11. J. E. Teitelbaum, B. Bird, R. Greenfield, A. Weiss, L. Muenz, and L. Gould, "Effective Treatment of Chronic Fatigue Syndrome (CFIDS) & Fibromyalgia (FMS): A Randomized, Double-Blind, Placebo-Controlled, Intent to Treat Study," *Journal of Chronic Fatigue Syndrome*, Vol. 8, Issue 2, 2001.

12. Jens Gaab, Ph.D., Dominik Hüster, MSc, Renate Peisen, MSc, Veronika Engert, BSc, Vera Sheitz, BSc, Tanja Schad, BSc, Thomas H. Schürmeyer, Ph.D., M.D., and Ulrike Ehlert, Ph.D., "Hypothalamic-Pituitary-Adrenal Axis Reactivity in Chronic Fatigue Syndrome and Health Under Psychological, Physiological, and Pharmacological Stimulation," *Psychosomatic Medicine* 64: 951–962 (2002).

13. E. N. Griep, J. W. Boersma, and E. R. de Kloet, "Altered Reactivity of the Hypothalamic-Pituitary-Adrenal Axis in the Primary Fibromyalgia Syndrome," *J Rheumatol* 1993; 20: 469–474.

14. A. J. Cleare, D. Blair, S. Chambers, and S. Wessely, "Urinary Free Cortisol in Chronic Fatigue Syndrome," *Am J Psychiatry* 158: 641–643, April 2001.

15. A. J. Cleare et al., "Hypothalamo-Pituitary-Adrenal Axis Dysfunction in Chronic Fatigue Syndrome, and the Effects of Low-Dose Hydrocortisone Therapy," *Journal of Clinical Endocrinology & Metabolism* 2001; 86 (8): 3545–3554.

16. A. J. Cleare et al., "Low-Dose Hydrocortisone in Chronic Fatigue Syndrome: A Randomized Crossover Trial," *The Lancet* 1999 February 6; 353 (9151): 455–458.

17. J. Gaab, D. Huster, R. Peisen, V. Engert, T. Schad, T. H. Schurmeyer, and U. Ehlert, "Low-Dose Dexamethasone Suppression Test in Chronic Fatigue Syndrome and Health," *Psychosom Med.* 2002 March–April; 64 (2): 311–318.

18. M. Altemus, J. K. Dale, D. Michelson, M. A. Demitrack, P. W. Gold, and S. E. Straus, "Abnormalities in Response to Vasopressin Infusion in Chronic Fatigue Syndrome," *Psychoneuroendocrinology* 2001 February 1; 26 (2): 175–188.

19. L. V. Scott, F. Svec, and T. Dinan, "A Preliminary Study of Dehydroepiandrosterone Response to Low-Dose ACTH in Chronic Fatigue Syndrome and in Healthy Subjects," *Psychiatry Res* 2000 December 4; 97 (1): 21–28.

20. L. V. Scott, J. Teh, R. Reznek, A. Martin, A. Sohaib, and T. G. Dinan, "Small Adrenal Glands in Chronic Fatigue Syndrome: A Preliminary Computer Tomography Study," *Psychoneuroendocrinology* 1999 October; 24 (7): 759–768.

21. C. Heim, U. Ehlert, and D. H. Hellhammer, "The Potential Role of Hypocortisolism in the Pathophysiology of Stress-Related Bodily Disorders," *Psychoneuroendocrinology* 2000 January; 25 (1).

22. L. V. Scott, S. Medbak, and T. G. Dinan, "Desmopressin Augments Pituitary-Adrenal Responsivity to Corticotropin-Releasing Hormone in Subjects with Chronic Fatigue Syndrome and in Healthy Volunteers," *Biol Psychiatry* 1999 June 1; 45 (11): 1447–1454.

23. P. de Becker, K. de Meirleir, E. Joos, I. Campine, E. van Steenberge, J. Smitz, and B. Velkeniers, "Dehydroepiandrosterone (DHEA) Response to IV ACTH in Patients with Chronic Fatigue Syndrome," *Horm Metab Res* 1999 January; 31 (1): 18–21.

24. L. Crofford, "The Hypothalamic-Pituitary-Adrenal Stress Axis in Fibromyalgia and Chronic Fatigue Syndrome," *J Rheumatol* 1998; 57 supplement 2: 67–71.

25. H. Kuratsune, K. Yamaguti, M. Sawada, S. Kodate, T. Machii, Y. Kanakura, and T. Kitani, "Dehydroepiandrosterone Sulfate Deficiency in Chronic Fatigue Syndrome," *Int J Mol Med* 1998 January; 1 (1): 143–146.

26. L. V. Scott, S. Medbak, and T. G. Dinan, "The Low-dose ACTH Test in Chronic Fatigue Syndrome and in Health," *Clin Endocrinol* (Oxf) 1998 June; 48 (6): 733–737.

27. L. V. Scott, S. Medbak, and T. G. Dinan, "Blunted Adrenocorticotropin and Cortisol Responses to Corticotropin-Releasing Hormone Stimulation in Chronic Fatigue Syndrome," *Acta Psychiatr Scand* 1998 June; 97 (6): 450–457.

28. P. Strickland, R. Morriss, A. Wearden, and B. A. Deakin, "Comparison of Salivary Cortisol in Chronic Fatigue Syndrome, Community Depression and Healthy Controls," *J Affect Disord* 1998 January; 47 (1–3): 191–194.

29. P. Strickland, R. Morriss, A. Wearden, and B. A. Deakin, "Comparison of Salivary Cortisol in Chronic Fatigue Syndrome, Community Depression and Healthy Controls," *J Affect Disord* 1998 January; 47 (1–3): 191–194.

30. W. Jefferies, "Mild Adrenocortical Deficiency, Chronic Allergies, Autoimmune Disorders and the Chronic Fatigue Syndrome: A Continuation of the Cortisone Story," *Med Hypotheses* 1994, Issue 3, Vol. 42, pp. 183–189, ISSN: 0306–9877.

31. A. J. Cleare, J. Bearn, T. Allain, A. McGregor, S. Wessely, R. M. Murray, and V. O'Keane, "Contrasting Neuroendocrine Responses in Depression and Chronic Fatigue Syndrome," *J Affect Disord* 1995 Aug. 18, Issue 4, Vol. 34, pp. 283–289.

32. M. Moutschen, J. M. Triffaux, J. Demonty, J. J. Legros, and P. J. Lefèbvre, "Pathogenic Tracks in Fatigue Syndromes," *Acta Clin Belg* 1994, Issue 6, Vol. 49, pp. 274–289, ISSN: 0001–5512.

33. Carruthers et al., "Myalgic Encepalomyelitis/Chronic Fatigue Syndrome: Clinical Working Case Definition, Diagnostic and Treatment Protocols," *Journal of Chronic Fatigue Syndrome*, Vol. 11 (1) 2003.

34. M. A. Demitrack and L. J. Crofford, "Evidence for and Pathophysiologic Implications of Hypothalamic-Pituitary-Adrenal Axis Dysregulation in Fibromyalgia and Chronic Fatigue Syndrome," *Ann N Y Acad Sci* 1998 May 1; 840: 684–697.

35. W. Jefferies, "Cortisol and Immunity," *Medical Hypotheses* 1991; 34: 198–208.

37. A. J. Cleare, D. Blair, S. Chambers, and S. Wessely, "Urinary Free Cortisol in Chronic Fatigue Syndrome," *Am J Psychiatry* 158: April 2001, 641–643.

38. M. A. Demitrack, J. K. Dale, S. E. Straus, L. Laue, S. J. Listwak, M.J.P. Kruesi, et al., "Evidence for Impaired Activation of the Hypothalamic-Pituitary-Adrenal Axis in Patients with Chronic Fatigue Syndrome," *J Clin Endocrinol Metab* 1991; 73: 1224–1234.

39. K. Tordjman, A. Jaffe, and N. Grazas, et al., "The Role of the Low-Dose (1 mg) Adrenocorticotropin Test in the Evaluation of Patients with Pituitary Diseases," *J Clin Endocrinol Metab* 1995; 80: 1301–1305.

40. G. Dickstein, C. Schechner, W. E. Nicholson, et al., "Adrenocorticotropin Stimulation Test: Effects of Basal Cortisol Level, Time of the Day, and Suggested New Sensitive Low Dose Test," *J Clin Endocrinol Metab* 1991; 72: 773–778.

41. S. Crowley, P. C. Hindmarsh, J. W. Honour, C.G.D. Brook, "Reproducibility of the Cortisol Response to Stimulation with a Low Dose of ACTH (1–24): The Effect of Basal Cortisol Levels and Comparison of Low Dose with High Dose Secretory Dynamics," *J Endocrinol* 1993; 136: 167–172.

42. J. Baraia-Etxaburu Artetxe, B. Astigarraga Aguirre, R. Elorza Olabegova, et al., "Primary Adrenal Failure and AIDS: Report of Eleven Cases and Review of the Literature," *Rev Clin Esp* 1998; 198: 74–79.

43. M. Zarkovic, J. Ciric, M. Stojanovic, et al., "Optimizing the Diagnostic Criteria for Standard (250-mg) and Low Dose (1-mg) Adrenocorticotropin Tests in the Assessment of Adrenal Function," *J Clin Endocrinol Metab* 1999; 84: 3170–3173.

44. T. A. Abdu, T. A. Elhadd, R. Neary, and R. N. Clayton, "Comparison of the Low-Dose Short Synacthen Test (1 mg), the Conventional Dose Short Synacthen Test (250 mg), and the Insulin Tolerance Test for Assessment of the Hypothalamo-Pituitary-Adrenal Axis in Patients with Pituitary Disease," *J Clin Endocrinol Metab* 1999; 84: 838–843.

45. Samuel A. McLean, David A. Williams, Richard E. Harris, Willem J. Kop, Kimberly H. Groner, Kirsten Ambrose, Angela K. Lyden, Richard H. Gracely, Leslie J. Crofford, Michael E. Geisser, Ananda Sen, Pinaki Biswas, and Daniel J. Clauw, "Momentary Relationship Between Cortisol Secretion and Symptoms in Patients with Fibromyalgia," *Arthritis & Rheumatism* Vol. 52, No. 11, November 2005, pp. 3660–3669.

46. W. Jefferies, "Mild Adrenocortical Deficiency, Chronic Allergies, Autoimmune Disorders and Chronic Fatigue Syndrome: A Continuation of the Cortisone Story," *Medical Hypotheses* 1994; 42, 183–189.

47. W. Jefferies, "Cortisol and Immunity," *Medical Hypotheses* 1991; 34: 198–208.

48. Riccardo Baschetti, "Investigations of Hydrocortisone and Fludrocortisone in the Treatment of Chronic Fatigue Syndrome," *Journal of Clinical Endocrinology & Metabolism* Vol. 84, No. 6, 2263–2264.

49. R. A. Anderson et al., "Chromium and Hypoglycemia," abstract, *American Journal of Clinical Nutrition* 41 (4) (April 1985): 841.

50. W. M. Jefferies, "Low-Dosage Glucocorticoid Therapy: An Appraisal of Its Safety and Mode of Action in Clinical Disorders, Including Rheumatoid Arthritis," *Archives of Internal Medicine* 119 (3) (March 1967): 265–278.

51. R. McKenzie, A. O'Fallon, J. Dale, et al., "Low-Dose Hydrocortisone for Treatment of Chronic Fatigue Syndrome: A Randomized Controlled Trial," *Journal of the American Medical Association* 280 (12) (23–30 September 1998): 1061–1066.

52. J. E. Teitelbaum, B. Bird, A. Weiss, et al., "Low Dose Hydrocortisone for Chronic Fatigue Syndrome," *Journal of the American Medical Association* 281 (1999): 1887–1888.

53. A. J. Cleare, E. Heap, G. S. Malhi, et al., "Low-Dose Hydrocortisone in CFS: A Randomized Crossover Trial," *The Lancet* 353 (9151) (6 February 1999): 455–458.

54. A. Cleare et al., "Hypothalamo-Pituitary-Adrenal Axis Dysfunction in Chronic Fatigue Syndrome, and the Effects of Low-Dose Hydrocortisone Therapy," *Journal of Clinical Endocrinology & Metabolism* 2001; 86 (8): 3545–3554.

55. J. A. Da Silva, J. W. Jacobs, J. R. Kirwan, M. Boers, K. G. Saag, L. B. Ines, E. J. de Koning, F. Buttgereit, M. Cutolo, H. Capell, R. Rau, J. W. Bijlsma, "Safety of Low Dose Glucocorticoid Treatment in Rheumatoid Arthritis: Published Evidence and Prospective Trial Data," *Ann Rheum Dis.* 2006 March; 65 (3): 285–293, E-published August 17, 2005.

56. *Principles and Practice of Endocrinology and Metabolism*, 3rd ed., Kenneth Becker, ed. (Philadelphia: Lippincott, Williams & Wilkins, 2001).

57. P. M. J. Zelissen, R. J. Croughs, P. P. van Rijk, et al., "Effect of Glucocorticoid Replacement Therapy on Bone Mineral Density in Patients with Addison Disease," *Annals of Internal Medicine* 120 (3) (1 February 1994): 207–210.

58. A. Susmano, A. S. Volgman, and T. A. Buckingham, "Beneficial Effects of Dextro-Amphetamine in the Treatment of Vasodepressor Syncope," *Pacing and Clinical Electrophysiology* 16 (1993): 1235–1239.

59. B. P. Grubb, D. A. Wolfe, D. Samoil, et al., "Usefulness of Fluoxetine Hydrochloride for Prevention of Resistant Upright Tilt Induced Syncope," *Pacing and Clinical Electrophysiology* 16 (1993): 458–464.

60. B. P. Grubb, D. Samoil, D. Kosinski, et al., "Use of Sertraline Hydrochloride in the Treatment of Refractory Neurocardiogenic Syncope in Children and Adolescents," *Journal of the American College of Cardiology* 24 (1994): 490–494.

61. P. C. Rowe, I. Bou-Holaigah, J. S. Kan, et al., "Is Neurally Mediated Hypotension an Unrecognized Cause of Chronic Fatigue?" *The Lancet* 345 (8950) (11 March 1995): 623–624.

62. O. Ozerbil, N. Okudan, H. Gokbel, and F. Levendoglu, "Comparison of the Effects of Two Antidepressants on Exercise Performance of the Female Patients with Fibromyalgia," *Clin Rheumatol* 2005 November 3: 1–3 (E-published ahead of print).

63. D. Blockmans, P. Persoons, B. van Houdenhove, and H. Bobbaers, "Does Methylphenidate Reduce the Symptoms of Chronic Fatigue Syndrome?" *Am J Med* 2006 February; 119 (2): 167.

64. A. W. Meikle, R. A. Daynes, B. A. Araneo, et al., "Adrenal Androgen Secretion and Biologic Effects," *Endocrine and Metabolic Clinics of North America* 20 (2) (June 1991): 381–421.

65. L. N. Parker, "Control of Adrenal Androgen Secretion," *Endocrine and Metabolic Clinics of North America* 20 (2) (June 1991): 401–421.

66. E. Barrett-Connor, R. T. Khaw, and S. C. Yen, "A Prospective Study of DHEA, Mortality and Cardiovascular Disease," *New England Journal of Medicine* 315 (1986): 1519–1524.

67. M. L. Lydic, M. McNurlan, et al., "Chromium Picolinate Improves Insulin Sensitivity in Obese Subjects with Polycystic Ovary Syndrome," *Fertil Steril*, 2006; 86 (1): 243–246.

68. G. R. Skinner, R. Thomas, M. Taylor, et al., "Thyroxine Should Be Tried in Clinically Hypothyroid but Biochemically Euthyroid Patients," *British Medical Journal* 314 (7096) (14 June 1997): 1764.

69. G. R. B. Skinner, D. Holmes, A. Ahmad, et al., "Clinical Response to Thyroxine Sodium in Clinically Hypothyroid but Biochemically Euthyroid Patients," *Journal of Nutritional and Environmental Medicine* 10 (2) (June 2000): 115–125.

70. R. A. Nordyke, T. S. Reppun, L. D. Madanay, et al., "Alternative Sequences of Thyrotropin and Free Thyroxine Assays for Routine Thyroid Function Testing: Quality and Cost," *Archives of Internal Medicine* 158 (3) (9 February 1998): 266–272.

70A. L. Hallberg, "Does Calcium Interfere with Iron Absorption?" editorial, *American Journal of Clinical Nutrition* 68 (1) (July 1998): 3–4.

71. J. G. Travell and D. G. Simons, *Myofascial Pain and Dysfunction: The Trigger Point Manual*, Vol. 1 (Baltimore, MD: Williams & Wilkins, 1983), pp. 103–164.

72. J. C. Lowe, R. L. Garrison, A. J. Reichman, et al., "Effectiveness and Safety of T_3 Therapy for Euthyroid Fibromyalgia: A Double-Blind, Placebo-Controlled Response Driven Crossover Study," *Clinical Bulletin of Myofascial Therapy* 2 (2/3) (1997): 31–58.

73. J. C. Lowe, A. J. Reichman, and J. Yellin, "The Process of Change During T_3 Treatment for Euthyroid Fibromyalgia: A Double-Blind, Placebo-Controlled, Crossover Study," *Clinical Bulletin of Myofascial Therapy* 2 (2/3) (1997): 91–124.

74. E. Vliet, *Screaming to Be Heard: Hormonal Connections Women Suspect . . . and Doctors Ignore* (New York: M. Evans and Co., 2001).

75. T. G. Travison, A. B. Araujo, A. B. O'Donnell, et al., "A Population-Level Decline in Serum Testosterone Levels in American Men," *J Clin Endocrin Metab*, first published ahead of print October 24, 2006 as doi: 10.1210.

76. http://www.dartmouth.edu/~news/releases/2003/april/040703a.html

77. Unpublished data from our research center.

78. http://www.medscape.com/viewarticle/544182

79. H. Burger, "How Effective Is Testosterone Replacement Therapy in Premenopausal Women with Severe Androgen Deficiency?" *Nat Clin Pract Endocrinol Metab.* 2006; 2 (8): 432–433.

80. http://www.medscape.com/viewarticle/544182

81. H. Burger, "How Effective Is Testosterone Replacement Therapy in Premenopausal Women with Severe Androgen Deficiency?" *Nat Clin Pract Endocrinol Metab.* 2006; 2 (8): 432–433.

82. Shores, *M Arch Intern Med* 2006; 166: 1660–1665.

83. http://www.medscape.com/viewarticle/543797

84. http://www.ncbi.nlm.nih.gov/entrez/query.fcgi?cmd=Retrieve&db=pubmed&dopt=Abstract&list_uids=11034937

85. http://www.ncbi.nlm.nih.gov/entrez/query.fcgi?cmd=Retrieve&db=pubmed&dopt=Abstract&list_uids=8222891

86. E. Rhoden, *BJU International* 2005; 98: 867–870.

87. C. J. Malkin, "Testosterone Therapy in Men with Moderate Severity Heart Failure: A Double-Blind Randomized Placebo Controlled Trial," *Eur Heart J*, 2006; 27 (1): 57–64, 44567 (4/2006).

88. C. C. Carson, "Prostate Cancer: Is Testosterone Replacement Therapy a Safety Issue?" *Medical Clinics of North America*, 90 (1) September 2006, 23–27.

89. C. S. Cooper, P. J. Perry, A. E. Sparks, J. H. MacIndoe, W. R. Yates, R. D. Williams, "Effect of Exogenous Testosterone on Prostate Volume, Serum and Semen Prostate Specific Antigen Levels in Healthy Young Men," *J Urol* 1998 February; 159 (2): 441–443.

90. O. N. Pamuk and N. Cakir, "The Variation in Chronic Widespread Pain and Other Symptoms in Fibromyalgia Patients: The Effects of Menses and Menopause," *Clin Exp Rheumatol* 2005 November-December; 23 (6): 778–782.

91. J. S. Jenkins, "The Role of Oxytocin: Present Concepts," *Clinical Endocrinology* 34 (1991): 515–525.

92. M. L. Vance, "Hypopituitarism," *New England Journal of Medicine* 330 (23) (9 June 1994): 1651–1662.

93. S. Pillemer, L. A. Bradley, L. J. Crofford, et al., "The Neuroscience and Endocrinology of FMS—[An NIH] Conference Summary," *Arthritis and Rheumatism* 40 (11) (November 1997): 1928–1939.

94. A. M. O. Bakheit, P. O. Behan, W. S. Watson, et al., "Abnormal Arginine-Vasopressin Secretion and Water Metabolism in Patients with Postviral Fatigue Syndrome," *Acta Neurologica Scandinavica* 87 (3) (March 1993): 234–238.

95. P. C. Rowe, H. Calkins, K. DeBusk, et al., "Fludrocortisone Acetate to Treat Neurally Mediated Hypotension in Chronic Fatigue Syndrome: A Randomized Controlled Trial," *Journal of the American Medical Association* 285 (1) (3 January 2001): 52–59.

ARTICLE ON SAFETY OF BIOIDENTICAL HORMONES AT THE END OF CHAPTER 4

1. H. J. Chang and T. T. Y. Lee, et al., "Influences of Percutaneous Administration of Estradiol and Progesterone on Human Breast Epithelial Cell Cycle in Vivo," *Fertil Steril* 1995; 63: 785–791.

2. L. A. Fitzpatrick et al. "Comparison of Regimens Containing Oral Micronized Progesterone of Medroxyprogesterone Acetate on Quality of Life in Postmenopausal Women: A Cross-Sectional Survey," *J Womens Health Gen Based Med* 2000 May; 9(4): 381–387.

3. Gompel et al. "Antiestrogen Action of Progesterone in Breast Tissue," *Breast Cancer Res Treat* 1986; 8 (3): 179–188.

4. Van der Burg et al. "Effects of Progestins on the Proliferation of Estrogen-Dependent Human Breast Cancer Cells Under Growth Factor-defined Conditions," *J Steroid Biochem Mol Biol* 1992 June; 42 (5): 457–465.

5. J. A. Mol, E. van Garderen, G. R. Rutteman, and A. Rijnberk, "New Insights in the Molecular Mechanism of Progestin-Induced Proliferation of Mammary Epithelium: Induction of the Local Biosynthesis of Growth Hormone (GH) in the Mammary

Glands of Dogs, Cats and Humans," *J Steroid Biochem Mol Biol* 1996 January; 57 (1–2): 67–71.

6. B. S. Hulka, "Links Between Hormone Replacement Therapy and Neoplasia," *Fertil Steril* 1994 December; 62 (6 supplement 2): 168S–175S.

7. L. J. Hofseth, A. M. Raafat, J. R. Osuch, D. R. Pathak, C. A. Slomski, and S. Z. Haslam, "Hormone Replacement Therapy with Estrogen or Estrogen Plus Medroxyprogesterone Acetate Is Associated with Increased Epithelial Proliferation in the Normal Postmenopausal Breast." *J Clin Endocrinol Metab* 1999 December; 84 (12): 4559–4565.

8. J. M. Foidart, C. Colin, X. Denoo, J. Desreux, A. Beliard, S. Fournier, and B. de Lignieres, "Estradiol and Progesterone Regulate the Proliferation of Human Breast Epithelial Cells," *Fertil Steril* 1998 May; 69 (5): 963–969.

9. G. A. Colditz and B. Rosner, "Cumulative Risk of Breast Cancer to Age 70 Years According to Risk Factor Status: Data from the Nurses' Health Study," *Am J Epidemiol* 2000 November 15; 152 (10): 950–964.

10. R. K. Ross, A. Paganini-Hill, P. C. Wan, and M. C. Pike, "Effect of Hormone Replacement Therapy on Breast Cancer Risk: Estrogen Versus Estrogen Plus Progestin," *J Natl Cancer Inst* 2000 February 16; 92 (4): 328–332.

12. "Estrogen Replacement Therapy and Heart Disease: A Discussion of the PEPI Trial," Women's Health Information Center.

13. K. Miyagawa, J. Rosch, F. Stanczyk, and K. Hermsmeyer, "Medroxyprogesterone Interferes with Ovarian Steroid Protection Against Coronary Vasospasm," *Nat Med* 1997 March; 3 (3): 324–327.

14. G. M. Rosano, C. M. Webb, S. Chierchia, G. L. Morgani, M. Gabraele, P. M. Sarrel, D. de Ziegler, and P. Collins, "Natural Progesterone, but not Medroxyprogesterone Acetate, Enhances the Beneficial Effect of Estrogen on Exercise-Induced Myocardial Ischemia in Postmenopausal Women," *J Am Coll Cardiol* 2000 December; 36 (7): 2154–2159.

15. T. B. Clarkson, "Progestogens and Cardiovascular Disease: A Critical Review," *J Reprod Med* 1999 February; 44 (2 supplement): 180–184.

16. W. E. Feeman, "Thrombotic Stroke in an Otherwise Healthy Middle-aged Female Related to the Use of Continuous-Combined Conjugated Equine Estrogens and Medroxyprogesterone Acetate," *J Gend Specif Med* 2000 November-December; 3 (8): 62–64; discussion 64–65.

17. R. Sitruk-Ware, "Progestins and Cardiovascular Risk Markers," *Steroids* 2000 October-November; 65 (10–11): 651–658.

18. P. Y. Scarabin, M. Alhenc-Gelas, G. Plu-Bureau, P. Taisne, R. Agher, and M. Aiach, "Effects of Oral and Transdermal Estrogen/Progesterone Regimens on Blood

Coagulation and Fibrinolysis in Postmenopausal Women: A Randomized Controlled Trial," *Arterioscler Thromb Vasc Biol* 1997 November; 17 (11): 3071–3078.

19. G. A. Colditz, "Hormones and Breast Cancer: Evidence and Implications for Consideration of Risks and Benefits of Hormone Replacement Therapy," *J Womens Health* 1999 April; 8 (3): 354–357.

20. F. Zhang, Y. Chen, E. Pisha, L. Shen, Y. Xiong, R. B. van Breemen, and J. L. Bolton, "The Major Metabolite of Equilin, 4-hydroxyequilin, Autoxidizes to an O-quinone Which Isomerizes to the Potent Cytotoxin 4-hydroxyequilenin-O-quinone," *Chem Res Toxicol* 1999 February; 12 (2): 204–213.

21. E. Pisha, X. Lui, A. I. Constantinou, and J. L. Bolton, "Evidence that a Metabolite of Equine Estrogens, 4-hydroxyequilenin, Induces Cellular Transformation in Vitro," *Chem Res Toxicol* 2001 January; 14 (1): 82–90.

22. F. Zhang, S. M. Swanson, R. B. van Breemen, X. Liu, Y. Yang, C. Gu, and J. L. Bolton, "Equine Estrogen Metabolite 4-hydroxyequilenin Induces DNA Damage in the Rat Mammary Tissues: Formation of Single-Strand Breaks, Apurinic Sites, and Stable Adducts, and Oxidized Bases," *Chem Res Toxicol* 2001 December; 14 (12): 1654–1659.

23. V. A. Tzingounis, M. F. Aksu, and R. B. Greenblatt, "Estriol in the Management of the Menopause," *JAMA* 1978 April 21; 239 (16): 1638–1641.

24. H. M. Lemon, P. F. Kumar, C. Peterson, J. F. Rodriguez-Sierra, and K. M. Abbo, "Inhibition of Radiogenic Mammary Carcinoma in Rats by Estriol or Tamoxifen," *Cancer* 1989 May 1; 63 (9): 1685–1692.

25. H. M. Lemon, H. H. Wotiz, L. Parsons, and P. J. Mozden, "Reduced Estriol Excretion in Patients with Breast Cancer Prior to Endocrine Therapy," *JAMA* 1966 June 27; 196 (13): 1128–1136.

26. H. M. Lemon, "Pathophysiologic Considerations in the Treatment of Menopausal Patients with Oestrogens: The Role of Oestriol in the Prevention of Mammary Carcinoma," *Acta Endocrinol Supplement* 1980; 233: 17–27. DNH

27. A. H. Follingstad, "Estriol: The Forgotten Estrogen," *JAMA* January 2, 1978; 239 (1): 29–30.

28. S. Kim, S. M. Liva, M. A. Dalal, M. A. Verity, and R. R. Voskuhl, "Estriol Ameliorates Autoimmune Demyelinating Disease: Implications for Multiple Sclerosis," *Neurology* 1999 April 12; 52 (6): 1230–1238.

29. S. Bansil, H. J. Lee, S. Jindal, C. R. Holtz, and S. D. Cook, "Correlation Between Sex Hormones and Magnetic Resonance Imaging Lesions in Multiple Sclerosis," *Acta Neurol Scand* 1999 February; 99 (2): 91–94.

30. L. D. Cowan, L. Gordis, J. A. Tonascia, and G. S. Jones, "Breast Cancer Incidence in Women with a History of Progesterone Deficiency," *Am J Epidemiol* 1981 August; 114 (2): 209–217.

31. A. Inoh, K. Kamiya, Y. Fujii, and K. Yokoro, "Protective Effects of Progesterone and Tamoxifen in Estrogen-Induced Mammary Carcinogenesis in Ovariectomized W/Fu Rats," *Jpn J Cancer Res* 1985 August; 76 (8): 699–704.

32. M. Otsuki, H. Saito, X. Xu, S. Sumitani, H. Kouhara, T. Kishimoto, and S. Kasayama, "Progesterone, but not Medroxyprogesterone, Inhibits Vascular Cell Adhesion Molecule-1 Expression in Human Vascular Endothelial Cells," *Arterioscler Thromb Vasc Biol* 2001 February; 21 (2): 243–248.

33. H. A. Braunsberg, N. G. Coldham, and W. Wong, "Hormonal Therapies for Breast Cancer: Can Progestogens Stimulate Growth?" *Cancer Lett* 1986 February; 30 (2): 213–218.

34. "Effects of Estrogen or Estrogen/Progestin Regimens on Heart Disease Risk Factors in Postmenopausal Women," The Postmenopausal Estrogen/Progestin Interventions (PEPI) Trial. The Writing Group for the PEPI Trial, *JAMA* 1995 January 18; 273 (3): 199–208.

35. News conference at the American Heart Association Annual Meeting, November 17, 1994.

36. J. T. Hargrove et al., "Menopausal Hormone Replacement Therapy with Continuous Daily Oral Mircronized Progesterone," *Obstet Gyn* 1989; 73: 606–612.

37. J. T. Hargrove and K. G. Osteen, "An Alternative Method of Hormone Replacement Therapy Using the Natural Sex Steroids," *Infertile Repro Med Clinics North Am.* 1995; 6: 563–674. DNH

38. J. T. Hargrove and E. Eisenberg, *Menopause. Med. Clinics North Am* 1995; 79: 1337–1356.

39. H. M. Lemon, "Antimammary Carcinogenic Activity of 17-alpha-ethnyl Estriol," *Cancer* 1987; 60: 2873–2881.

40. J. Schneider, M. M. Huh, H. L. Bradlow, and J. Fishman, "Antiestrogen Action of 2-hydroxyestrone on MCF-7 Human Breast Cancer Cells," *J Biol Chem* 1984; 259: 4840–4845.

41. B. Vandewalle and J. Lefebvre, "Opposite Effects of Estrogen and Catechol Estrogen on Hormone-Sensitive Breast Cancer Cell Growth and Differentiation," *Mol Cell Endocrinol* 1989; 61: 239–246.

42. H. L. Bradlow, N. T. Telang, D. W. Sepkovic, and M. P. Osborne, "2-hydroxyestrone: The 'Good' Estrogen," *J Endocrinol* 1996; 150: Supplement S259–S265.

43. J. Fishman and C. Martucci, "Biological Properties of 16-alpha-hydroxyestrone: Implications in Estrogen Physiology and Pathophysiology," *J Clin Endocrinol Metab* 1980; 51: 611–615. DNH

44. J. Schneider, D. Kinne, A. Fracchia, V. Pierce, K. E. Anderson, H. L. Bradlow, and J. Fishman, "Abnormal Oxidative Metabolism of Estradiol in Women with Breast Cancer," *Proc Natl Acad Sci USA* 1982; 79: 3047–3051.DNH

45. M. P. Osborne, H. L. Bradlow, G. Y. C. Wong, and N. T. Telang, "Upregulation of Estradiol C16 Alpha-hydroxylation in Human Breast Tissue: A Potential Biomarker of Breast Cancer Risk," *J Natl Cancer Inst* 1993; 85: 1917–1920.

46. H. L. Bradlow, R. J. Hershcopf, C. P. Martucci, and J. Fishman, "Estradiol 16-hydroxylation in the Mouse Correlates with Mammary Tumor Incidence and Presence of Murine Mammary Tumor Virus: A Possible Model for the Hormonal Etiology of Breast Cancer in Humans," *Proc Natl Acad Sci USA* 1985; 82: 6295–6299.

47. N. T. Telang, A. Suto, G. Y. Wong, M. P. Osborne, and H. L. Bradlow, "Induction by Estrogen Metabolite 16 Alpha-hydroxyestrone of Genotoxic Damage and Aberrant Cell Proliferation in Mouse Mammary Epithelial Cells in Culture," *J Natl Cancer Inst* 1992; 82: 634–638.

48. G. C. Kabat, C. J. Chang, J. A. Sparano, D. W. Sepkovic, X. P. Hu, A. Khalil, R. Rosenblatt, and H. L. Bradlow, "Urinary Estrogen Metabolites and Breast Cancer: A Case-Control Study," *Cancer Epidemiol Biomark Prev* 1997; 6: 505–509.

49. B. de Lignieres, "Oral Micronized Progesterone," *Clin Ther* 1999 January; 21 (1): 41–60.

50. L. A. Fitzpatrick and A. Good, "Micronized Progesterone: Clinical Indications and Comparison with Current Treatment," *Fertil Steril* 1999 September; 72 (3): 389–397.

51. M. R. Adams, T. C. Register, D. L. Golden, J. D. Wagner, and J. K. Williams, "Medroxyprogesterone Acetate Antagonizes Inhibitory Effects of Conjugated Equine Estrogens on Coronary Artery Atherosclerosis," *Arterioscler Thromb Vasc Biol* 1997 January; 17 (1): 217–221 (ISSN: 1079–5642).

52. J. D. Wagner, M. A. Martino, M. J. Jayo, M. S. Anthony, T. B. Clarkson, and W. T. Cefalu, "The Effects of Hormone Replacement Therapy on Carbohydrate Metabolism and Cardiovascular Risk Factors in Surgically Postmenopausal Cynomolgus Monkeys," *Metabolism* 1996 October; 45 (10): 1254–1262.

53. R. L. Levine, S. J. Chen, J. Durand, Y. F. Chen, and S. Oparil, "Medroxyprogesterone Attenuates Estrogen-Mediated Inhibition of Neointima Formation After Balloon Injury of the Rat Carotid Artery," *Circulation* 1996 November 1; 94 (9): 2221–2227.

54. T. C. Register, M. R. Adams, D. L. Golden, and T. B. Clarkson, "Conjugated Equine Estrogens Alone, But not in Combination with Medroxyprogesterone Acetate, Inhibit Aortic Connective Tissue Remodeling After Plasma Lipid Lowering in Female Monkeys," *Arterioscler Thromb Vasc Biol* 1998 July; 18 (7): 1164–1171.

55. M. C. Pike and R. K. Ross, "Progestins and Menopause: Epidemiological Studies of Risks of Endometrial and Breast Cancers," *Steroids* 2000; 65: 659–664.

56. B. MacMahon, P. Cole, J. B. Brown, K. Aoki, T. M. Lin, R. W. Morgan, and N. Woo, "Oestrogen Profiles of Asian and North American Women," *The Lancet* 1971 October 23; 2 (7,730): 900–902.

57. H. M. Lemon, "Genetic Predisposition to Carcinoma of the Breast: Multiple Human Genotypes for Estrogen 16 alpha-hydroxylase Activity in Caucasians," *J Surg Oncol* 1972; 4 (3): 255–273.

58. H. M. Lemon, "Oestriol and Prevention of Breast Cancer." *The Lancet* 1973; March 10: 546–547.

59. R. D. Bulbrook, M. C. Swain, D. Y. Wang, J. L. Hayward, S. Kumaoka, O. Takatani, O. Abe, and J. Utsunomiya, "Breast Cancer in Britain and Japan: Plasma Oestradiol-17 beta, Oestrone and Progesterone, and Their Urinary Metabolites in Normal British and Japanese Women," *Eur J Cancer* 1976 September; 12 (9): 725–735.

60. L. Speroff, "The Breast As an Endocrine Target Organ," *Contemp Obst Gyn* 1977 9: 69–72. DNH

61. M. R. Adams, et al., "Inhibition of Coronary Artery Athrosclerosis by 17-beta Estradiol in Ovariectomized Monkeys: Lack of an Effect of Added Progesterone," *Arteriosclerosis* 1990; 10: 1051–1057.

62. W. N. Spellacy, "A Review of Carbohydrate Metabolism and the Oral Contraceptives," *Am J Obstet Gynecol* 1969 June 1; 104 (3): 448–460.

63. M. J. Tikkanen, T. Kuusi, E. A. Nikkila, and S. Sipinen, "Post-menopausal Hormone Replacement Therapy: Effects of Progestogens on Serum Lipids and Lipoproteins: A Review," *Maturitas* 1986 March; 8 (1): 7–17.

64. H. H. Newham, "Oestrogens and Atherosclerotic Vascular Disease: Lipid Factors," *Baillieres Clin Endo Metab* 1993; 7: 61–93.

65. R. A. Lobo, "The Role of Progestins in Hormone Replacement Therapy," *Am J Obstet Gynecol* 1992 June; 166 (6 Pt 2): 1997–2004.

66. I. I. Bolaji, H. Grimes, G. Mortimer, D. F. Tallon, P. F. Fottrell, and E. M. O'Dwyer, "Low-Dose Progesterone Therapy in Oestrogenised Postmenopausal Women: Effects on Plasma Lipids, Lipoproteins and Liver Function Parameters," *Eur J Obstet Gynecol Reprod Biol* 1993 January; 48 (1): 61–68.

67. S. Moorjani, A. Dupont, F. Labrie, B. De Lignieres, L. Cusan, P. Dupont, J. Mailloux, and P. J. Lupien, "Changes in Plasma Lipoprotein and Apolipoprotein Composition in Relation to Oral Versus Percutaneous Administration of Estrogen Alone or in Cyclic Association with Utrogestan in Menopausal Women," *J Clin Endocrinol Metab* 1991 August; 73 (2): 373–379.

68. R. D. Minshall, K. Miyagawa, C. C. Chadwick, M. J. Novy, and K. Hermsmeyer, "In Vitro Modulation of Primate Coronary Vascular Muscle Cell Reactivity by Ovarian Steroid Hormones," *FASEB J* 1998 October; 12 (13): 1419–1429.

69. R. D. Minshall, F. Z. Stanczyk, K. Miyagawa, B. Uchida, M. Axthelm, M. Novy, and K. Hermsmeyer, "Ovarian Steroid Protection Against Coronary Artery

Hyperreactivity in Rhesus Monkeys," *J Clin Endocrinol Metab* 1998 February; 83 (2): 649–659.

70. L. Fahraeus, U. Larsson-Cohn, and L. Wallentin, "L-norgestrel and Progesterone Have Different Influences on Plasma Lipoproteins," *Eur J Clin Invest* 1983 December; 13 (6): 447–453.

71. J. Jensen, B. J. Riis, V. Strom, L. Nilas, and C. Christiansen, "Long-term Effects of Percutaneous Estrogens and Oral Progesterone on Serum Lipoproteins in Postmenopausal Women," *Am J Obstet Gynecol* 1987 January; 156 (1): 66–71.

72. U. B. Ottosson, B. G. Johansson, and B. von Schoultz, "Subfractions of High-Density Lipoprotein Cholesterol During Estrogen Replacement Therapy: A Comparison Between Progestogens and Natural Progesterone," *Am J Obstet Gynecol* 1985 March 15; 151 (6): 746–750.

73. K. E. Elkind-Hirsch, L. D. Sherman, and R. Malinak, "Hormone Replacement Therapy Alters Insulin Sensitivity in Young Women with Premature Ovarian Failure," *J Clin Endocrinol Metab* 1993 February; 76 (2): 472–475.

74. T. L. Bush, E. Barrett-Connor, L. D. Cowan, M. H. Criqui, R. B. Wallace, C. M. Suchindran, H. A. Tyroler, and B. M. Rifkind, "Cardiovascular Mortality and Noncontraceptive Use of Estrogen in Women: Results from the Lipid Research Clinics Program Follow-up Study," *Circulation* 1987 June; 75 (6): 1102–1109.

75. I. F. Godsland, K. Gangar, C. Walton, M. P. Cust, M. I. Whitehead, V. Wynn, and J. C. Stevenson, "Insulin Resistance, Secretion, and Elimination in Postmenopausal Women Receiving Oral or Rransdermal Hormone Replacement Therapy," *Metabolism* 1993 July; 42 (7): 846–853.

76. A. K. Morey, A. Pedram, M. Razandi, B. A. Prins, R. M. Hu, E. Biesiada, and E. R. Levin, "Estrogen and Progesterone Inhibit Vascular Smooth Muscle Proliferation," *Endocrinology* 1997 August; 138 (8): 3330–3339.

77. W. S. Lee, J. A. Harder, M. Yoshizumi, M. E. Lee, and E. Haber, "Progesterone Inhibits Arterial Smooth Muscle Cell Proliferation," *Nat Med* 1997 September; 3 (9): 1005–1008.

78. G. A. Colditz, S. E. Hankinson, D. J. Hunter, W. C. Willett, J. E. Manson, M. J. Stampfer, C. Hennekens, B. Rosner, and F. E. Speizer, "The Use of Estrogens and Progestins and the Risk of Breast Cancer in Postmenopausal Women," *N Engl J Med* 1995 June 15; 332 (24): 1589–1593.

79. B. von Schoultz, G. Soderqvist, M. Cline, E. von Schoultz, and L. Skoog, "Hormonal Regulation of the Normal Breast," *Maturitas* 1996 May; 23 supplement: S23–S25.

80. Y. Chen, X. Liu, E. Pisha, A. I. Constantinou, Y. Hua, L. Shen, R. B. van Breemen, E. C. Elguindi, S. Y. Blond, F. Zhang, and J. L. Bolton, "A Metabolite of Equine

Estrogens, 4-hydroxyequilenin, Induces DNA Damage and Apoptosis in Breast Cancer Cell Lines," *Chem Res Toxicol* 2000 May; 13 (5): 342–350.

81. J. Desreux, F. Kebers, A. Noel, D. Francart, H. Van Cauwenberge, V. Heinen, J. L. Thomas, A. M. Bernard, J. Paris, R. Delansorne, and J. M. Foidart, "Progesterone Receptor Activation: An Alternative to SERMs in Breast Cancer," *Eur J Cancer* 2000 September; 36 supplement 4: S90–S91.

Chapter 5. I—Infections:
Destroy Your Body's Hidden Invaders

1. J. R. Quesada, M. Talpaz, A. Rios, et al., "Clinical Toxicity of Interferon in Cancer Patients: A Review," *Journal of Clinical Oncology* 4 (February 1986): 234–243; and F. Adams, J. R. Quesada, and J. U. Gutterman, "Neuropsychiatric Manifestations of Human Leukocyte Interferon Therapy in Patients with Cancer," *Journal of the American Medical Association* 252 (7) (17 August 1984): 938–941.

2. A. W. Meikle, R. A. Daynes, B. A. Araneo, et al., "Adrenal Androgen Secretion and Biologic Effects," *Endocrine and Metabolic Clinics of North America* 20 (2) (June 1991): 381–421.

3. E. Barker, S. F. Fujimura, M. B. Fadem, et al., "Immunologic Abnormalities Associated with Chronic Fatigue Syndrome," *Clinical Infectious Diseases* 18, supplement 1 (1994): 5,136–5,141.

4. T. Aoki, H. Miyakoshi, Y. Usuda, et al., "Low NK Syndrome and Its Relationship to Chronic Fatigue Syndrome," *Clinical Immunology and Immunopathology* 69 (December 1993): 253–265.

5. B. Evengard, "Comparison of the Composition of Intestinal Microflora of CFS Patients When in the Acute Phase of the Illness," Viral Immune Poster Session Abstract, IACFS Conference. Ft Lauderdale, FL, January 12, 2007.

6. J. E. Teitelbaum, and B. Bird, "Effective Treatment of Severe Chronic Fatigue: A Report of a Series of 64 Patients." *J Musculoskeletal Pain* 1995; 3 (4): 91–110.

7. William G. Crook, *The Yeast Connection and the Woman* (Jackson, TN: Professional Books, 1995).

8. J. Savolainen, K. Lammintausta, K. Kalimo, et al., "Candida Albicans and Atopic Dermatitis," *Clinical Experimental Allergy* 23 (4) (April 1993): 332–339.

9. G. Reid, K. Millsap, and A. P. Bruce, "Implantation of Lactobacillus casei var. Rhamnosus into Vagina," *The Lancet* 344 (8931): 1229.

10. J. Edman, J. D. Sobel, and M. L. Taylor, "Zinc Status in Women with Recurrent Vulvovaginal Candidiasis," *American Journal of Obstetrics and Gynecology* 155 (1986): 1082–1088.

11. S. Naylor, "Role of Fungi in Allergic Fungal Sinusitis and Chronic Rhinosinusitis," *Mayo Clinic Proceedings* 75 (5) (May 2000): 540–541.

12. J. Avorn, M. Monane, J. H. Gurwitz, et al., "Reduction of Bacteriuria and Pyuria After Ingestion of Cranberry Juice," *Journal of the American Medical Association* 271 (10) (9 March 1994): 751–754.

13. S. Toyota, Y. Fukushi, S. Katoh, S. Orikasa, and Y. Suzuki, "Anti-Bacterial Defense Mechanism of the Urinary Bladder, Role of Mannose in Urine" [Article in Japanese], *Nippon Hinyokika Gakkai Zasshi* 1989 December; 80 (12): 1816–1823.

14. "Effect of D-mannose and D-glucose on Escherichia coli Bacteriuria in Rats," *Urol Res* 11 (2): 1983; 97–102.

15. "Mannose-sensitive Adherence of Escherichia coli to Epithelial Cells from Women with Recurrent Urinary Tract Infections," *J Urol* 131 (5): May 1984; 906–910.

16. Procter and Gamble Pharmaceuticals, in-house research data.

17. D. A. Shoskes et al., "Quercetin in Men with Category 3 Chronic Prostatitis: A Preliminary Prospective, Double-Blind, Placebo-Controlled Trial," *Urology*, 1999; 54: 960–963.

18. R. J. Deckelbaum, "ELISA More Accurate Than Microscopy for Giardia," *Infectious Diseases in Children*, October 1993, p. 30.

19. L. Galland, M. Lee, H. Bueno, et al., "Giardia as a Cause of Chronic Fatigue," *Journal of Nutritional Medicine* 1 (1990): 27–32.

20. Ann Louise Gittleman, *Guess What Came to Dinner: Parasites and Your Health* (Garden City Park, NY: Avery Publishing Group, 1993).

21. J. G. Travell and D. G. Simons, *Myofascial Pain and Dysfunction: The Trigger Point Manual*, Vol. I (Baltimore, MD: Williams & Wilkins, 1983), pp. 103–164.

22. J. Dylewski et al., "Absence of Detectable IgM Antibody During Cytomegalovirus Disease in Patients with AIDS," *New England Journal of Medicine* 1985: 309: 493.

23. Carruthers et al., "Myalgic Encephalomyelitis/Chronic Fatigue Syndrome: Clinical Working Case Definition, Diagnostic and Treatment Protocols," *Journal of Chronic Fatigue Syndrome*, Vol. 11 (1) 2003.

24. D. V. Ablashi, C. Zompetta, C. Lease, S. F. Josephs, N. Balachandran, A. L. Komaroff, G. R. F. Krueger, B. Henry, J. Luka, and S. Z. Salahuddin, "Human Herpesvirus-6 (HHV–6) and Chronic Fatigue Syndrome (CFS)," *Canada Disease Weekly Report* 1991; 17SE: 33–40.

25. M. Zorenzenon, G. Rukh, G. A. Botta, et al., "Active HHV–6 Infection in Chronic Fatigue Syndrome Patients from Italy: New data," *J Chron Fatigue Syndr* 1996; 2 (4): 3–12.

26. K. K. Knox, J. H. Brewer, and D. R. Carrigan, "Persistent Active Human Herpesvirus-6 (HHV–6) Infections in Patients with Chronic Fatigue Syndrome," *J Chron Fatigue Syndr* 1999; 5: 245–246.

27. J. H. Brewer, K. K. Knox, and D. R. Carrigan, "Longitudinal Study of Chronic Active Human Herpesvirus-6 (HHV-6) Viremia in Patients with Chronic Fatigue Syndrome," Abstract, IDSA, 37th Annual Meeting, November 18–21, 1999, Philadelphia, PA.

28. Wagner et al., "Chronic Fatigue Syndrome: A Critical Evaluation of Testing for Active Human Herpesvirus-6 Infection. Review of Data of 107 cases," *Journal of Chronic Fatigue Syndrome*; 2 (4) 1996.

29. G. R. F. Krueger, D. V. Ablashi, and R. C. Gallo, "Persistent Herpesvirus Infections: Current Techniques in Diagnosis," *J Virol Methods* 21: 1988; 1–326.

30. R. F. Gerhard et al., "Clinical Correlates of Infection with Human Herpesvirus-6," *In Vivo* 1994; 8: 457–486.

31. D. V. Ablashi et al., "Human Herpes Virus and Chronic Fatigue Syndrome," *Canad Dis Weekly Rep* 1991; 17S1: 33–40.

32. D. V. Albashi et al., "Human, Lymphotropic Virus (Human Herpesvirus-6)," *J Virol Methods* 1988; 21: 29–48.

33. S. F. Josephs et al., "HHV-6 Reactivation in Chronic Fatigue Syndrome," *The Lancet* 1991; 1346–1347.

34. J. Dylewski, S. Chou, and T. C. Merigan, "Absence of Detectable IgM Antibody During Cytomegalovirus Disease in Patients with AIDS," *New England Journal of Medicine*, 1985; 309: 493.

35. G. R. F. Krueger et al., "Overview of Immunopathology of Chronic Active Herpesvirus Infection," *J Virol Methods* 1988; 21: 11–18.

36. J. K. S. Chia, "The Role of Enterovirus in Chronic Fatigue Syndrome," *Journal of Clinical Pathology* 2005; 58: 1126–1132; doi: 10.1136/jcp.2004.020255 2005.

37. J. Brewer, "Treatment of Active HHV-6 Infection with HHV-6 Specific Transfer Factor in Patients with Chronic Fatigue Syndrome," *American Association for Chronic Fatigue Syndrome*, Spring 2004; 203–208.

38. D. Viza, J. M. Vich, J. Phillips, et al., "Orally Administered Specific Transfer Factor for the Treatment of Herpesvirus Infections," *Lymphok Res* 1985; 4: 27–30.

39. H. Fudenberg and G. Pizza, "Transfer Factor 1993: New Frontiers," *Progress in Drug Res* 1994; 42: 309–400.

40. I. Lang, H. Nekam, P. Gergely, et al., "Effect of In Vivo and In Vitro Treatment with Dialyzable Leukocyte Extracts on Human Natural Killer Cell Activity," *Clin Immunol and Immunopathol* 1982; 25: 139–144.

41. G. L. Nicolson, R. Gan, and J. Haier, "Multiple Coinfections (Mycoplasma, Chlamydia, Human Herpes Virus-6) in Blood of Chronic Fatigue Syndrome Patients: Association with Signs and Symptoms," *APMIS*, 2003 May; 111 (5): 557–566.

42. D. Buchwald et al., "A Chronic Illness Characterized by Fatigue, Neurological and Immunological Disorders, and Active Human Herpes Virus 6 Infection," *Annals of Internal Medicine* 1992; 116: 103–113.

43. "HHV-6 Biology, Viruses, and Immunology in Chronic Fatigue Syndrome," IACFS Research Conference, Ft. Lauderdale, FL, January 12–14, 2007.

44. Montoya et al., "Use of Valganciclovir [Valcyte] in Patients with Elevated Antibody Titers Against Human Herpesvirus-6 (HHV-6) and Epstein-Barr Virus (EBV) Who Were Experiencing Central Nervous System Dysfunction Including Long-standing Fatigue," *Journal of Clinical Virology*, December 2006; also presented at the IACFS Research Conference. Fort Lauderdale, FL, January 12–14, 2007.

45. http://www.sciencedaily.com/releases/2005/11/051109181127.htm

Chapter 6. N–Nutrition:
Optimizing Your Body's Ability to Heal

1. R. M. Marston and B. B. Peterkin, "Nutrient Content of the National Food Supply," *National Food Review*, Winter 1980, pp. 21–25.

2. William G. Crook, *The Yeast Connection and the Woman* (Jackson, TN: Professional Books, 1995).

3. R. M. Marston and B. B. Peterkin, op. cit.; and J. H. Nelson, "Wheat: Its Processing and Utilization," *American Journal of Clinical Nutrition* 41, supplement (May 1985): 1070–1076.

4. H. A. Schroeder, "Losses of Vitamins and Trace Minerals Resulting from Processing and Preservation of Foods," *American Journal of Clinical Nutrition* 24 (5) (May 1971): 562–573.

5. H. C. Trowell, ed., *Western Diseases: Their Emergence and Prevention* (Cambridge, MA: Harvard University Press, 1981).

6. S. B. Eaton and N. Konner, "Paleolithic Nutrition. A Consideration of Its Nature and Current Implications," *New England Journal of Medicine* 312 (5) (31 January 1985): 283–289.

7. W. Mertz, ed., "Beltsville 1 Year Dietary Intake Survey," *American Journal of Clinical Nutrition* 40, supplement (December 1984): 1323–1403.

8. B. Bartali et al., "Low Micronutrient Levels as a Predictor of Incident Disability in Older Women," *Arch Intern Med* 2006; 166: 2335–2340.

9. "The Relationship Between Dietary Intake and the Number of Teeth in Elderly Japanese Subjects," *Gerodontology* 2005; 22 (4): 211–218.

10. J. G. Travell and D. G. Simons, *Myofascial Pain and Dysfunction: The Trigger Point Manual*, Vol. I (Baltimore, MD: Williams & Wilkins, 1983), pp. 103–164.

11. S. Ozgocmen, H. Ozyurt, S. Sogut, O. Akyol, O. Ardicoglu, and H. Yildizhan, "Antioxidant Status, Lipid Peroxidation and Nitric Oxide in Fibromyalgia: Etiologic and Therapeutic Concerns," *Rheumatol Int* 2005 November 10; 1–6 (E-pub ahead of print).

12. A. A. Litonjua, S. L. Rifas-Shiman, et al., "Maternal Antioxidant Intake in Pregnancy and Wheezing Illnesses in Children at 2 y of Age," *American Journal of Clinical Nutrition*, 2006; 84 (4): 903–911.

13. S. Hercberg et al., *Arch Intern Med* 2004; 164: 2335–2342.

14. H. J. Kim, M. K. Kim, et al., "Effect of Nutrient Intake and Helicobacter Pylori Infection on Gastric Cancer in Korea: A Case-Control Study," *Nutr Cancer* 2005; 52 (2): 138–146.

15. J. Medina and R. Moreno-Otero, "Pathophysiological Basis for Antioxidant Therapy in Chronic Liver Disease," *Drugs* 2005; 65 (17): 2445–2461.

16. J. Zhang, R. G. Munger, et al., "Antioxidant Intake and Risk of Osteoporotic Hip Fracture in Utah: An Effect Modified by Smoking Status," *Am J Epidemiol* 2006; 163 (1): 9.

17. M. Takumida and M. Anniko, "Radical Scavengers: A Remedy for Presbyacusis: A Pilot Study," *Acta Otolaryngol* 2005; 135 (12): 1290–1295.

18. R. van Leeuwen, S. Boekhoorn, et al., "Dietary Intake of Antioxidants and Risk of Age-Related Macular Degeneration," *JAMA* 2005; 294 (24): 3101–3107.

19. http://www.medscape.com/viewarticle/520823

20. I. S. Kwun, K. H. Park, et al., "Lower Antioxidant Vitamins (A, C and E) and Trace Minerals (Zn, Cu, Mn, Fe and Se) Status in Patients with Cerebrovascular Disease," *Nutr Neurosci*, 2005; 8 (4): 251–257.

21. J. A. Pasco, M. J. Henry, et al., "Antioxidant Vitamin Supplements and Markers of Bone Turnover in a Community Sample of Nonsmoking Women," *J Womens Health* (Larchmont), 2006; 15 (3): 295–300.

22. S. Das, R. Ray, et al., "Effect of Ascorbic Acid on Prevention of Hypercholesterolemia Induced Atherosclerosis," *Mol Cell Biochem* 2006 February 14.

23. http://www.medicalnewstoday.com/medicalnews.php?newsid=40914

24. M. Akmal, J. Q. Qadri, et al., "Improvement in Human Semen Quality After Oral Supplementation of Vitamin C," *J Med Food* 2006; 9 (3): 440–442.

25. S. Sasazuki, S. Sasaki, et al., "Effects of Vitamin C on Common Cold: Randomized Controlled Trial," *European Journal of Clinical Nutrition*, August 24, 2005 (e-published ahead of print).

26. http://www.medscape.com/viewarticle/493649

27. B. T. Drewel, D. W. Giraud, et al., "Less Than Adequate Vitamin E Status Observed in a Group of Preschool Boys and Girls Living in the United States," *The J of Nutr Biochem* 2006; 17 (2): 132–138.

28. http://www.abcnews.go.com/Health/wireStory?id=544848

29. M. P. Malafa, F. D. Fokum, et al., "Vitamin E Succinate Suppresses Prostate Tumor Growth by Inducing Apoptosis," *Int J Cancer* 2005 (E-published ahead of print).

30. P. W. Sylvester and S. J. Shah, "Mechanisms Mediating the Antiproliferative and Apoptotic Effects of Vitamin E in Mammary Cancer Cells," *Front Biosci* 2005 January 1; 10: 699–709.

31. A. Cherubini, A. Martin, et al., "Vitamin E Levels, Cognitive Impairment and Dementia in Older Persons: The InCHIANTI Study," *Neurobiol Aging* 2005; 26 (7): 987–994.

32. Z. El-Akawi, N. Abdel-Latif, et al., "Does the Plasma Level of Vitamins A and E Affect Acne Condition?" *Clin Exp Dermatol* 2006; 31 (3): 430–433.

33. A. L. Ray, R. D. Semba, et al., "Low Serum Selenium and Total Carotenoids Predict Mortality Among Older Women Living in the Community: The Women's Health and Aging Studies," *J Nutr* 2006; 136 (1): 172–176.

34. J. Marniemi, "Dietary and Serum Vitamins and Minerals as Predictors of Myocardial Infarction and Stroke in Elderly Subjects," *Nutr Metab Cardiovasc Dis* 2005 June; 15 (3): 188–197. 43761 (10/2005)

35. S. A. Hanninen, P. B. Darling, et al., "The Prevalence of Thiamin Deficiency in Hospitalized Patients with Congestive Heart Failure," *Journal of the American College of Cardiology* 2006; 47: 354–361.

36. *Neuropsychology* 1995; 32: 98–105.

37. "Thiamine Supplementation, Mood and Cognitive Functioning," *Psychopharmacology* 1997; 129: 66–71. #26997

38. "Red Cell Transketolase Studies in a Private Practice Specializing in Nutritional Correction," *Journal of the American College of Nutrition* 1988; 7 (1): 61–67, and Interview in *Medical Pearls* with Kirk Hamilton #29204.

39. M. Gold, "Plasma and Red Blood Cell Thiamin Deficiency in Patients with Dementia of the Alzheimer's Type," *Archives of Neurology*, November 1995; 52: 1081–1085. #23739

40. Y. Miyake, S. Sasaki, et al., "Dietary Folate and Vitamins B_{12}, B_6, and B_2 Intake and the Risk of Postpartum Depression in Japan: The Osaka Maternal and Child Health Study," *J Affect Disord* 2006 June 29 (E-published ahead of print).

41. http://www.my.webmd.com/content/Article/90/100791.htm

42. Y. Osono, N. Hirose, K. Nakajima, and Y. Hata, "The Effects of Pantethine on Fatty Liver and Fat Distribution," *J Atheroscler Thromb* 2000; 7 (1): 55–58.

43. C. H. Cheng, S. J. Chang, et al., "Vitamin B_6 Supplementation Increases Immune Responses in Critically Ill Patients," *Eur J Clin Nutr* 2006; 60 (10): 1207–1213.

44. P. T. Lin, C. H. Cheng, et al., "Low Pyridoxal 5´Phosphate Is Associated with Increased Risk of Coronary Artery Disease," *Nutrition* 2006 October 9 (E-published ahead of print).

45. http://www.medscape.com/viewarticle/506337; *Gastroenterology* June 2005; 128: 1830–1837.

46. J. Lindenbaum, E. B. Healton, D. G. Savage, et al., "Neuropsychiatric Disorders Caused by Cobalamin Deficiency in the Absence of Anemia or Macrocytoses," *New England Journal of Medicine* 318 (26) (30 June 1988): 1720–1728.

47. J. Lindenbaum, I. H. Rosenberg, P. W. Wilson, et al., "Prevalence of Cobalamin Deficiency in the Framingham Elderly Population," *American Journal of Clinical Nutrition* 60 (1) (July 1994): 2–11.

48. W. S. Beck, "Cobalamin and the Nervous System," editorial, *New England Journal of Medicine* 318 (1988): 1752–1754.

49. D. S. Karnaze and R. Carmel, "Low Serum Cobalamin Levels in Primary Degenerative Dementia: Do Some Patients Harbor Atypical Cobalamin Deficiency States?" *Archives of Internal Medicine* 147 (3) (March 1987): 429–431.

50. B. Regland, M. Andersson, L. Abrahamsson, et al., "Increased Concentrations of Homocysteine in the Cerebrospinal Fluid in Patients with Fibromyalgia and Chronic Fatigue Syndrome," *Scandinavian Journal of Rheumatology* 26 (4) (1997): 301–307.

51. V. Lerner, "Vitamin B_{12} and Folate Serum Levels in Newly Admitted Psychiatric Patients," *Clin Nutr*, 2006 February; 25 (1): 60–67. E-published 2005 October 10. 44868 (6/2006).

52. R. A. Dhonukshe-Rutten et al. "Homocysteine and Vitamin B_{12} Status Relate to Bone Turnover Markers, Broadband Ultrasound Attenuation, and Fractures in Healthy Elderly People," *J Bone Miner Res* 2005 June; 20 (6): 921–929; and M. S. Morris, P. F. Jacques, and J. Selhub, "Relation Between Homocysteine and B-vitamin Status Indicators and Bone Mineral Density in Older Americans," *Bone* 2005; 37 (2).

53. J. Robertson, F. Iemolo, et al., "Vitamin B_{12}, Homocysteine and Carotid Plaque in the Era of Folic Acid Fortification of Enriched Cereal Grain Products," *CMAJ* 2005; 172 (12): 1569–1573.

54. D. E. Diaz, A. M. Tuesta, M. D. Ribo, et al., "Low Levels of Vitamin B_{12} and Venous Thromboembolic Disease in Elderly Men," *Journal of Internal Medicine* 2005; 258 (3): 244–249.

55. M. Lajous et al., "Folate, Vitamin B_6, and Vitamin B_{12} Intake and the Risk of Breast Cancer Among Mexican Women," *Cancer Epidemiology Biomarkers & Prevention*, Vol. 15, March 2006, 443–448.

56. http://www.latimes.com/news/nationworld/nation/wire/ats-ap_health10jun 20,1,7209352.story?coll=sns-ap-tophealth&ctrack=1&cset=true

57. G. Ravaglia, P. Forti, et al., "Homocysteine and Folate as Risk Factors for Dementia and Alzheimer's Disease," *American Journal of Clinical Nutrition* 2005; 82 (3): 636–643; and http://www.lef.org/protocols/prtcl-006.shtml

58. S. Kono and K. Chen, "Genetic Polymorphisms of Methylenetetrahydrofolate Reductase and Colorectal Cancer and Adenoma," *Cancer Science* 2005; 96 (9): 535–542.

59. M. F. Holick, "High Prevalence of Vitamin D Inadequacy and Implications for Health," *Mayo Clin Proc* 2006; 81 (3): 353–373.

60. http://www.medscape.com/viewarticle/529426; and E. Giovannucci, Y. Liu, E. B. Rimm, B. W. Hollis, C. S. Fuchs, M. J. Stampfer, and W. C. Willett, "Prospective Study of Predictors of Vitamin D Status and Cancer Incidence and Mortality in Men," *J Natl Cancer Inst* 2006; 98: 451–459.

61. M. Berwick, *Journal of the National Cancer Institute*, February 2, 2005; Vol. 97: pp. 195–199.

62. Smedby K. Ekström, *Journal of the National Cancer Institute*, February 2, 2005; Vol. 97: pp. 199–209.

63. K. M. Egan, *Journal of the National Cancer Institute*, February 2, 2005; Vol. 97: pp. 161–163.

64. http://www.my.webmd.com/content/Article/101/106006.htm

65. Berube et al., "Cancer Epidemiology Biomarkers & Prevention: Vitamin D and Calcium Intakes from Food or Supplements and Mammographic Breast Density," *Cancer Epidemiol Biomarkers Prev* 2005; 14 (7): 1653–1659.

66. http://www.medicalnewstoday.com/medicalnews.php?newsid=62413

67. C. Palmieri, T. Macgregor, et al., "Serum 25 Hydroxyvitamin D Levels in Early and Advanced Breast Cancer," *J Clin Pathol* 2006 October 17; listed (E-published ahead of print).

68. 2005 Multidisciplinary Prostate Cancer Symposium, cosponsored by the American Society of Clinical Oncology, the Prostate Cancer Foundation, the American Society for Therapeutic Radiology and Oncology, and the Society of Urologic Oncology, Orlando, FL, February 17–19, 2005. News release, Brigham and Women's Hospital and Harvard University School of Public Health.

69. Reuters Sun, "Vitamin D Helps Lung Cancer Survival—Study," Monday, April 18, 2005.

70. C. F. Garland, F. C. Garland, et al., "The Role of Vitamin D in Cancer Prevention," *Am J Public Health* 2005 December 27 (E-published ahead of print).

71. http://www.abcnews.go.com/Health/wireStory?id=997923

72. S. Gaugris, R. P. Heaney, et al., "Vitamin D Inadequacy Among Postmenopausal Women: A Systematic Review," *QJM* 2005; 98 (9): 667–676.

73. M. K. Javaid, S. R. Crozier, et al., "Maternal Vitamin D Status During Pregnancy and Childhood Bone Mass at Age 9 Years: A Longitudinal Study," *The Lancet* 2006; 367 (9504): 36–43.

74. Cooper et al., *The Lancet* 2006; 367: 36–43; and http://www.medscape.com/viewarticle/520990

75. Merlino et al., *Arthritis Rheum* 2004: 50: 72–77.

76. H. M. Pappa et al., *Pediatrics* 2006 November; 118 (5): 1950–1961.

77. Chiu et al., *American Journal of Clinical Nutrition* 2004; 79: 820–825; Liu, "Dietary Calcium, Vitamin D, and the Prevalence of Metabolic Syndrome in Middle-aged and Older U.S. Women," *Diabetes Care* 2005; 28 (12): 2926–2932.

78. Mathieu et al., "Vitamin D and Diabetes," *Diabetologia* 2005; 48 (7): 1247–1257.

79. P. Pozzilli, S. Manfrini, et al., "Low Levels of 25-hydroxyvitamin D-3 and 1,25-dihydroxyvitamin D-3 in Patients with Newly Diagnosed Type 1 Diabetes," *Hormone and Metabolic Research*, 2005; 37 (11): 680–683.

80. http://www.medscape.com/viewarticle/528837

81. http://www.medscape.com/viewarticle/529076

82. R. Scragg and Chest, "Relationship Between Serum 25-hydroxyvitamin D and Pulmonary Function in the Third National Health and Nutrition Examination Survey," *Black PN*, 2005; 128 (6): 3792–3798.

83. E. Xystrakis, S. Kusumakar, et al., "Reversing the Defective Induction of IL10 Secreting T-regulatory Cells in Glucocorticoid-resistant Asthma Patients," *Journal of Clinical Investigation* 2005 8 December.

84. http://www.medpagetoday.com/Pulmonary/Asthma/tb2/2796. "Vitamin D Deficiency During Pregnancy Also Contributes to Low Birth Weights."

85. http://news.bbc.co.uk/1/hi/health/4938932.stm

86. W. G. John, K. Noonan, et al., "Hypovitaminosis D is Associated with Reductions in Serum Apolipoprotein A-I But not with Fasting Lipids in British Bangladeshis," *American Journal of Clinical Nutrition* 2005; 82 (3): 517–522.

87. J. Marniemi, "Dietary and Serum Vitamins and Minerals as Predictors of Myocardial Infarction and Stroke in Elderly Subjects," *Nutr Metab Cardiovasc Dis* 2005 June; 15 (3): 188–197. 43761 (10/2005)

88. H. A. Bischoff-Ferrari et al., *Am J Clin Nutr* 2006; 84: 18–28.

89. http://www.medscape.com/viewarticle/541149

90. L. Rejnmark, P. Vestergaard, et al., "No Effect of Vitamin K_1 Intake on Bone Mineral Density and Fracture Risk in Perimenopausal Women," *Osteoporos Int* 2006 May 9 (E-published ahead of print).

91. http://www.reutershealth.com/en/index.html

92. N. Leone and D. Courbon, "Zinc, Copper, and Magnesium and Risks for All-cause, Cancer, and Cardiovascular Mortality," *Epidemiology* 2006; 17 (3): 308–314.

93. C. Skibola, *Journal of Nutrition*, February 2005; Vol. 135: pp. 296–300. News release, University of California, Berkeley.

94. R. Pokan et al., "Oral Magnesium Therapy, Exercise Heart Rate, Exercise Tolerance, and Myocardial Function in Coronary Artery Disease Patients," *British Journal of Sports Medicine* 6 July 2006; 40: 773–778; doi:10.1136/bjsm.2006.027250

95. M. S. Seelig, "The Requirement of Magnesium by the Normal Adult," *American Journal of Clinical Nutrition* 14 June 1964: 342–390.

96. M. J. Hoes, "Plasma Concentrations of Magnesium and Vitamin B_1 in Alcoholism and Delirium Tremens. Pathogenic and Prognostic Implications," *Acta Psychiatrica Belgica* 81 (1) (January-February 1981): 72–84.

97. N. Leone and D. Courbon, op. cit.

98. Massachusetts Institute of Technology news release, December 2, 2004. Study published in the December 2, 2004, issue of *Neuron*.

99. http://www.medscape.com/viewarticle/504408 and http://www.medscape.com/viewarticle/504441

100. http://www.medscape.com/viewarticle/528661

101. R. M. van Dam, *Diabetes Care* 2006; 29: 2238–2243.

102. K. M. Ryder, et al., "Magnesium Intake from Food and Supplements Is Associated with Bone Mineral Density in Healthy Older White Subjects," *J Am Geriatr Soc* 2005; 53 (11): 1875–1880.

103. T. O. Carpenter, M. C. Delucia, et al., "A Randomized Controlled Study of Effects of Dietary Magnesium Oxide Supplementation on Bone Mineral Content in Healthy Girls," *J Clin Endocrinol Metab* 2006; 91 (12): 4866–4872.

104. D. King, "Magnesium Supplement Intake and C-reactive Protein Levels in Adults," *Nutrition Research* 2006; 26 (5): 193–196. 44508 (9/2006)

105. A. R. Folsom and C. P. Hong, "Magnesium Intake and Reduced Risk of Colon Cancer in a Prospective Study of Women," *Am J Epidemiol* 2006; 163 (3): 232–235.

106. C. Gontijo-Amaral, M. A. Ribeiro, et al., "Oral Magnesium Supplementation in Asthmatic Children: A Double-Blind Randomized Placebo-Controlled Trial," *Eur J Clin Nutr* 2006 June 21 (E-published ahead of print).

107. A. Peikert et al., "Prophylaxis of Migraine with Oral Magnesium: Results from a Prospective, Multi-center, Placebo-Controlled and Double-Blind Randomized Study," *Cephalgia*, 1996 June; 16 (4): 257–263.

108. F. Facchinetti et al., "Magnesium Prophylaxis of Mention Migraine: Effects on Intracellular Magnesium," *Headache*, 1991 May; 31 (5): 298–301.

109. M. Mousain-Bosc, M. Roche, et al., "Improvement of Neurobehavioral Disorders in Children Supplemented with Magnesium-Vitamin B_6. II. Pervasive Developmental Disorder-Autism," *Magnes Res* 2006; 19 (1): 46–52.

110. E. T. Jacobs, R. Jiang, D. S. Alberts, E. R. Greenberg, E. W. Gunter, M. R. Karagas, E. Lanza, L. Ratnasinghe, M. E. Reid, A. Schatzkin, S. A. Smith-Warner, K. Wallace, and M. E. Martinez, "Selenium and Colorectal Adenoma: Results of a Pooled Analysis," *J Natl Cancer Inst* 2004 November 17; 96 (22): 1669–1675.

111. N. T. Akbaraly, J. Arnaud, et al., "Selenium and Mortality in the Elderly: Results from the EVA Study," *Clin Chem* 2005; 51 (11): 2117–2123.

112. A. L. Ray, R. D. Semba, et al., "Low Serum Selenium and Total Carotenoids Predict Mortality among Older Women Living in the Community: The Women's Health and Aging Studies," *J Nutr* 2006; 136 (1): 172–176.

113. J. Arnaud, "Selenium and Mortality in the Elderly: Results from the EVA Study," *Clin Chem* 2005 November; 51 (11): 2117–2123 (E-published 2005 August 25. 44052 (3/2006)

114. J. G. Penland, April 4 at the Experimental Biology 2005 meeting in San Diego.

115. http://www.reutershealth.com/en/index.html

116. J. K. Virtanen, S. Voutilainen, et al., "High Dietary Methionine Intake Increases the Risk of Acute Coronary Events in Middle-aged Men," *Nutr Metab Cardiovasc Dis* 2006; 16 (2): 113–120.

117. Y. Matuszczak, M. Farid, et al., "Effects of N-Acetyl-L-Cysteine on Glutathione Oxidation and Fatigue During Handgrip Exercise," *Muscle Nerve*, 2005; 32 (5): 633–638.

118. D. Yesilbursa, A. Serdar, et al., "Effect of N-Acetyl-L-Cysteine on Oxidative Stress and Ventricular Function in Patients with Myocardial Infarction," *Heart Vessels* 2006; 21 (1): 33–37.

119. D. L. Lafleur, C. Pittenger, et al., "N-Acetyl-L-Cysteine Augmentation in Serotonin Reuptake Inhibitor Refractory Obsessive-Compulsive Disorder," *Psychopharmacology* (Berl), 2006; 184 (2): 254–256.

120. S. Ersan, S. Bakir, et al., "Examination of Free Radical Metabolism and Anti-oxidant Defence System Elements in Patients with Obsessive-Compulsive Disorder," *Prog Neuropsychopharmacol Biol Psychiatry* 2006 May 6 (E-published ahead of print).

121. D. C. Rushton, I. D. Ramsay, J. J. Gilkes, et al., "Ferritin and Fertility," letter to the editor," *The Lancet* 337 (8757) (22 June 1991): 1554.

122. http://www.webmd.com/content/Article/122/114601.htm

123. L. B. Trost, *Journal of the American Academy of Dermatology* May 2006; Vol. 54: pp. 824–844.

124. J. Marniemi, "Dietary and Serum Vitamins and Minerals as Predictors of Myocardial Infarction and Stroke in Elderly Subjects," *Nutr Metab Cardiovasc Dis* 2005 June; 15 (3): 188–197. 43761 (10/2005)

125. M. Maes, I. Mihaylova, and J. C. Leunis, "In Chronic Fatigue Syndrome, the Decreased Levels of Omega-3 Polyunsaturated Fatty Acids Are Related to Lowered Serum Zinc and Defects in T cell Activation," *Journal: Neuro Endocrinol Lett* 2005 December 28; 26 (6) (E-published ahead of print).

126. B. K. Puri, "The Use of Eicosapentaenoic Acid in the Treatment of Chronic Fatigue Syndrome: Prostaglandins Leukot Essential Fatty Acids." 2004 April; 70 (4): 399–401.

127. G. Fontani, F. Corradeschi, et al., "Cognitive and Physiological Effects of Omega-3 Polyunsaturated Fatty Acid Supplementation in Healthy Subjects," *Eur J Clin Invest* 2005; 35 (11): 691–699.

128. C. Bouzan, J. T. Cohen, et al., "A Quantitative Analysis of Fish Consumption and Stroke Risk," *Am J Prev Med* 2005; 29 (4): 347–352.

129. B. Miljanovic and K. A. Trivedi, "Relation Between Dietary N-3 and N-6 Fatty Acids and Clinically Diagnosed Dry Eye Syndrome in Women," *Am J Clin Nutr*, 2005; 82 (4): 887–893.

130. http://www.my.webmd.com/content/Article/90/100860.htm; and E. Oken, R. O. Wright, K. P. Kleinman, et al., "Maternal Fish Consumption, Hair Mercury, and Infant Cognition in a U.S. Cohort," *Environ Health Perspect* 2005; 113 (10): 1376–1380.

131. M. T. Salam, Y. F. Yi, et al., "Maternal Fish Consumption During Pregnancy and Risk of Early Childhood Asthma," *J Asthma* 2005; 42 (6): 513–518.

132. http://www.npicenter.com/anm/templates/newsATemp.aspx?articleid=14384&zoneid=41

133. M. Peet and C. Stokes, "Omega-3 Fatty Acids in the Treatment of Psychiatric Disorders," *Drugs* 2005; 65 (8): 1051–1059.

134. S. Frangou, M. Lewis, and P. McCrone, "Efficacy of Ethyl-Eicosapentaenoic Acid in Bipolar Depression: Randomized Double-Blind Placebo-Controlled Study," *Br J Psychiatry* 2006; 188: 46–50.

135. A. Elvin, A. K. Siosteen, A. Nilsson, and E. Kosek, "Decreased Muscle Blood Flow in Fibromyalgia Patients During Standardised Muscle Exercise: A Contrast Media Enhanced Colour Doppler Study," *Eur J Pain* 2006 February; 10 (2): 137–144.

Chapter 7. Natural and Prescription Pain Relief for Fibromyalgia

1. S. Chrubasik et al., "Treatment of Low Back Pain Exacerbations with Willow Bark Extract: A Randomized Double-Blind Study," *American Journal of Medicine* 2000 July; 109 (1): 9–14.

2. S. Chrubasik, O. Kunzel, et al., "Potential Economic Impact of Using a Proprietary Willow Bark Extract in Outpatient Treatment of Low Back Pain: An Open Non-Randomized Study," *Phytomedicine* 2001 July; 8 (4): 241–251.

3. R. W. Marz and F. Kemper, "Willow Bark Extract—Effects and Effectiveness: Status of Current Knowledge Regarding Pharmacology, Toxicology and Clinical Aspects" (Article in German), *Wien Med Wochenschr*, 2002;152 (15–16): 354–359.

4. B. Schmid et al., "Efficacy and Tolerability of a Standardized Willow Bark Extract in Patients with Osteoarthritis: Randomized Placebo-Controlled, Double Blind Clinical Trial." *Phytother Res* 2001 June; 15 (4): 344–350.

5. E. S. Highfield and K. J. Kemper, "White Willow Monograph," Longwood Herbal Task Force. Accessed on June 7, 2004. Available at: http://www.mcp.edu/herbal/willowbark/willow.pdf

6. T. Hedner and B. Everts, "The Early Clinical History of Salicylates in Rheumatology and Pain," *Clinical Rheumatology* 1998; 17: 17–25.

7. S. Chrubasik and E. Eisenberg, "Treatment of Rheumatic Pain with Herbal Medicine in Europe," *Pain Digest* 1998; 8: 231–236.

8. B. Meier, O. Sticher, and R. Julkunen-Tiitto, "Pharmaceutical Aspects of the Use of Willows in Herbal Remedies," *Planta Medica* 1988: 559–560.

9. G. B. Singh et al., *Agents and Actions* 1986; 18: 407.

10. M. L. Sharma et al., *Agents and Actions* 1988; 24: 161.

11. M. L. Sharma et al., *International Journal Immunopharm*, 1989; 11: 647.

12. A. Kar and M. K. Menon, *Life Sciences* 1969; 8: 1023.

13. M. K. Menon and A. Kar, *Planta Medica* 1971; 19: 333.

14. O. Sander, G. Herborn, and R. Rau, "[Is H15 (Resin Extract of Boswellia serrata, "incense") a Useful Supplement to Established Drug Therapy of Chronic Polyarthritis? Results of a Double-Blind Pilot Study]," *Z Rheumatol* 1998; 57: 11–16. German.

15. M. L. Sharma et al., *Agents and Actions* 1988; 24: 161.

16. R. Etzel, *Phytomedicine* 1996; 3 (1): 91–94.

17. N. Kimmatkar, V. Thawani, L. Hingorani, et al., *Phytomedicine* 2003; 10 (1): 3–7.

18. H. Safayhi et al., "Inhibition by Boswellic Acids of Human Leukocyte Elastase," *Journal of Pharmacological Experimental Therory* 1997 April; 281 (1): 460–463.

19. I. Gupta et al., "Effects of a Boswellia Resin in Patients with Bronchial Asthma: Results of a Double-Blind, Placebo-Controlled, Six Week Clinical Study," *European Journal of Medical Research*, 1998; 3: 511–514.

20. I. Gupta et al., "Effects of Gum Resin of Boswellia Serrata in Patients with Chronic Colitis," *Planta Medica* 2001 July; 67 (5): 391–395.

21. K. Hostanska et al., "Cytostatic and Apoptosis-Inducing Activity of Boswellic Acids Toward Malignant Cell Lines in Vitro," *Anticancer Res*, 2002 September-October; 22 (5): 2853–2862.

22. M. T. Huang et al., "Anti-tumor and Anti-carcinogenic Activities of Triterpenoid, Beta-Boswellic Acid," *Biofactors* 2000; 13 (1–4): 225–230.

23. N. P. Seeram et al., "Cyclooxygenase Inhibitory and Antioxidant Cyanidin Glycosides in Cherries and Berries," *Phytomedicine* 2001 September; 8 (5): 362–369.

24. S. Y. Kang et al., "Tart Cherry Anthocyanins Inhibit Tumor Development in Apc(Min) Mice and Reduce Proliferation of Human Colon Cancer Cells," *Cancer Letter* 2003 May 8; 194 (1): 13–19.

25. L. W. Blau, "Cherry Diet Control for Gout and Arthritis," *Tex Report on Biol Medicine* 1950; 8: 309–311.

26. K. C. Srivastava and T. Mustafa, "Ginger (Zingiber officinale) in Rheumatism and Musculoskeletal Disorders," *Medical Hypotheses* 39 (4) (December 1992): 342–348.

27. V. Challapalli, I. W. Tremont-Lukats, E. D. McNicol, J. Lau, and D. B. Carr, "Systemic Administration of Local Anesthetic Agents to Relieve Neuropathic Pain," *Cochrane Database Syst Rev* 19; (4): CD003345, 2005.

28. M. C. Rowbotham, L. A. Reisner-Keller, and H. L. Fields, "Both Intravenous Lidocaine and Morphine Reduce the Pain of Postherpetic Neuralgia," *Neurology* 1991, 41: 1024–1028.

29. J. Sorenson, A. Bengtsson, E. Backman, K. G. Henriksson, and M. Bengtsson, "Pain Analysis in Patients with Fibromyalgia: Effects of Intravenous Morphine, Lidocaine and Ketamine," *Scan J Rheumatol* 1995, 24: 360–365.

30. M. I. Bennett and Y. M. Tai, "Intravenous Lignocaine in the Management of Primary Fibromyalgia Syndrome," *Int J Clin Pharm Res* 1995, 15: 115–119.

Chapter 8. More Natural Remedies

1. Juneja et al., *Trends in Food Sci Tech* 1999; 199–204.

    Kobayashi et al., *Nippon Nogeikagaku Kaishi* 1998; 72: 153–157.

2. Kakuda et al., 2000; 64: 287–293.

3. Y. N. Singh and M. Blumenthal, "Kava: An Overview," *Herbalgram* 39 (Spring 1997): 33–55.

4. G. Piscopo, "Kava Kava: Gift of the Islands," *Alternative Medicine Review* 2 (5) (1997): 355–364.

5. E. Grassel, "Effect of Ginkgo Biloba Extract on Mental Performance," *Fortschritte der Medizin* 110 (5) (February 1992): 73–76.

6. W. Hopfenmuller, "Proof of the Therapeutic Effectiveness of a Ginkgo Biloba Extract—A Meta Analysis of 11 [Placebo-Controlled] Trials in Aged Patients with Cerebral Insufficiency," *Arzneimittel-Forschung* 44 (9) (September 1994): 1005–1010.

7. I. Hindmarch, "Activity of Ginkgo Biloba Extract on Short Term Memory," *Presse Medicale* 15 (31) (September 1986): 1592–1594.

7A. A. Tamborini and R. Taurelle, "Value of Standardized Ginkgo Biloba Extract (EGb 761) in the Management of Congestive Symptoms of Premenstrual Syndrome," Revue Francaise de gynecologie et d'Obstetrique 88 (7–9) (July-September 1993): 447–457.

8. J. P. Haguenauer, F. Cantenot, H. Koskas, et al., "Treatment of Equilibrium Disturbances with Ginkgo Biloba—A Multicenter, Placebo Controlled Study," *Presse Medicale* 15 (31) (25 September 1986): 1569–1572.

9. P. F. Smith and C. L. Darlington, "Can Vestibular Compensation Be Enhanced by Drug Treatment? A Review of Recent Evidence" review, *Journal of Vestibular Research* 4 (3) (May-June 1994): 169–179.

10. D. F. Neri, D. Wiegmann, R. R. Stanny, et al., "The Effects of Tyrosine on Cognitive Performance During Extended Wakefulness," *Aviation, Space, and Environmental Medicine* 66 (4) (1995): 313–319.

11. R. H. Wolbling et al., "Local Therapy of Herpes Simplex with Dried Extract From Melisa Officianalis," *Phyto Medicine* 1 (1994): 25–31.

12. P. J. Meunier et al., "Strontium Ranelate: Dose-Dependent Effects on Established Postmenopausal Vertebral Osteoporosis—a Two-Year Randomized Placebo-

Controlled Trial," *Journal of Clinical Endocrinology and Metabolism*, May 2002; 87 (5): 2060–2066.

13. P. J. Meunier et al., "The Effects of Strontium on the Risk of Vertebral Fracture in Women with Postmenopausal Osteoporosis," *New England Journal of Medicine*, 2004, January 29; 350 (5): 459–468.

14. F. E. McCaslin et al., "The Effect of Strontium Lactate in the Treatment of Osteoporosis," *Proceedings of the Staff Meetings of the Mayo Clinic* 34: 1959; 329–334.

Chapter 9. Other Areas to Explore

1. S. B. Miller, "IgG Food Allergy Testing by ELISA/EIA—What Do They Really Tell Us?" *Townsend Letter for Doctors and Patients*, January 1998, pp. 62–66, 106.

2. R. M. Jaffe, "A Novel Treatment for Fibromyalgia Improves Clinical Outcomes in a Community Based Study," study presented before the American Association for the Advancement of Science, Baltimore, MD, 9 February 1996.

3. R. Shoemaker and D. E. House, "Sick Building Syndrome (SBS) and Exposure to Water-Damaged Buildings," *Neurotoxicology and Teratology* 28 (2006) 573–588. Available online at www.sciencedirect.com.

4. B. Hurwitz et al., "Therapeutic Effect of Epoetin Alpha on RBC Volume, Perceived Fatigue and Susceptibility to Syncope in CFS," IACFS Conference abstract and presentation. Ft. Lauderdale, FL, January 12–14, 2007.

5. R. Shoemaker and M. S. Maizel, "Treatment of CFS patients with Elevated C4A Using Low Dose Erythropoietin Corrects Abnormalities in CNS Metabolites and Restores Executive Cognitive Functioning," IACFS Conference abstract, Ft. Lauderdale, FL, January 12–14, 2007.

6. S. Ruhrmann and S. Kasper, "Seasonal Depression," *Medizinische Monatsschrift für Pharmazeuten* 15 (1992): 293–299.

7. J. Liebermann and D. S. Bell, "Serum Angiotensin-Converting Enzyme as a Marker for the Chronic Fatigue-Immune Dysfunction Syndrome: A Comparison to Serum Angiotensin-Converting Enzyme in Sarcoidosis," *American Journal of Medicine* 95 (1993): 407–412.

8. J. Goldstein, "Fibromyalgia Syndrome: A Pain Modulation Disorder Related to Altered Limbic Function?" *Bailliere's Clinical Rheumatology* 8 (November 1994): 777–800.

9. S. Rogers, *Tired or Toxic* (Syracuse, NY: Prestige Publishing, 1990).

S. Rogers, "Chemical Sensitivity: Breaking the Paralyzing Paradigm, Part I," *Internal Medicine World Report* 7 (3): 1.

10. T. H. Park, "Comprehensive Treatments with IVIG for CFS," IACFS Conference abstract, Ft. Lauderdale, FL, January 12–14, 2007.

Chapter 10. Am I Crazy?
Understanding the Mind-Body Connection

1. E. K. Axe et al., "Major Depressive Disorder in Chronic Fatigue Syndrome: A CDC Surveillance Study," *Journal of Chronic Fatigue Syndrome*, Vol. 12 (3) 2004.

2. I. Castro, F. Barrantes, M. Tuna, G. Cabrera, C. Garcia, M. Recinos, L. R. Espinoza, and A. Garcia-Kutzbach, "Prevalence of Abuse in Fibromyalgia and Other Rheumatic Disorders at a Specialized Clinic in Rheumatic Diseases in Guatemala City," *Clin Rheumatol* 2005 June; 11 (3): 140–145.

3. http://www.medscape.com/viewarticle/544942 ECNP 19th Congress: Presentation S.13.05. Presented September 18, 2006.

Appendix G: For Physicians

1. F. Wolfe, K. Ross, J. Anderson, et al., "The Prevalence and Characteristics of Fibromyalgia in the General Population," *Arthritis and Rheumatism* 38 (1) (January 1995): 19–28.

2. J. E. Teitelbaum and B. Bird, "Effective Treatment of Severe Chronic Fatigue: A Report of a Series of 64 Patients," *Journal of Musculoskeletal Pain* 3 (4) (1995): 91–110.

3. J. E. Teitelbaum, B. Bird, R. M. Greenfield, et al., "Effective Treatment of CFS and FMS: A Randomized, Double-Blind Placebo-Controlled Study," *Journal of Chronic Fatigue Syndrome* 8 (2) (2001). The full text of the study can be found at www.vitality101.com.

4. M. A. Demitrack, K. Dale, S. E. Straus, et al., "Evidence for Impaired Activation of the Hypothalamic-Pituitary-Adrenal Axis in Patients with Chronic Fatigue Syndrome," *Journal of Clinical Endocrinology and Metabolism* 73 (6) (December 1991): 1223–1234.

5. J. E. Teitelbaum, "Estrogen and Testosterone in CFIDS/FMS," *From Fatigued to Fantastic!* newsletter, February 1997.

6. P. O. Behan, "Post-viral Fatigue Syndrome Research," in *The Clinical and Scientific Basis of Myalgic Encephalitis and Chronic Fatigue Syndrome*, Byron Hyde, Jay Goldstein, and Paul Levine, eds. (Ottawa, Ontario, Canada: Nightingale Research Foundation, 1992), p. 238.

7.   J. E. Teitelbaum, "Mitochondrial Dysfunction [in CFS/FMS]," *From Fatigued to Fantastic!* newsletter 1 (2) (1997). Contains numerous references on this topic.

8.   F. Wolfe et al., "The American College of Rheumatology 1990 Criteria for the Classification of Fibromyalgia: Report of the Multicenter Criteria Committee," *Arthritis and Rheumatology* 33 (1990): 160–172.

9.   H. Blatman, editorial, *Journal of the American Academy of Pain Management*, April 2002.

10. Conference on the Neuroscience and Endocrinology of Fibromyalgia Syndrome, sponsored by the National Institutes of Health, 16–17 July 1996.

11. T. Fleming, ed., "Jamaican Dogwood" PDR for herbal medicines, 1998 pp. 428–429.

12. "Humulus Lupus," Monograph. *Alternative Medicine Review*, 8 (2) 2003, 190–192.

13. J. R. Cronin, "Passionflower—Reigniting Male Libido and Other Potential Uses," *Alternative and Complementary Therapies* April 2003, pp. 89–92.

14. K. Dhawan et al., "Reversal of Morphine Tolerance and Dependence by Passiflora Incarnata," *Pharmaceutical Biology* 2002; 40 (8): 576–580.

15. S. Hadley et al. "Valerian," *American Family Physician* 2003; 67 (8): 1755–1758.

16. M. B. Yunus and J. C. Aldag, "Restless Leg Syndrome and Leg Cramps in Fibromyalgia Syndrome: A Controlled Study," *British Medical Journal* 312 (7042) (25 May 1996): 1339.

17. J. C. Lowe, R. L. Garrison, A. J. Reichman, J. Yellin, M. Thompson, and D. Kaufman, "Effectiveness and Safety of T_3 Therapy for Euthyroid Fibromyalgia: A Double-Blind, Placebo-Controlled Response Driven Crossover Study," *Clinical Bulletin of Myofascial Therapy* 1997: 2 (2/3): 31–58.

18. J. C. Lowe, A. J. Reichman, and J. Yellin, "The Process of Change During T_3 Treatment for Euthyroid Fibromyalgia: A Double-Blind, Placebo-Controlled, Crossover Study," *Clinical Bulletin of Myofascial Therapy* 1997; 2 (2/3): 91–124.

19. G. Faglia, L. Bitensky, A. Pinchera, et al., "Thyrotropin Secretion in Patients with Central Hypothyroidism: Evidence for Reduced Biological Activity of Immunoreactive Thyrotropin," *Journal of Clinical Endocrinology and Metabolism* 48 (6) (June 1979) 989–998.

20. G. R. B. Skinner, D. Holmes, A. Ahmad, et al., "Clinical Response to Thyroxine Sodium in Clinically Hypothyroid but Biochemically Euthyroid Patients," *Journal of Nutritional and Environmental Medicine* 10 (2) (June 2000): 115–125.

21. R. A. Nordyke, T. S. Reppun, L. D. Madanay, et al., "Alternative Sequences of Thyrotropin and Free Thyroxine Assays for Routine Thyroid Function Testing. Quality and Cost," *Archives of Internal Medicine* 158 (3) (9 February 1998): 266–272.

22.   E. N. Griep, J. N. Boersma, and E. R. de Kloet, "Altered Reactivity of the Hypo-thalamic-Pituitary Axis in the Primary Fibromyalgia Syndrome," *Journal of Rheumatology* 20 (3) (March 1993): 469–474.

23.   G. A. McCain and K. S. Tilbe, "Diurnal Hormone Variation in Fibromyalgia Syndrome and a Comparison with Rheumatoid Arthritis," *Journal of Rheumatology* 25 (1993): 469–474.

24.   W. M. Jefferies, *Safe Uses of Cortisol*, 2nd ed., monograph (Springfield, IL: Charles C. Thomas, 1996).

25.   W. M. Jefferies, "Low-Dosage Glucocorticoid Therapy. An Appraisal of Its Safety and Mode of Action in Clinical Disorders, Including Rheumatoid Arthritis," *Archives of Internal Medicine* 119 (3) (March 1967): 265–278.

26.   R. McKenzie, A. O'Fallon, J. Dale, et al., "Low-Dose Hydrocortisone for Treatment of Chronic Fatigue Syndrome: A Randomized Controlled Trial," *Journal of the American Medical Association* 280 (12) (23–30 September 1998): 1061–1066.

27.   J. E. Teitelbaum, B. Bird, A. Weiss, et al., "Low Dose Hydrocortisone for Chronic Fatigue Syndrome," *Journal of the American Medical Association* 281 (1999): 1887–1888.

28.   A. J. Morales, J. J. Nolan, J. C. Nelson, et al., "Effects of Replacement Dose of Dehydroepiandrosterone in Men and Women of Advancing Age," *Journal of Clinical Endocrinology and Metabolism* 78 (6) (June 1994): 1360–1367.

29.   Elizabeth Lee Vliet, *Screaming to Be Heard: Hormone Connections Women Suspect . . . and Doctors Ignore* (New York, NY: M. Evans and Company, 1995).

30.   J. V. Wright and L. Lenard, *Maximize Your Vitality and Potency, for Men Over 40*, Smart Publications; 1999 (an excellent reference for those who would like to explore the topic further).

30A.   L. S. Marks et al., "Effect of Testosterone Replacement Therapy on Prostate Tissue in Men with Late-Onset Hypogonadism: A Randomized Controlled Trial," *JAMA* 2006; 296 (19): 2351–2361 (ISSN: 1538–3598).

30B.   *Arch Intern Med* 2006; 166: 1660–1665.

31.   R. S. Ivker, *Sinus Survival* (New York, NY: Tarcher/Putnam, 2000).

32.   W. M. Becker, J. B. Reece, M. F. Poenie, et al., *The World of the Cell*, 3rd ed. (San Francisco, CA: Benjamin Cummings, 1996).

33.   B. Regland, M. Andersson, L. Abrahamsson, et al., "Increased Concentrations of Homocysteine in the Cerebrospinal Fluid in Patients with Fibromyalgia and Chronic Fatigue Syndrome," *Scandinavian Journal of Rheumatology* 26 (4) (1997), 301–307.

34. J. Lindenbaum, I. H. Rosenberg, P. W. Wilson, et al., "Prevalence of Cobalamin Deficiency in the Framingham Elderly Population," *American Journal of Clinical Nutrition* 60 (1) July 1994; 2–11.

35. J. Lindenbaum, E. B. Healton, D. G. Savage, et al., "Neuropsychiatric Disorders Caused by Cobalamin Deficiency in the Absence of Anemia or Macrocytoses," *New England Journal of Medicine* 318 (26) (30 June 1988): 1720–1728.

36. W. S. Beck, "Cobalamin and the Nervous System," editorial, *New England Journal of Medicine* 318 (26), (30 June 1988): 1752–1754.

37. Ibid.; and S. Chrubasik, et al., "Treatment of Low Back Pain Exacerbations with Willow Bark Extract: A Randomized Double-Blind Study," *American Journal of Medicine*, 2000 July; 109 (1): 9–14.

38. S. Chrubasik, O. Kunzel, et al., "Potential Economic Impact of Using a Proprietary Willow Bark Extract in Outpatient Treatment of Low Back Pain: An Open Non-randomized Study," *Phytomedicine*, 2001 July; 8 (4): 241–251.

39. R. W. Marz and F. Kemper, "Willow Bark Extract—Effects and Effectiveness. Status of Current Knowledge Regarding Pharmacology, Toxicology and Clinical Aspects," [Article in German] *Wien Med Wochenschr* 2002; 152 (15–16): 354–359.

40. B. Schmid et al., "Efficacy and Tolerability of a Standardized Willow Bark Extract in Patients with Osteoarthritis: Randomized Placebo-Controlled, Double Blind Clinical Trial," *Phytother Res*, 2001 June; 15 (4): 344–350.

41. E. S. Highfield and K. J. Kemper, "White willow monograph." Longwood Herbal Task Force. Available at: http://www.mcp.edu/herbal/willowbark/willow.pdf.

42. T. Hedner and B. Everts, "The Early Clinical History of Salicylates in Rheumatology and Pain," *Clinical Rheumatology*, 1998; 17: 17–25.

43. S. Chrubasik and E. Eisenberg, "Treatment of Rheumatic Pain with Herbal Medicine in Europe," *Pain Digest*, 1998; 8: 231–236.

44. B. Meier, O. Sticher, and R. Julkunen-Tiitto, "Pharmaceutical Aspects of the Use of Willows in Herbal Remedies," *Planta Medica* 1988: 559–560.

45. G. B. Singh and C. K. Atal, *Agents and Actions* 1986; 18: 407.

46. M. L. Sharma et al., *Agents and Actions* 1988; 24: 161.

47. M. L. Sharma et al., *International Journal Immunopharm*, 1989; 11: 647.

48. A. Kar and M. K. Menon, *Life Sciences* 1969; 8: 1023.

49. M. K. Menon and A. Kar, *Planta Medica* 1971; 19: 333.

50. O. Sander, G. Herborn, and R. Rau, "[Is H15 (Resin Extract of Boswellia serrata, "incense") a Useful Supplement to Established Drug Therapy of Chronic Poly-

arthritis? Results of a Double-Blind Pilot Study], *Z Rheumatol,* 1998; 57: 11–6. German.

51.   M. L. Sharma et al., *Agents and Actions* 1988; 24: 161.

52.   R. Etzel, *Phytomedicine* 1996; 3 (1): 91–94.

53.   N. Kimmatkar, V. Thawani, L. Hingorani, et al., *Phytomedicine* 2003; 10 (1): 3–7.

54.   H. Safayhi et al., "Inhibition by Boswellic Acids of Human Leukocyte Elastase," *Journal of Pharmacological Experimental Therory,* 1997 April; 281 (1): 460–463.

55.   P. C. Rowe, I. Bou-Holaigah, J. S. Kan, et al., "Is Neurally Mediated Hypotension an Unrecognized Cause of Chronic Fatigue?" *The Lancet* 345 (8950) (11 March 1995): 623–624.

Index